Homemaker/Home Health Aide

Fourth Edition

Homemaker/Home Health Aide

Fourth Edition

Helen Huber, BA
Audree Spatz, MEd, BSN, RN

Revised by Suzann Balduzzi, MEd, BSN, RN

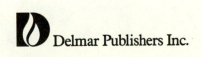

Delmar Publishers Inc.

I(T)P™

NOTICE TO THE READER

Cover credit: Three Communication Design

Delmar staff:

Associate Editor: Adrianne C. Williams
Developmental Editor: Marjorie A. Bruce
Project Editor: Melissa A. Conan
Production Coordinator: Mary Ellen Black
Art and Design Coordinator: Brian Yacur/Mary Siener

For information, address
Delmar Publishers Inc.
3 Columbia Circle, Box 15015
Albany, NY 12203-5015

Printed in the United States of America
Published simultaneously in Canada
by Nelson Canada,
a division of The Thomson Corporation

1 2 3 4 5 6 7 8 9 10 XXX 00 99 98 97 96 95 94

Library of Congress Cataloging-in-Publication Data

Huber, Helen.
    Homemaker/Home health aide / Helen Huber, Audree Spatz. -- 4th ed.
        p.   cm.
    Includes index.
    ISBN 0-8273-5270-0 (textbook)
        1. Home health aides.   2. Visiting housekeepers.   3. Home nursing.
    I. Spatz, Audree.   II. Title.
    RA645.3.H8   1993
    649.8--dc20   92-40574
                                                            CIP

Contents

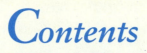

Part 1 Basic Principles

Section 1
Becoming a Home Health Aide   3

Unit 1
Home Health Services   4

The beginning of home care services   5
Increase in need for home care services   5
DRGs   6
Role of the home health aide   7
Programs and other important issues
　　influencing health care   8

Unit 2
Developing Good Habits and Practices   11

Learning procedures   12
Working with others   12
Developing self-understanding   14
Personal health and hygiene   15
Attitude   16
The health care team   16

Unit 3
Role Responsibilities and Ethical Standards   19

Career adjustments   20
Observing   24
Reporting   26
Documenting   26
Confidentiality   27
Liability   30
Ethics   31
Client's rights   33
Home health aide's rights   34
Case Study: Client Confidentiality   34
Client Abuse   35
Case Study: Job Ethics and Confidentiality   35

Unit 4
Developing Effective Communication Skills   38

Basic components of communication   39
Verbal communication   40
Nonverbal communication   41
Written communication   42
Medical terminology   42
Communication with clients   43
Case Study: Communication   45

Unit 5
Understanding Differences: Individuals, Families, and Cultures   50

The family unit—past and present   51
General background about contrasts
　　creating family differences   54
Racial prejudice and discrimination   57

Section 2
Basic Anatomy and Physiology   61

Unit 6
Functions and Disorders of the Body Systems   62

Integumentary system   64
Musculoskeletal system   67
Nervous system   71
Circulatory system   73
Respiratory system   77
Digestive system   79
Urinary system   81
Reproductive system   82
Endocrine system   85
The remarkable body   85
Factors that influence body development   87

Section 3
Understanding Human Development and Age-Related Health Problems   91

Unit 7
Infancy to Adolescence   92

Pregnancy   93
Labor and delivery   93
Normal infant growth and development   93
Common health problems in infancy   94
Responsibilities of the home health aide   96
Todlers and preschoolers   96
School-age children   96
Adolescence   97
Child abuse, maltreatment, and neglect   100

Unit 8
Early and Middle Adulthood   103

Early adulthood   104
Middle adulthood   105
Effects of exercise   105
Acceptance of illness or disability   106
Emotional needs   106
Retirement   107

Unit 9
Late Adulthood   109

Effects of aging on the body systems   110
Chronic illness, physical health problems, and aging   112
Emotional and psychological effects of aging   116
Case Study 1: Spouse Dependency   119
Alzheimer's disease   121
Case Study 2: Client Alone   122
Validation therapy   126
Reality orientation   130

Section 4
Promoting Health and Understanding Illness   133

Unit 10
Mental Health   134

Understanding emotions   135

Defense mechanisms   137
Effects of emotions on health   138

Unit 11
Nutritional Guidelines   141

Food guide pyramid   142
Developing good eating habits   145
General guidelines for meal planning   148
Diet therapy   151

Unit 12
Principles of Safety and Body Mechanics   157

Common hazards   159
Principles of good body mechanics   175
Physical restraints   179

Unit 13
Understanding Illness   181

Internal disorders   182
Observing signs and symptoms   183
Cardinal signs   183
Height and weight   186
Conscious and unconscious clients   186
Need for rehabilitation   187
Diversion and recreation   189

Unit 14
Preventing the Spread of Disease   191

Microorganisms   192
Cleanliness in the home   194
Controlling the spread of illness   195
Universal precautions   195
Isolation   196
Infection control measures   197

Unit 15
Caring for the Client with an Infectious Disease   199

Infectious diseases   200
Special precautions   201
Immune deficiencies   202
How to protect against AIDS   204
Caring for the AIDS client   204

Section 5
Caring for Clients with Acute and Chronic Disorders   209

Unit 16
Caring for Clients with Diabetes — 210

Diabetes mellitus — 211
Facts and figures — 211
Classifications — 211
Signs and symptoms — 211
Testing — 212
Emergency treatment — 212
   1: Testing Blood — 213
Diet — 214
Exercise — 215
Drug therapy — 215
Long-term complications — 216
Special nursing care — 217
Identification tag — 219

Unit 17
Caring for Clients with Circulatory Disorders — 221

Risk factors — 222
Disorders of the heart and circulatory system — 222

Unit 18
Caring for Clients with Arthritis — 235

Definition of arthritis — 236
Management of clients with arthritis — 238

Unit 19
Caring for Clients with Cancer — 242

Cancer treatments — 243
Caring for clients with cancer — 244
Cancer of the female reproductive system — 245
Cancer of the respiratory system — 246
Gastrointestinal cancer — 248
Skin cancer — 249

Unit 20
Caring for the Client who is Terminally Ill — 251

Cultural differences — 252
Stages of adjustment to dying and death — 253
Religious and cultural influences — 254

Part 2   Practical Applications

Section 6
Homemaking Services — 261

Unit 21
Principles of Household Management — 262

Planning and organization — 264
Preventing injuries in the home — 267
Combining client care and household tasks — 268

Unit 22
Maintaining a Clean Environment in the Home — 270

Daily cleaning tasks — 271
Weekly cleaning tasks — 272
Periodic cleaning tasks — 272
Kitchen maintenance and cleaning — 273
Bathroom maintenance and cleaning — 276

Unit 23
Marketing and Meal Preparation — 279

Menus and shopping lists — 280
Purchasing food — 280
Storing food — 282
Meal preparation — 282

Unit 24
Laundry Duties — 287

Sorting clothes and linens — 288
Loading the washing machine — 288
Drying, ironing, and mending — 290

Section 7
Health Care Services — 293

Unit 25
Introduction to Client Care Procedures — 294

Unit 26
Infection Control and Universal Precautions — 299

Client care procedures
   2: Handwashing — 300

3: Gloving   301
4: Putting on and Removing Personal
   Protective Equipment   302
5: Collecting Specimen in Isolation   304

Unit 27
Restorative Care   305

6: Maintaining Body Alignment   306
7: Turning the Client Toward You   307
8: Moving the Client Up in Bed Using the
   Drawsheet   308
9: Log Rolling the Client   309
10: Positioning the Client in Supine Position 310
11: Positioning the Client in Lateral/
    Side-lying Position   310
12: Positioning the Client in Prone Position 311
13: Positioning the Client in Fowler's
    Position   312
14: Assisting the Client from Bed to Chair   313
15: Assisting the Client from Chair to Bed   314
16: Transferring the Client from Wheelchair
    to Toilet/Commode   314
17: Performing Passive Range of Motion
    Exercises   315
18: Assisting the Client to Walk with
    Crutches, Walker, or Cane   319
19: Lifting the Client Using a Mechanical
    Lift   321

Unit 28
Bathing   322

20: Assisting with Tub Bath or Shower   323
21: Giving a Bed Bath   326
22: Giving a Partial Bath   328
23: Giving a Back Rub   328
24: Giving Female Perineal Care   329
25: Giving Male Perineal Care   330
26: Special Skin Care and Pressure Sores   330

Unit 29
Daily Care   332

27: Assisting with Routine Oral Hygiene   333
28: Caring for Dentures   334
29: Shaving the Male Client   337
30: Dressing and Undressing the Client   338
31: Applying Elasticized Stockings   339
32: Making an Unoccupied Bed   340
33: Making an Occupied Bed   343

34: Giving Nail Care   344
35: Shampooing the Client's Hair in Bed   344
36: Assisting the Client with Self-
    administered Medications   346
37: Inserting a Hearing Aid   347
38: Caring for an Artificial Eye   348

Unit 30
Feeding and Toileting   350

39: Feeding the Client   351
40: Measuring and Recording Fluid Intake
    and Output   353
41: Giving and Emptying the Bedpan   354
42: Giving and Emptying the Urinal   356

Unit 31
Collecting Specimens and Catheter Care   357

43: Collecting a Clean-catch Urine
    Specimen   358
44: Caring for a Urinary Catheter   359
45: Connecting the Leg Bag   360
46: Emptying a Drainage Unit   361
47: Retraining the Bladder   362
48: Collecting a Sputum Specimen   363

Unit 32
Vital Signs and Measurement   364

49: Taking an Oral Temperature   365
50: Taking a Rectal Temperature   367
51: Taking an Axillary Temperature   368
52: Taking the Radial and Apical Pulse   369
53: Counting Respirations   371
54: Taking a Blood Pressure   371
55: Measuring Weight and Height   374

Unit 33
Hot and Cold Applications   375

56: Applying an Ice Bag, Cap, or Collar   376
57: Applying a K-Pad—Moist or Dry   377
58: Performing a Warm Foot Soak   378

Unit 34
Rectal Care   379

59: Giving a Commercial Enema   380
60: Giving a Rectal Suppository   381
61: Training and Retraining Bowels   382

62: Applying Adult Briefs 383
63: Collecting a Stool Specimen 383

Unit 35
Special Treatment 385

64: Applying Unsterile Dressing and
Ointment to Unbroken Skin 386
65: Caring for Casts 388
66: Assisting with Changing an Ostomy Bag 390
67: Assisting the Client with Oxygen
Therapy 392
68: Assisting with Cough and Deep
Breathing Exercises 394

Unit 36
Infant Care 396

69: Assisting with Breast-feeding and
Breast Care 397
70: Giving the Infant a Sponge Bath 398
71: Bottle-feeding the Infant 400

Section 8
Employment 403

Unit 37
Job-seeking Skills 404

Trends affecting employment 405
Contacting prospective employers 405
The job interview and application form 406

Appendices 413

A Temperature Conversion Chart 415
B Sample of Weekly Time Sheet 416
C Daily and Weekly Scheduling Chart 417
D Living Will and Durable Power
of Attorney 418
E Prefixes and Suffixes Commonly Used in
Medical Terminology 422

Glossary 425

Index 443

Index of Procedures

1. Testing Blood — 213
2. Handwashing — 300
3. Gloving — 301
4. Putting on and Removing Personal Protective Equipment — 302
5. Collecting Specimen in Isolation — 304
6. Maintaining Body Alignment — 306
7. Turning the Client Toward You — 307
8. Moving the Client Up in Bed Using the Drawsheet — 308
9. Log Rolling the Client — 309
10. Positioning the Client in Supine Position — 310
11. Positioning the Client in Lateral/Side-lying Position — 310
12. Positioning the Client in Prone Position — 311
13. Positioning the Client in Fowler's Position — 312
14. Assisting the Client from Bed to Chair — 313
15. Assisting the Client from Chair to Bed — 314
16. Transferring the Client from Wheelchair to Toilet/Commode — 314
17. Performing Passive Range of Motion Exercises — 315
18. Assisting the Client to Walk with Crutches, Walker, or Cane — 319
19. Lifting the Client Using a Mechanical Lift — 321
20. Assisting with Tub Bath or Shower — 323
21. Giving a Bed Bath — 326
22. Giving a Partial Bath — 328
23. Giving a Back Rub — 328
24. Giving Female Perineal Care — 329
25. Giving Male Perineal Care — 330
26. Special Skin Care and Pressure Sores — 330
27. Assisting with Routine Oral Hygiene — 333
28. Caring for Dentures — 334
29. Shaving the Male Client — 337
30. Dressing and Undressing the Client — 338
31. Applying Elasticized Stockings — 339
32. Making an Unoccupied Bed — 340
33. Making an Occupied Bed — 343
34. Giving Nail Care — 344
35. Shampooing the Client's Hair in Bed — 344
36. Assisting the Client with Self-administered Medications — 346
37. Inserting a Hearing Aid — 347
38. Caring for an Artificial Eye — 348
39. Feeding the Client — 351
40. Measuring and Recording Fluid Intake and Output — 353
41. Giving and Emptying the Bedpan — 354
42. Giving and Emptying the Urinal — 356
43. Collecting a Clean-catch Urine Specimen — 358
44. Caring for a Urinary Catheter — 359
45. Connecting the Leg Bag — 360
46. Emptying a Drainage Unit — 361
47. Retraining the Bladder — 362
48. Collecting a Sputum Specimen — 363
49. Taking an Oral Temperature — 365
50. Taking a Rectal Temperature — 367
51. Taking an Axillary Temperature — 368
52. Taking the Radial and Apical Pulse — 369
53. Counting Respirations — 371
54. Taking a Blood Pressure — 371
55. Measuring Weight and Height — 374
56. Applying an Ice Bag, Cap, or Collar — 376
57. Applying a K-Pad—Moist or Dry — 377
58. Performing a Warm Foot Soak — 378
59. Giving a Commercial Enema — 380
60. Giving a Rectal Suppository — 381
61. Training and Retraining Bowels — 382
62. Applying Adult Briefs — 383
63. Collecting a Stool Specimen — 383
64. Applying Unsterile Dressing and Ointment to Unbroken Skin — 386
65. Caring for Casts — 388
66. Assisting with Changing an Ostomy Bag — 390
67. Assisting the Client with Oxygen Therapy — 392
68. Assisting with Cough and Deep Breathing Exercises — 394
69. Assisting with Breast-feeding and Breast Care — 397
70. Giving the Infant a Sponge Bath — 398
71. Bottle-feeding the Infant — 400

Preface

Introduction

Homemaker/Home Health Aide, 4th edition, is a comprehensive textbook that is designed for use in basic home health aide training programs and also as a reference book in required continuous in-service courses for home health aides.

The book is divided into two parts. Part 1 introduces the basic principles and theory involved in caring for a variety of clients in their homes. Topics in Part 1 include clients' rights; communication skills; observation and reporting skills; anatomy and physiology; human development from birth through the elder adult; the aging process; infection control; diseases such as AIDS, Alzheimer's, arthritis, cancer, diabetes, hepatitis, and tuberculosis. Part 2 is concerned with the practical application of procedures that are required not only by OBRA, but are commonly performed by home health aides, including homemaker tasks. The procedures are listed in a step-by-step format for ease of readability. The procedures are well-illustrated with photographs to show students the correct methods for performing tasks.

The demand for home health aides is expected to increase due to changing health care patterns related to increasing health care costs. This text has been designed to train new individuals entering the field to be caring, dedicated, and skilled paraprofessionals. Although the skills required today for home health aides are different compared to those required early in this century when home health aides first provided care to clients in their homes, the goal has not changed: to give safe, competent care to the client.

The Fourth Edition

This text was revised to include all the topics and procedures required by federal legislation that became effective on April 1, 1992 for training home health aides. The topics of clients' rights, universal precautions, restorative care, and safety are stressed throughout the text. The major changes for this edition are as follows.

- Emphasis on the role of the home health aide as a valuable member of the health care team.
- Greater emphasis on universal precautions; more content on the use of measures to prevent the spread of disease in the client's home. Procedure steps were changed to adapt to these new requirements.
- In-depth information on diabetes and arthritis.
- Infectious diseases, such as tuberculosis, AIDS, and hepatitis condensed into one unit.
- Ethical and professional conduct for the home health aide is clearly stated.
- More illustrations of the anatomy and physiology of the human body; full color insert of anatomy drawings.
- Expanded information on body mechanics, including the ten basic rules.
- Introduction of the role of the case manager in the home health care team.
- New photographs throughout the text; step-by-step photos for essential procedures.
- New procedures for:

  use of a gait belt
  gloving
  positioning clients in supine, lateral, prone,
    and Fowler's positions

dangling a client
giving male and female perineal care
inserting a hearing aid
caring for an artificial eye
bladder retraining
applying adult briefs
connecting a urinary leg bag
collecting a sputum specimen
collecting a stool specimen for occult blood
taking an apical pulse
measuring height and weight
giving a warm foot soak
applying nonsterile dressing
applying over-the-counter ointment to
   broken skin
coughing and deep breathing exercises

- Expanded questions at the end of each unit in Part 1.
- New content relating to child abuse, cultural diversity, skin care, types of families, communicating with the hard-of-hearing client, and postmortem care.
- Addition of the food pyramid and diet modifications to meet current guidelines.
- Illustrations and photographs of assistive and restorative aids.
- New content on advanced directives, including living wills and durable power of attorney.

Supplements

A new instructional system/package has been developed to achieve two goals:

1. To assist students in learning essential information to permit them to function as a home health care provider.
2. To assist instructors in planning and implementing their instructional approach for the most efficient use of time and resources.

Instructor's Guide

The expanded Instructor's Guide provides the instructor with valuable resources to simplify the planning and implementation of the instructional program. The content of the Instructor's Guide includes:

- Teaching tips and strategies
- Teaching resources
- Course syllabi
- Unit lesson plans
- Class activities
- Answers to text/workbook questions
- Quizzes and final examination with answers
- Competency checklists for text procedures
- Transparency masters

Workbook

The new student workbook provides additional questions, practice exercises, quizzes, and case studies. This material is designed to help the student master the text content and skills. The workbook content includes the following:

- Overview of units (unit objectives, unit summary, terms to define)
- Application exercises
- Quizzes
- Case studies with questions
- Competency checklists for text procedures

Acknowledgments

The authors wish to thank:

- Bruce Van Dyke of Van Dyke Photography, Camarillo, CA, for his skill, patience, and expertise during the long photography sessions that provided several hundred new photographs for the fourth edition of this text.
- Harry L. McNamara, Administrator, staff, and residents at Bay Harbor Rehabilitation Center, Torrance, CA, for their enthusiastic cooperation and assistance during the photo session at the facility.
- Jane Spaeter, President, Chris Cubar, and the staff of Just Right Home Care, for the use of their models and classrooms for photographs.
- Administrator, Donna Hesse, staff, and clients of Canterbury, Rancho Palos Verdes, CA, for their cooperation and eagerness to assist the photography team.
- Joyce Burke, Jane Cochran, Bob Barger, and Margaret Ohleyer, Elizabeth and Alexandria

White, for the use of their homes and for serving as models for photographs.

- Adrianne Williams, Associate Editor, Marjorie A. Bruce, Developmental Editor, and Melissa Conan, Project Editor, for their assistance and for sharing their expertise throughout the writing and editing of the fourth edition.

The authors and the project team at Delmar Publishers also wish to express their appreciation to a dedicated group of professionals who reviewed and provided commentary on the manuscript at various stages.

Jane A. Moore, RN, MS (Director of Patient Care for a proprietary home health agency, Dallas, TX)

Janice L. Hodges, MBA (Special Care Home Health, Inc., Pompano Beach, FL)

Suzann Balduzzi, MEd, BSN, RN (Western Wisconsin Technical College, La Crosse, WI)

Patricia L. Kuhns, MSN, MPH (Management Consultant, Stamford, CT)

Shirley Hoeman, PhD, RN (Consultant, Long Valley, NJ)

Judie Franko, RN, BSN (St. Paul Technical College, St. Paul, MN)

Gene Hamrick Campbell (State Specialist, Montgomery, AL)

Shirley Hohorst, RN (Consultant, Virginia Beach, CA)

Patricia A. Bittinger, RN, BS, MS (Salina, KS)

Dolly Finkelstein (Norrell Home Care, Queens, NY)

PART 1

Basic Principles

Sections

1 Becoming a Home Health Aide

2 Basic Anatomy and Physiology

3 Understanding Human Development and Age-Related Health

4 Promoting Health and Understanding Illness

5 Caring for Clients with Acute and Chronic Disorders

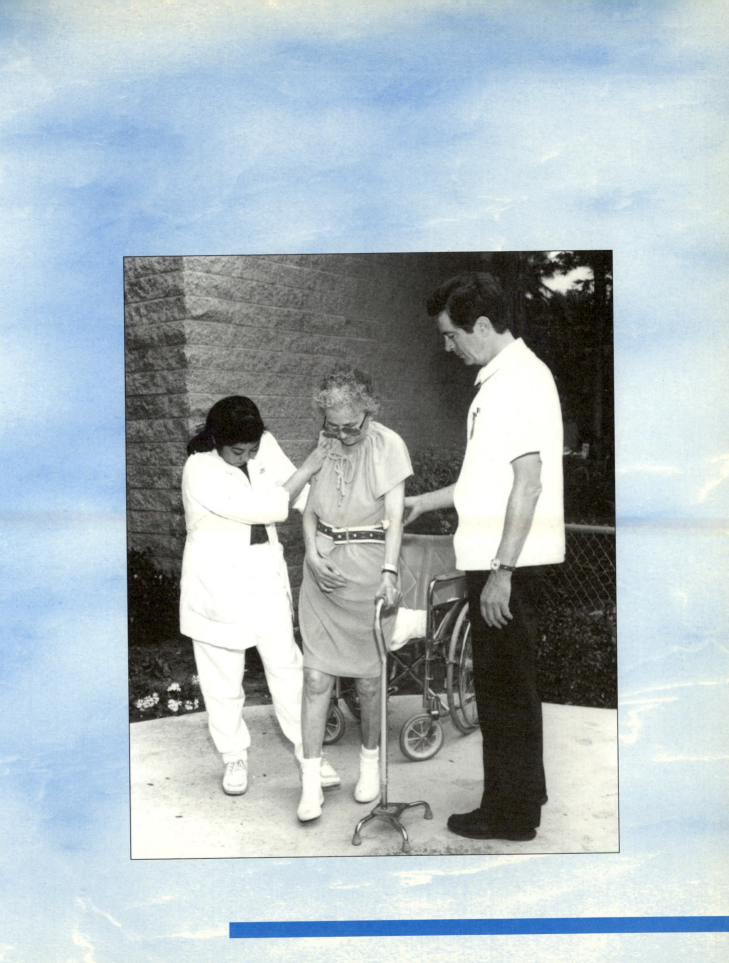

Section 1

Becoming a Home Health Aide

Units

1 Home Health Services

2 Developing Good Habits and Practices

3 Role Responsibilities and Ethical Standards

4 Developing Effective Communication Skills

5 Understanding Differences: Individuals, Families, and Cultures

Unit **1** Home Health Services

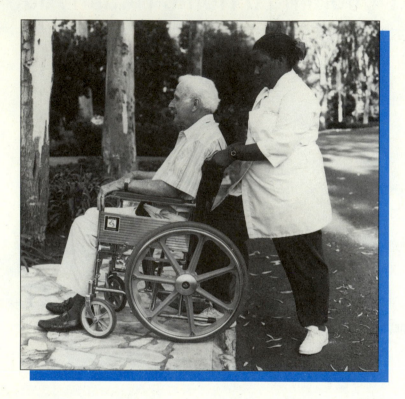

KEY TERMS
....

acute illness
CHAP
chronic illness
developmentally disabled
home care aide

home health aide
homemaker
homemaker/home health aide
long-term care facilities

Medicaid
Medicare
OBRA
personal care worker

LEARNING OBJECTIVES
....

After studying this unit, you should be able to:

- Name three reasons why the trend toward home care has returned.
- Name the two services provided by the home health aide.
- Explain the difference between acute and chronic illness.

- Define DRGs.
- List two differences between Medicare and Medicaid.
- List one purpose of the CHAP program.
- Define OBRA.

Illness has always been a part of the human condition. Care has been given according to the folkways and beliefs of society. Care also depends on the knowledge and kinds of treatments available. In many early societies, home remedies using herbs and plants found in the woods were used as medicine. Attending to the personal needs of the ill was most often performed by members of the family. Even then one special person was often called to help with medical emergencies. In some communities a midwife came to the home during the birth of a child. For labor or delivery problems the midwife was the only trained person available. In remote areas of the country, doctors were not easy to reach. There were fewer hospitals and nursing homes than there are today. Each family had to assume the task of nursing its own family members within the home. When the mother was ill, activities in the home were usually disrupted and home services were needed to provide families with help.

The Beginning of Home Health Services

The first homemaker service was established by a social service agency in the United States in 1903. Its main purpose was to provide child care. In the early 1920s employment agencies advertised for mature, practical women experienced in child care and household management. During the 1930s the Works Projects Administration (WPA) funded a program to train "housekeeping aides." They received preservice training and some on-the-job training as well. Later, in 1959 the National Conference on Homemaker Service met in Chicago. It was decided that homemaker service should be given to families with children, chronically ill persons, or aged members. It was advised that these individuals should receive care in the home whenever possible, without regard to family income. In 1960, at another conference, personal and health care was seen as an added duty of a homemaker's job; the term **home health aide** came into use. Home health aides were expected to work only under direct nursing supervision.

Increase in Need for Home Care Services

In 1976, laws were passed in a few states setting minimum standards for home health aides. In 1987, the Omnibus Budget Reconciliation Act, known as **OBRA,** was passed, which includes minimum training and competency requirements for the home health aide. Because services requested and needed by clients vary tremendously, the home health field has expanded to try to address all of these various needs. A few clients want a bath once a week, whereas another client might need 24-hour-a-day services mainly for companionship. Home care agencies have tried to accommodate these requests from clients by providing different categories of care providers.

A brief description of the types of care providers follows:

Homemaker: Performs household duties such as laundry and cooking
Personal care worker: Assists with a minimal level of daily living activities such as companionship and meal preparation
Home health aide: Performs personal and nursing care skills such as bathing the client (supervised by a registered nurse)
Homemaker/home health aide: Assists in general household tasks, personal care, and simple nursing duties such as feeding and bathing the client
Home care aide: Works with a client with the goal of assisting the client with independent living under professional supervision (title promoted by the National Association for Home Care)
Registered nurse (RN): Directs and supervises client care and activities. Can provide direct care to clients, i.e., treatments and medications. Assesses client problems and coordinates care with other health care providers. Licensed by the state.
Licensed vocational nurse (LVN); Licensed practical nurse (LPN): Provides direct client care, i.e., medication and treatments. Licensed by the state.

To answer a need, home health personnel may practice in various roles in a client's home.

They can be employed solely to bathe a client or to cook for the client. The role of a home health aide depends on the amount of training and the classification on the state registry. The home health aide is a necessary link to keep clients in their own home rather than a hospital or **long-term care facility.**

There are several reasons for the trend back to home care. One is the high cost of hospital care and early discharge of patients from hospitals. Hospital care is expensive and even with adequate insurance, a long stay in a hospital could cause a heavy financial burden for the individual.

A second reason for the increase in home care is that it is more readily available to individuals and can provide a wide range of services for individuals. Home care agencies can provide a variety of services ranging from cooking a meal to operating a kidney dialysis machine. These services may be needed only one day a week or 24 hours a day, 365 days a year.

A third reason for the increase in home care is that most individuals prefer to be attended to in the privacy and security of their own home. Clients usually prefer to be in a familiar environment, rather than in a strange one, such as a long-term care facility. A positive mental outlook is important for improvement in a physical disorder. It is often better for a person to stay in familiar surroundings than to be moved. This means being near loved ones, friends, and relatives. Try to imagine how clients might feel about being taken from their home, not knowing if they will ever return.

A fourth reason for the trend toward providing home care is the vastly increased number of aged persons. Modern health care and advanced technology have resulted in a longer average life span for Americans. The majority of the aged individuals are affected by one or more chronic illnesses. A **chronic illness** is a long-term health problem such as arthritis or diabetes, which is not generally expected to be cured. An **acute illness** is one that arises quickly, requires immediate care, and can be expected to go away, such as a common cold, flu, or appendicitis. Other individuals now cared for in their own homes rather than in institutions are mentally, physically, and developmentally disabled individuals. The term **developmentally**

disabled means a severe chronic disability of a person such as individuals with cerebral palsy or Down syndrome.

The need of quality care and assistance for frail individuals has placed a strong demand on society to find alternative ways of providing care. The number of long-term care facilities is inadequate to accommodate all persons in need. Many long-term care facilities are filled to capacity and have long waiting lists. Most of the needy do not require the high level of care provided by a skilled long-term care facility and in reality would prefer to stay in their homes than to be placed in one of these facilities. This has caused a great demand for home care providers.

The health care field is one of the top growth industries in the nation. For example, spending on home health care has grown by 18% in 1990, more than any other segment of the health care industry.

The older population, persons 65 years or older, numbered 31.0 million in 1989. This group represents 12.5% of the United States, about one in every eight Americans. Approximately 23% of these mature people need assistance with personal care activities and 27% have difficulty in home management activities.

Meeting the needs of the disabled and frail is a challenging task. A few of these individuals may live in group homes, others in their own home or apartment, whereas others may live with grown children. The decision to seek assistance for personal or health care needs can be made by the client, family members, or friends. In many instances, the family or spouse can do some of the care but not all of it. Many grown children are working and cannot be gone from their jobs to maintain care on a 24-hours-a-day, 7-days-a-week basis. In other cases, the family member may not have the necessary skills to provide the required care. The home health aide may be the person hired to help both the client in need of care and the family coping with the illness, whether it be an acute or chronic illness.

DRGs

In the interest of lowering medical costs to Medicaid and private carriers, a system was devised called **Diagnostic Related Groupings (DRGs).** Under this system, careful studies were made of the number of days of hospitalization required for various medical conditions. Each specific ailment was then allocated a fixed reimbursement amount based on statistics compiled by hospitals throughout the country. The purpose was to lower medical costs to the insurance carrier and to get patients out of the hospital as soon as possible. This made hospital beds available and returned patients to their normal environments where it was expected that recovery would be hastened.

Anyone who has spent time in a hospital will realize that this plan has a great deal of merit. Hospitals must maintain a rather rigid schedule. Aides and nurses start very early with the morning routine of waking patients, bathing, changing linens, giving medications, taking blood and urine samples, bringing bedpans, and feeding. Although everyone is wakened at an early hour, the number of aides and nurses is limited. Thus, some patients are not given their baths and do not have their beds changed until late in the afternoon. These persons feel that they have had their rest disturbed for no good reason.

It is also true that most people are happier in familiar surroundings and it is reasonable to expect that being at home would speed recovery. There is not the regimentation of a hospital and tasks may be done at the client's own pace. This allows the person to feel more relaxed, more comfortable, and less fearful. After all, if the doctor sends you home, it must mean that you are getting better!

You can see that DRGs have some very positive benefits. However, the negative aspects must be mentioned. Some people heal faster than others. Some do not want to leave the safe environment of a hospital. There have been cases where the person left the hospital too soon and complications developed. For that reason, hospitals and doctors have been very cautious and conservative with the DRGs and if they feel there is any chance of complications, they will reassess the patient and change the grouping to allow for more days in the hospital. This reassessment is very important because a person who is released too soon and has a severe setback might sue the hospital, doctors, and nurses for malpractice.

Before a patient is released from the hospital, a detailed care plan is prepared by the medical team and a discharge planner. One reason for making such a careful plan is to make sure that the home care team will have full information as to how to deal with normal recovery, will know how to recognize a problem, and will know what to do if one occurs. This is for the welfare of the person as well as for the protection of the hospital and medical team. Included in the release plan should be schedules for physical therapy, occupational therapy, any special or unusual treatment plans, and medication schedules as well as a complete dietary plan prepared by a dietitian or nutritional therapist.

A good discharge plan simplifies the job of a home health aide because there will be no doubts about what care is required for the client. The release plan will be discussed with the health care agency so that the aide's supervisor will be fully aware of all aspects of the care plan. Thus, if an aide on the job does have questions, he or she will be able to contact the agency supervisor for advice.

Role of the Home Health Aide

The duties of the home health aide may fall into many categories, ranging from homemaking to simple nursing care in the home, Figure 1-1. Homemaking duties involve assisting with the upkeep of the home and daily household operations. Doing the client's laundry, preparing meals, and going to the market may all be part of the aide's duties, Figure 1-2. A home health aide is not expected to do heavy cleaning such as washing windows or walls, waxing floors, or moving heavy furniture. However, the home must be kept clean and tidy. Guidelines will be presented throughout the text to help understand what is expected.

Another main duty of the home health aide is to provide personal and nursing care skills within the home, Figure 1-3. This is performed under the supervision of another member of the health care team. The two health care members who generally supervise the home health aide are either a registered nurse (RN) or a case manager (CM). The supervisor will design a care plan for you to follow once a client is assigned. The care plan

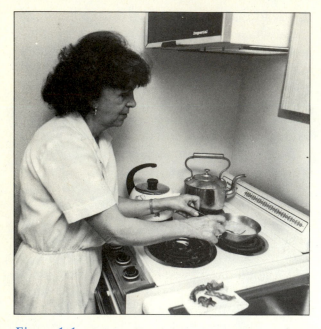

Figure 1-1   A home health aide preparing a meal

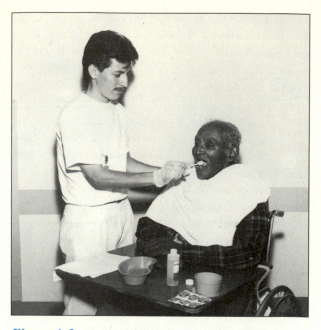

Figure 1-3   A home health aide assisting a client with his personal care

will specifically outline the responsibilities of the home health aide while working in the client's home.

The single most important task of a home health aide is to treat each client with respect, dignity, and kindness. This sounds simple; however, in truth, it is easy in some situations but difficult in others. Each person needing an aide

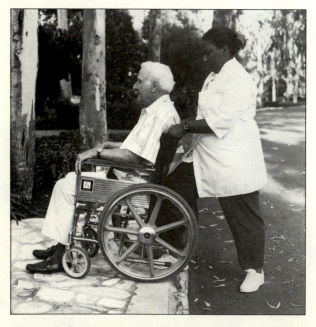

Figure 1-2   A home health aide pushing a client in a wheelchair outside

has his or her own set of special needs. An aide needs to be aware of the cultural differences, physical needs, diet requirements, family situations, and emotional support needed by each and every client, Figure 1-4.

Each case will be different and challenging, but also very rewarding and fulfilling. A home health aide will meet a variety of clients with many different personalities. Some clients will respond positively to the care you give them, but others will not.

In each unit of this text you will find new words to master and new techniques to learn. As your knowledge grows, so does your confidence as an individual. In becoming a home health aide you can be proud of your newly acquired skills. Satisfaction comes in being able to serve those who need your skills.

Programs and Other Important Issues Influencing Health Care

Community Health Accreditation Program (CHAP)

The Community Health Accreditation Program, Inc. **(CHAP)** has become the first private accreditation body to be recommended for "deemed status" by the United States Department of

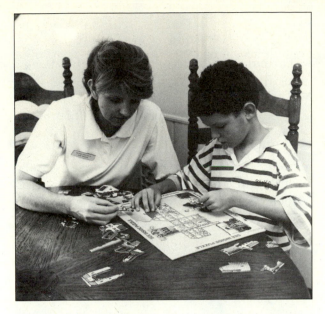

Figure 1-4 A home care aide assisting a young child put a puzzle together

Health and Human Services. Deemed status means that home health agencies that meet CHAP's accreditation standards will be considered to have met the federal government conditions for participation in the Medicare program.

People at home require a highly personal and devoted level of care. Medicare and CHAP provide rigid controls attempting to ensure that home health agencies are effectively managed and that they employ qualified, well-trained staff. CHAP works closely with consumers, those who use the services, to make sure that their needs are being met in the best and most cost-effective way, in their own homes. CHAP sets high standards of care instead of just requiring that minimum safety and care guidelines be met. CHAP's philosophy is that consumers have the right to know which agencies provide the highest quality of home care services.

Medicare and Medicaid

At the present time, everyone in the United States who has paid into Social Security is enti-

tled to Medicare insurance once they are disabled or become 65 years of age. **Medicare** is a federally funded program in which an individual most enroll and pay a monthly fee to participate. There are two reimbursement parts to the program. One is for the physician services (called Part A) and the other is for other services such as diagnostic tests and hospital stays (called Part B). Medicare insurance pays for part of the costs of health care, but not all.

Medicaid is also a federally funded program that pays for health care service for persons whose income is below a certain amount. The coverage provided to recipients and the minimum income level that makes one eligible varies from state to state. A person can qualify for both Medicare and Medicaid benefits.

Whenever governmental funding is involved, the federal or state government can regulate the health care industry and demand that certain standards be maintained with regard to health care facilities, health care workers, and educational requirements. The home health aide must be aware of these standards.

Omnibus Budget Reconciliation Act (OBRA)

In 1987, the federal government implemented the Omnibus Budget Reconciliation Act (OBRA), which mandates federal Medicare and Medicaid standards for nursing homes and home health agencies. A variety of topics and issues concerning health care for the elderly and developmentally disabled were covered in this legislation, such as the use of restraints, nursing assistant training guidelines, and rights of clients. A mutual goal of the OBRA, Medicare, and Medicaid regulations is to improve care for individuals in long-term care facilities and in their own homes.

SUMMARY

- The need for educated, dedicated home health aides continues to grow, and it is expected that as our population ages, more and more individuals will require health care services in the home.
- The home health aide is expected to give safe and proper care to the client. The aide should be able to provide skilled care.
- To observe and report accurately is important to the other members of the health team.

- The aide should cooperate with other family members as well as the client.
- Federal standards require home health aides to be on the local state registry if they work for a federally accredited home health agency.
- Medicare and Medicaid funds assist the elderly and disabled to pay part of the cost of their health care.

REVIEW

1. List three reasons for the increasing trend toward home care.
2. List two main services provided by the home health aide.
3. Explain the term chronic illness.
4. List two positive benefits of DRGs.
5. Name two differences between Medicare and Medicaid.
6. Explain the differences between CHAP and the OBRA Medicare and Medicaid regulations.
7. Payment for the home health aide services is collected by the agency that assumes responsibility for your client. These payments may come from:
   a. Medicare
   b. Medicaid
   c. The client
   d. Any of the above
8. Home health aide care involves:
   a. Client care and housekeeping activities
   b. Supervising client's care
   c. Laundry and wallpapering
   d. Client care and giving injections
9. One of the reasons for the increased home care is that patients are discharged from the hospital very early and need assistance with their care.
   a. true
   b. false
10. The name of the system that allocates fixed reimbursement amounts on a specific ailment when an individual is hospitalized is called:
    a. CHAP
    b. OBRA
    c. DRGs
    d. ADLs
11. An aide needs to be aware of the client's:
    a. Cultural differences
    b. Physical needs
    c. Family situations
    d. All of the above

Unit 2 Developing Good Habits and Practices

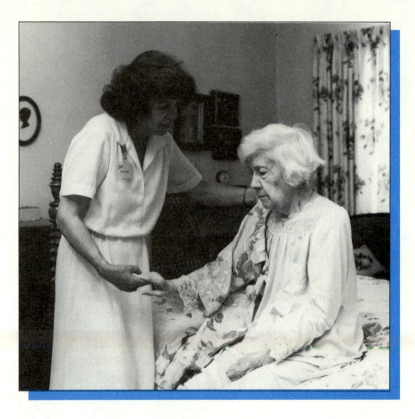

KEY TERMS

attitude · case manager · components · evaluation · hygiene · interaction · interpersonal relationships · LPN · offensive · oral hygiene · practice · procedure · RN · theory

attitude
case manager
components
evaluation
hygiene

interaction
interpersonal relationships
LPN
offensive
oral hygiene

practice
procedure
RN
theory

LEARNING OBJECTIVES

After studying this unit, you should be able to:

- Define interpersonal relationships and interaction.
- Give an example of self-understanding.
- Identify the need for evaluation.

- State the difference between theory and practice.
- Give four examples of good personal hygiene.
- Identify five members of the health care team.

11

At first glance, the role of a home health aide may appear to be quite simple. It is made up of everyday tasks: keeping a house in order, preparing and cleaning up after meals, and providing for the comfort and safety of a client. Students may feel that they already know how to take care of a house. Most people have been doing housekeeping tasks since early childhood. Often it is thought that there is nothing new to learn about familiar jobs. The student may ask, "Why don't we get to the important things? After all, I want to care for the sick. Why should I waste time learning homemaking skills?"

Everyone can benefit by learning new ways to do certain jobs. Once the new method is learned, the aide can compare it with the old way and may discover a more efficient technique.

By learning to focus on the components of a task, the aide will find understanding comes more easily. **Components** are the separate parts that make up a whole. Learning how to do something, when to do it, and what should be done first will add up to a more complete understanding. Students must learn how and when to do all the tasks that need to be done. They also learn what tasks are most important. In this way, the student completing the course will become a useful and successful home health aide.

Learning Procedures

There are many ways to do some tasks, for example, prepare a meal. There will be certain essential components of the task that if not completed correctly and in the right order will mean the task has been done wrong. For example, you need to wash your hands and you need to do that first. You need to follow client's dietary requirements, but you may prepare any of a variety of foods. You can toast the bread before or after you slice the tomato, but you must put ingredients away and clean up after preparing food. Other tasks, however, have rigid procedures and only one way to proceed, such as washing hands and taking an oral temperature. A **procedure** is a list of steps used to complete a task. A procedure can be either a nursing task or a homemaking task. The judging is known as an **evaluation.**

The student will need to demonstrate a designated list of procedures satisfactorily in front of an instructor. Each procedure will be demonstrated by the instructor before the student performs the procedure. The instructor will give the student a copy of the procedure with all the required steps listed. Use these procedure guidelines in practicing each procedure in the laboratory. Written tests are also given for evaluation purposes, Figure 2-1. Evaluation helps the student know which areas require extra study or practice.

There are usually two parts to the instruction given to the home health aide. The first is called theory. **Theory** is the information that forms a basis for action. In classroom lectures and in the assigned readings, the student learns theory. The second component is devoted to practice. **Practice** is the actual performance of the procedures. Practice is combined with the theory to enable the student to build skills in both areas at the same time. The home health aide learns client care procedures and homemaking procedures.

Forming Study Habits

Study habits differ from person to person. Some people need more time for study than others. Some are able to perform certain tasks more easily than others. Students must recognize their own needs in forming study habits.

Working with Others

Nurses and home health aides are employed in the service of giving care to ill persons. Delivering this service makes it necessary for the home health aide to work closely with family members. Conflicts and arguments among family members sometimes occur. Everyone has probably observed or been a part of a family dispute. What happens when an outsider enters into a family argument? In some cases, the family will band together and turn against the outsider. The family could turn away or show anger if the aide interfered in a family matter. Consider, for instance, the following situation:

> You are assigned to a home by the agency for whom you work. There are two children (ages 4 and 6) and a new baby. Your job is to keep the house in

Students should become familiar with the common testing methods. Examples of the most common types are presented below:

True-False

Directions: Circle T for true and F for false.

Example:

T   F   The duties of the home health aide may fall in many categories ranging from homemaking to simple nursing care in the home.

Brief Answer

Directions: Briefly answer the following questions.

Example: List one reason for the recent expansion of home care.

Multiple Choice

Directions: Fill in the blank with the correct word or phrase.

Example:

An example of a chronic disease is:

    a. diabetes

    b. flu

    c. cold

    d. pneumonia

Matching

Directions: Match items in Column I with the correct descriptions in Column II.

Example:

Column I	Column II
___ mental abuse	a. humiliating the client
___ involuntary seclusion	b. locking a client up without client's permission
___ negligence	c. bathing a client in too hot water
___ sexual abuse	d. making sexual advances toward your client

Essay

Directions: In 20 to 30 words, answer the following question.

Example: Explain the difference between an acute illness and a chronic illness.

Figure 2-1   Examples of common test questions

order, prepare meals, and give care to the children and the mother. The mother is sitting in the kitchen having coffee; you are at the stove making formula for the baby. The two children burst into the room, fighting over a toy. One child falls against you, the aide; the baby's bottle of formula drops. Formula and broken glass cover the floor.

What would be your reaction? What reaction is likely to bring the best results? Concern for the safety of the children should be the first response of the home health aide. The children should be told that you are glad that no one was hurt. Then take them from the kitchen and clean up the broken glass and spilled formula.

In most instances, discipline must be left to the mother or other adult family member. If you should come up against special problems about child behavior, you should call your supervisor for advice. If you have cause to think that a child is being beaten or otherwise mistreated, you should report to your supervisor immediately. Do not try to interfere, but report such information at once.

Interpersonal Relationships

When people live, work, or play together, one person acts and the other reacts or responds to the act. This process is called an **interaction.** Figure 2-2 shows that several persons may be involved in a situation—the arrows point to all the possible interactions.

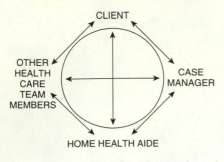

Figure 2-2   A home health aide needs to interact with all members of the health care team and is an important member of the team.

People are expected to handle interactions as a part of everyday life. The feeling and understanding that result from the interactions between two or more persons form what are called **interpersonal relationships.** To the person entering a service occupation, interpersonal relationships can determine success or failure. Each of the persons involved in these relationships is entitled to be treated with dignity. Everyone should follow the golden rule—treat others as you would like to be treated. This helps to establish good interpersonal relationships.

In Figures 2-2, 2-3, and 2-4, look at the combinations of relationships that may develop for the home health aide. The home health aide must remember that he/she is entering a home where an illness or a problem already exists. An illness or problem may cause the family members to be unhappy or disorganized. Anger, fear, and other emotional reactions may be present. The client may be in pain, cranky, sad, or depressed. The home health aide who is aware of the source of the problem often finds it easier to accept the family's behavior. As a result, awkward interpersonal relationships can often be avoided.

Developing Self-understanding

The secret of understanding others begins with self-understanding. You know what makes you feel good. When others are kind to you, compliment you on a job well done, tell you how well you look, don't you suddenly feel terrific? Think how you have felt when you have been criticized or when you have had a really "bad" day. Everyone shares those feelings. All individuals have the same basic needs, Figure 2-5. The physical needs are food, shelter, clothing, sleep, and, of course, good health.

All people also have psychological and emotional needs. These include the need for love, having a feeling of belonging, and a feeling of well-being, to name a few. When these needs are not met, an individual may not function at his or her highest level. This can lead to stress and even illness. The person who is sensitive to his or her own needs and desires is better able to relate to others. This can be an asset to someone entering the health care field. All people must be treated with respect!

Some people have a very low opinion of themselves. They always "put themselves down."

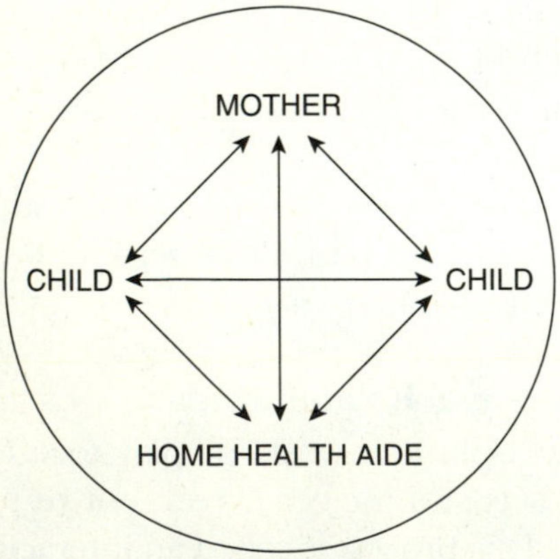

Figure 2-3   Many interactions may take place between the home health aide and family members.

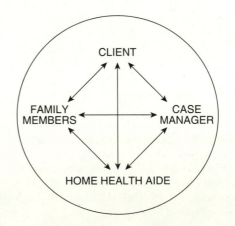

Figure 2-4   Learning to handle relationships is part of the home health aide's job.

PHYSICAL	MENTAL
1. Hygiene	1. Sexual
2. Comfort	2. Spiritual
3. Safety	3. Cultural
4. Body alignment	4. Self-esteem/love, affection
5. Mobility	5. Belonging
6. Rest and sleep	6. Stimulation
7. Nutrition	7. Loss and death
8. Elimination	8. Knowledge
9. Respiration and circulation	9. Coping mechanisms
10. Fluid balance	10. Growth and development
11. Growth and development	11. Intellectual achievement
	12. Relationships
	13. Self-actualization

Figure 2-5   Basic human needs as defined by Abraham Maslow, the well-known expert on human behavior.

They say such things as, "I'm so dumb," "I'm so fat," "Nobody likes me," or "I know I'll fail." At the other extreme are those who brag about where they have been, who they know, and how important they are. Most people are comfortable around those individuals who are secure but modest about their success. Unfortunately, it is often much easier to judge others than to judge oneself.

Self-understanding is a growth process that continues throughout life. People who have found a goal and get pleasure from their work probably feel good about themselves. As a result, they develop feelings of self-esteem. This usually makes them less critical of others and they are better able to understand others. Part of self-understanding is accepting one's own failures and weaknesses. Accepting others becomes easier after admitting that no one is perfect.

Personal Health and Hygiene

A home health aide must observe the personal **hygiene** standards expected of any health team member, Figure 2-6. When working in other people's homes, the aide should reflect the highest standards. This means being clean and well groomed each workday. The person who goes on a job unbathed, with dirty hair and nails, and wearing wrinkled, spotted clothes makes a bad impression. A sloppy appearance implies that the person also has a poor self-image and sloppy working habits.

An aide should wear a clean uniform, clean undergarments, and comfortable, polished shoes.

An aide who is appropriately dressed or in the proper uniform creates a more professional appearance and makes the client feel more comfortable. Home care agencies vary greatly in their dress codes. A few agencies do require a designated uniform, whereas others may allow the

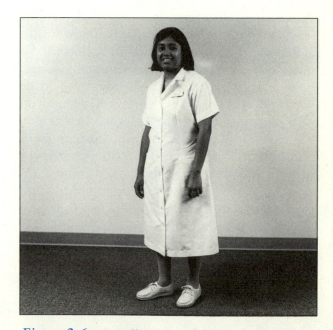

Figure 2-6   A well-groomed home health aide. Note the smile on her face and her neat appearance. Also note that aide wears little makeup or jewelry and that she wears a name tag on her uniform.

aide to wear comfortable, clean, untattered street clothes. Most agencies do not allow their home health aides to wear blue jeans or shorts. In all situations, the aide must follow the agency's dress code or uniform requirement, Figure 2-6.

It is also important for the home health aide to wear a name tag at all times. The name tag gives the name of the aide and the proper title.

Bathing, brushing the teeth, and wearing a neat hair style is also part of good grooming. Fingernails should be short, smooth, and clean. Jewelry should be limited to a watch and a wedding band. Small post earrings for pierced ears are usually acceptable. Bracelets and dangling necklaces are not worn because they may catch on bedding or furniture. A ring might scratch the client or become lost.

Good grooming is important not only for appearance but also for safety reasons. Jewelry and rough fingernails could cause scratches. The danger of infection is always present if the skin has been scratched. Dirt and germs may easily enter an opening in the skin. Infected wounds heal more slowly among clients who are affected with other serious illnesses. The home health aide must not add pain or discomfort to the client by being careless.

Personal cleanliness is also necessary to prevent and remove body odors. A home health aide is in close contact with clients; odors can be quite **offensive.** Remember, some clients may be allergic to perfumes. Body odors should be removed with soap and water, not covered up with perfume. A considerate home health aide will check mouth odor as well. Brushing teeth regularly and using mouthwash helps prevent mouth odors. Eating garlic and onions and smoking cigarettes increases the need for oral hygiene. **Oral hygiene** means keeping the mouth clean and healthy. One important way to improve oral hygiene is to have annual dental checkups. It must be emphasized that an aide should not smoke while on duty unless the client has given permission. Be sure to check your agency's policy on smoking in clients' homes. The aide must recognize that a client with a lung disease, allergies, respiratory illness, or personal distaste for the smell of smoke has the right to refuse to allow the aide to smoke within the home.

Attitude

Have you ever said, "I don't like your attitude"; or, "That one really has an attitude"? **Attitude** refers to state of mind, behavior, or conduct about some matter. A home health aide who has "a bad attitude" will not be able to do good work. Such an aide might seem angry when performing personal tasks for a client and thereby make the client uncomfortable and embarrassed. For example, when a client must use a bedside commode for a bowel movement, there will be an unpleasant smell in the room. If a home health aide is unwilling to accept dealing with such conditions, the client may be aware of the aide's attitude. This does not lead to a pleasant working relationship.

When you decide to become a home health aide, you must prepare yourself to face some tasks that are very personal and not always pleasant. Your client may be demanding and even disagreeable. As a professional home health aide, you must develop a positive attitude toward all your clients. You will have to work with a variety of clients in a variety of homes. You must take pride in helping each of them feel better. With the right attitude, your work will be satisfying to you and to your clients. A healthy attitude about yourself and your work will make you a more professional home health aide.

The Health Care Team

A home health aide is one member of the health care team. Although working in a home creates physical distance between an aide and other members, the team concept still exists. For the aide to work best within the team, the duties of other members should be clearly understood. Special trained health care personnel who are part of the health care team may include:

Nurses and home care aides
Physicians
Case managers
Speech therapists
Occupational therapists
Physical therapists
Social workers

Respiratory therapists
Dietitians
Pharmacists
Chiropractors
Medical laboratory technicians

The physician orders the medications and special treatments for the client. A client who has many health problems may also have many physicians. The client usually has a family doctor, also called a general practitioner. For a specific problem, however, the client may have a specialist. The home health aide should be aware of the names of the various medical specialties.

At all levels of nursing, a state examination is required to be completed with a passing grade before a nurse may practice. Licensed practical nurses (**LPNs**) or licensed vocational nurses (LVNs) study for approximately 12 months; registered nurses (**RNs**) may study in a 2-, 3-, or 4-year educational program. Generally, a home health nurse who has a 4-year degree supervises the home health aide. The home health aide works most closely with the agency supervisors and reports directly to them.

Recently, due to the expansion of home care, a new member of the health team has emerged. This new member is called a **case manager.** The case manager may have a social work or RN background and coordinates all the services the client may require. In addition, the case manager may assist the client with their financial situation. The case manager tries to see that all the client's needs are met in the most cost-efficient way. Activities within the case manager's scope range from aiding the client with transportation to the local clinic or locating safe and appropriate housing to arranging a food program such as Meals on Wheels.

Because of the frequent and personal contact the aide has with the client, the aide may be the first to observe any changes in the client's condition. Such changes must be documented and reported immediately to the case manager or nursing supervisor. Most often the nursing supervisor will contact the doctor or family member if it is necessary. Each client and each home is unique. The home health aide must fully understand the assignment. Submitting a complete report to the appropriate person is also an important part of the home health aide's responsibility. Each aide must know who and when to call. It is better to call for advice than make an error in the client's care.

A caring and dedicated home health aide will continue to learn new skills and be ready to face the challenges of home care as more is learned about illness and its effect on the client, the family, and the health team. For that reason, home health aides should attend the required in-service programs through their agencies. The more an aide knows, the better care the aide can provide.

SUMMARY

- A practicing home health aide will be faced with many new learning situations. The aide will have new skills to learn and will need to continue to increase his or her knowledge about working with ill or disabled clients.
- Students learn by doing, by studying, and by observing. The person who develops good study habits now is laying a foundation for good work habits later.
- Successful home health aides are sensitive to the emotional and physical needs of their clients.

- Student home health aides need to learn about interpersonal relationships and apply the knowledge learned to their own families, classmates, instructors, and clients with whom they will work. The greater the self-understanding, the greater a student may understand relationships with others.
- As a member of the health care team, the home health aide must also be concerned about the image conveyed to others by his or her personal grooming. An aide's own health habits have an effect on how he or she is accepted by others. Poor grooming habits and

a messy appearance may affect others negatively. Personal cleanliness and a neat appearance reflect a positive self-image and give the aide a head start toward success on the job.

- The work of a home health aide combines an active knowledge of personal care, simple client care tasks, and homemaking procedures. Although the health care needs are the first consideration, keeping the client's environment clean is also important.

- An aide must be flexible and well organized in each situation. Work hours, conditions, and settings will vary greatly with each case.
- COURTESY, KINDNESS, and GENTLENESS are always expected attributes of a home health aide.
- The home health aide is an important member of the health care team.

REVIEW

1. What is the difference between theory and practice?

2. What is an interpersonal relationship?

3. Define a procedure.

4. Why are evaluations helpful?

5. Give four examples of good personal hygiene.

6. List five members of the health care team.

7. Place the letter from Column II, which describes a nursing action that would be appropriate for meeting a specific need, as identified by Abraham Maslow, that is named in Column I.

Column I	Column II
___1. security and safety	a. provide proper food for the client
___2. self-esteem	b. allow client to make choices, so client can feel in control
___3. physical	c. encourage visits with neighbors and family
___4. self-actualization	d. keep your promises to clients and do not lie to them, so that
___5. love/social	they can trust those who care for them
	e. address client by proper name and title, i.e., "Good afternoon, Mr. Clinton."

8. A case manager may _____ for a client.
   a. assist in planning care
   b. arrange for Meals on Wheels
   c. assist with financial matters
   d. all of the above

9. The home health team consists of:
   1. doctor
   2. case manager
   3. home health aide
   4. pharmacist
   5. physical therapist

   a. all of the above
   b. 2 and 3
   c. all but 4
   d. all but 1

10. When you work in the home, you will be:
    a. responsible for making decisions without help
    b. working under the supervision of a case manager
    c. away from your agency and unable to contact your supervisor
    d. expected to call the client's doctor with information

11. A home health aide must attend in-service educational programs on an ongoing basis once employed by a home care agency.
    a. true   b. false

Unit *3* Role Responsibilities and Ethical Standards

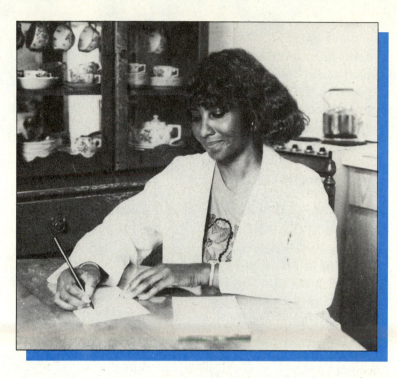

KEY TERMS

. . . .

abuse
career
confidentiality
documentation
ethics

flexible
intrafamily
liability
manipulation

negligence
observation
reporting
time organization

LEARNING OBJECTIVES

. . . .

After studying this unit, you should be able to:

- Identify two career adjustments required of a home health aide.
- Name two client care responsibilities.
- Define ethics and identify two examples of ethical practice.
- Explain why accurate observation, reporting, and documentation are important tasks for the home health aide.

- Define the term "confidentiality."
- Explain what is meant by "liability" and give five examples of actions to avoid.
- List five "rights" of the client.
- List three "rights" of the home health aide.
- Define client abuse and list four types of client abuse.

A **career** is the occupation or profession for which one has been specially educated. In every new field of employment it is necessary to make adjustments, both mentally and physically, to gain satisfaction from the job.

Career Adjustments

The home health aide will encounter irregular working hours and must be able to adjust to a variety of assignments, settings, and equipment. The aide must also learn to follow instructions and adhere to established policies. Setting up a workable schedule and learning client care responsibilities and limitations are also adjustments the home health aide must make.

Working Hours

Working hours may be irregular. Primarily the working hours will be during the day, but occasionally a home health aide may be required to work during the night. The aide may be asked to work on varying shifts or on weekends. It is common for a home health aide to be assigned several part-time cases. Three different clients might be visited in one day or on different days of the week. Due to this irregularity of assignments, a home health aide must be **flexible** and have access to transportation. This means being able to quickly adjust from one type of situation to another and being able to feel comfortable meeting new people.

Variety of Assignments

The aide must adjust to different family situations and varied health care needs of the clients. In one home, the aide might be expected to care for infants, preschool children, and teenagers. In another, there may be only middle-aged or elderly people. No two family situations are the same. This means the aide will have to establish new interpersonal relationships in each case. The medical conditions can range from ill infants to terminally ill clients. The aide must be prepared to give safe and proper care in each situation.

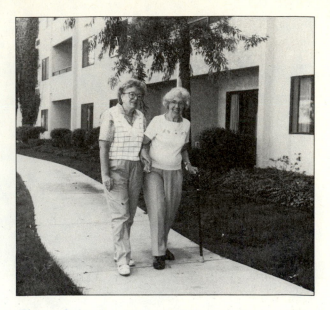

Figure 3-1   An aide ambulating a client outside of her apartment

Variety of Settings and Equipment

The aide must also adapt to homes that are not as well equipped as others. Some homes have modern equipment and beautiful furnishings. Others offer the bare necessities of life. The home health aide must not make judgments about people based on their belongings. Some clients prefer simple living. The aide should also remember that most people who live in poverty do not do so by choice. The home health aide will be expected to treat all clients with dignity regardless of their financial position. Each human being is entitled to respectful and dignified care. That is the only kind of care for which a home health aide is trained to perform, Figure 3-1.

Following Instructions and Policies

Another career adjustment is learning to carry out the assignment according to instructions. The aide must follow the directions of the supervisor. The comfort and well-being of the client should always take top priority. This means that it is the most important part of client care. In case of an emergency or any unexpected problem developing, the aide should immediately report to the agency supervisor or the employer. Before taking a case, a home health aide should be sure to ask for all vital information. In addition, the supervisor will provide a home care plan for the client, outlining the specific care to be provided and the aide's responsibilities. This includes duties, client needs, and the name and phone number of the person to be contacted in emergencies.

A successful aide possesses good organization skills. An aide must manage time well to be able to complete all the tasks required in the allotted time. The instructions may include: light housekeeping, laundry and ironing, meal preparation, marketing, and personal care of the client. The aide will have to decide the best way to plan each day's activities. This will require flexibility, practical judgment, and **time organization.** Some pitfalls to avoid are:

- Not replacing or ordering supplies when needed from your case manager
- Gossiping with the client or family member instead of working
- Watching a favorite television show
- Jumping from one job to another and one room to another without organizing priorities
- Putting off unpleasant tasks because they are disagreeable
- Talking to friends on the phone or doing personal business
- Stopping frequently for a cup of coffee or a cigarette
- Trying to do too much in one day, and doing nothing well

The best way to deal with a new set of circumstances is to look the situation over carefully and get organized. On entering a new situation, it is human nature to think about the end result. Often one is tempted to try to do everything in one day. This leads to frustration and nothing gets done well. Begin by asking where supplies are stored. Communicate with the client or family and supervisor to find out exactly what is expected. Prepare a written plan each day for the cases assigned, Figure 3-2. At the end of the working day, see what did not get done. Revise the plan for the next day. It is best to select only one big project for each day. After the routine tasks and client care procedures are done for the day, tackle the larger job. These

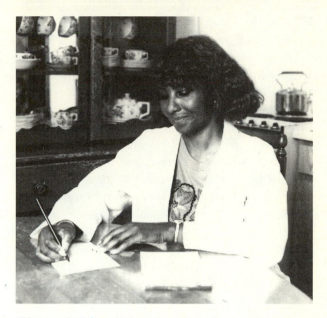

Figure 3-2A   Aide planning her assignment before the start of her work day

tasks can be planned for periods when the client does not require your full attention. The household often will function better as a result of preplanning and organization.

A home health aide may be assigned to work with several clients each week. The aide should prepare a schedule for each assignment. In this way the aide's time can be used most effi-

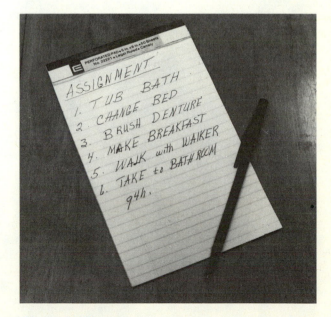

Figure 3-2B   This is a sample list of tasks to be completed by the aide.

ciently. Each daily plan should be flexible enough to allow for the unexpected. The supervisor can make suggestions and help define the duties in each case. The aide must perform these duties in the time allotted.

When beginning a new job, the aide must adjust to the client's or family's routine. Aides should not reorganize the entire house or daily schedule to suit themselves. Major changes should be made only with the approval of the client or a responsible family member. An aide's job is to make the family comfortable and to assist them, not to change their life-style. A well-organized home health aide saves time and effort by planning ahead and anticipating possible problems.

Knowledge of Role and Responsibility

Home health aides must keep in mind the purpose of their job and employment, Figure 3-3.

If you are employed to do just personal care, then complete this task in the allotted time with the best quality work possible. If you are employed in the home to do homemaking tasks only, do the tasks the best you can in the allotted time. Occasionally an aide is employed to do both the personal care tasks and the homemaking tasks. It is important for the aide to prioritize the tasks; do the essentials first and then complete the other tasks in the time allotted. Before starting an assignment, the aide should look over the assignment list and review the order in which the tasks need to be done. When reviewing the list, the aide should prioritize from the most important and essential to the least important, Figure 3-4. If possible, the aide should do the most important tasks first and then go to the least important tasks. Then, if something unexpected happens in the middle of the assignment, adjustments can be made more readily.

CLIENT CARE RESPONSIBILITIES*

Give simple emotional and psychological support to the client and other household members.
Encourage the client to become as independent as possible within the care plan guidelines.
Make occupied or unoccupied bed.
Provide personal care:

Mouth care	Shower or tub
Daily shave	Bedpan or urinal as requested or scheduled
Nail care	Assistance with bathroom use
Shampoo	Assistance with dressing
Hair care	Denture care
Bed bath—complete or partial	

Transfer client from bed to chair and return client back to bed.
Take and record:

Temperature	Intake
Pulse	Output
Respirations	Weight
Blood pressure	Height

Assist with oral medications that are self-administered.
Accompany client to doctor's office or to areas outside the home, if permitted.
Assist client with medically recommended physical activities.
Carry out procedures assigned and demonstrated by supervisor including:

Range of motion	Prosthesis application
Collecting specimens	Special skin care
Bowel and bladder retraining	Minor dressing changes
Diet preparation	

*(Procedures listed here will be explained later in the text.)

Figure 3-3   Client care services are given under the directions of a nursing supervisor or case manager.

A. Routine home health aide functions include the following:
1. With guidance from the nurse or agency supervisor, arranging the schedule so that the client follows the care plan such as increased physical activity and other activities of daily living
2. Keeping an aide care plan as part of the client record
3. Taking temperature, pulse, and respiration
4. Assisting the client on and off the bedpan, commode, or toilet
5. Assisting with bathing of the client in bed, in the tub, or in the shower as determined by the doctor, nurse, or agency supervisor
6. Assisting with the care of teeth and mouth
7. Assisting with grooming—care of hair, including shampooing; shaving; and the ordinary care of the nails
8. Assisting the client with dressing
9. Assisting the client with eating
10. Assisting the client in moving from bed to chair or wheelchair and assisting the client in walking
11. Accompanying the client to obtain medical care (when practical)
12. Preparing and serving meals according to instructions
13. Washing dishes as needed
14. Making or changing the bed
15. Reminding clients to take medications on schedule
16. Doing light housekeeping; i.e., dusting and vacuuming the rooms the client uses
17. Listing needed supplies
18. Shopping for the client if no other arrangement is possible
19. Doing the client's personal laundry if no family member is available or able; may include necessary ironing and mending
20. Notifying supervisor or case manager to whom you report of any change in the client's condition

B. Special home health aide functions:
With permission of the case manager or supervisor, the home health aide may do the following procedures:
1. Reinforcing dressings and changing simple nonsterile dressings
2. Applying prescribed ice cap or ice collar
3. Applying TED hose
4. Assisting with prescribed skin care
5. Taking the blood pressure
6. Assisting with the change of ostomy bags
7. Measuring intake and output, as ordered
8. Preparing modified diets, as prescribed by the physician
9. Assisting the client with prescribed exercises that have been taught by appropriate professional personnel
10. Helping the client relearn household skills
11. Assisting with rehabilitation measures

Figure 3-4   Home health aides functions approved by most states

Clients may ask the aide to perform skills that have not been included in the instructions, Figure 3-5. How can the aide inform the client that what has been requested is not part of the assigned duties? Anger and hostility accomplish nothing. The aide should say, "This procedure was not included in my studies, and it would not be right for me to take unneces-sary risks. Shall I call the supervisor?" If the request involves a housekeeping task, the aide might say, "There are many things I can do, and am ready to do. However, my assignment does not state it."

The following list summarizes the guidelines the home health aide is to observe in all assignments:

CLIENT CARE LIMITATIONS

- Do not assist with medication without permission of your case manager.
- Do not insert an indwelling catheter.
- Do not insert feeding tubes.
- Do not change sterile dressings.
- Do not omit, neglect, or change the doctor's orders.
- Do not give injections.

Figure 3-5   Limitations are set for the protection of the client and the home health aide.

1. Follow your client's plan of care.
2. Work carefully.
3. Be sure you are insured if you are expected to transport your client to clinics or doctor's visits in your car.
4. Provide only those services for which you have been trained.
5. Call your local emergency number if emergency medical care is needed.
6. Only give first aid for which you have been trained.
7. Do not provide more or less of duties.
8. Report unsafe working conditions to your case manager.
9. Always call your case manager if you have any questions.

What you do for the client and how you do it are important. Much of the information in this book is directed toward teaching you the "what" and "how" of being a home health aide. Your technical knowledge and skills are what the client wants and needs. An equally important part of your job responsibility involves some activities that are not seen by the client. These responsibilities include observing, reporting, documenting, following rules of ethics and confidentiality, and understanding liability.

Because the home health aide usually spends more time with the client than any other member of the health care team does, he or she is often able to see actions or reactions that no one else sees, and to make other unique observations. What the home health aide does with this information is very important to the total care of the client.

Observing

All five senses (seeing, hearing, touching, smelling, and tasting) should be used in the day-to-day work of the home health aide. Let's consider each sense:

1. Seeing
   Look at the client carefully, watching for any changes since your last visit. Some of the things you might note are facial expression, posture, skin color and cleanliness, rashes, discharges, redness, swelling, evenness of facial features, way of walking (gait), steadiness, stains on clothing, Figure 3-6.

   Look at the home for safety hazards (frayed electric cords, wet floors, slippery throw rugs, loose steps), cleanliness, medications sitting out, food supply, spots, stains and spills on clothing, furniture, or floors.

2. Hearing
   Listen to the client. What is being said? How is it being said? Is the client's speech clear or slurred? Is it logical or nonsensical? Are the words sad, angry, friendly, or hostile? Do you hear wheezing, coughing, or gasping for breath?

   Listen to the home. Does the faucet drip? Does the refrigerator vibrate? Is the radio or TV volume too loud to permit conversation? Are the telephone and doorbells loud enough for the client to hear?

3. Touching
   Does the client's skin feel hot, cold, or moist? Is it rough, or puffy? What is the pulse rate?

   Are the sheets dry? Is the diaper wet? Is the bread dried out? Are the crackers soggy? Is the bath water too hot?

4. Smelling
   Does the client have bad breath or body odor? Does the odor smell like perspiration, urine, feces, alcohol, or fruit? Is there an odor from a wound or dressing?

   How does bathroom, bedroom, and kitchen smell? How does the inside of the

refrigerator smell? Have items of food spoiled?
5. Tasting
   Is the food too salty or too spicy?

Develop the habit of paying attention to everything you see, hear, touch, smell, and taste in the home. Ask yourself at each visit, "Is anything different today from what it was the last time I was here?" If you don't take the time to be a careful observer, you may overlook some small but important signs of change.

Changes in the client's physical or mental condition, social support system, or household environment may occur suddenly. Some examples of sudden changes to look for:

Physical: cuts, fractures, paling of the skin, bluish color of the lips
Mental: a previously cheerful and cooperative person doesn't seem to recognize you today or appears disoriented
Social support: loss of spouse, loss of close neighbors
Household: a broken water pipe floods the kitchen

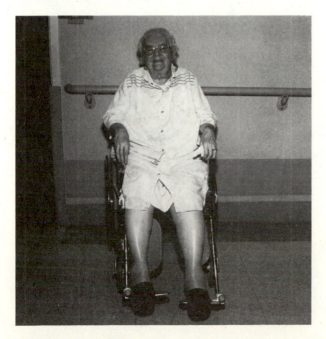

Figure 3-6 Edema of the ankles is an abnormal sign that is important to report and record.

These sudden changes are usually easy to observe and describe. Sudden changes are usually of a severe nature and require an immediate **intervention** (an action to improve the situation).

More often, however, changes occur gradually. These changes are not as obvious to the home health aide who sees the client frequently as they may be to someone else, such as the supervisor, who sees the person infrequently. You've probably heard someone say, "My goodness, you've grown so tall since I saw you last!" or "Hasn't Aunt Maude failed since her operation?" In each of these cases, the people living with the child or Aunt Maude were unaware of the changes.

It is in regard to slow changes that the home health aide needs to use skill in observation. As you work in the home over a period of time, you will become familiar with the client's life-style, habits, social activities, and place of residence. If you fail to be alert to gradual changes, you may miss them. Some examples of gradual changes to look for:

Physical: Client moves more slowly or holds onto furniture; client doesn't watch TV as much; hair color changes and becomes dull; appetite decreases; weight loss occurs
Mental: increasing "forgetfulness"; crying; suspicion of longtime friends
Social support: family or friends visit less frequently or write less often
Household: carpet becomes frayed; refrigerator doesn't keep food as cold; electric cords fray; chair joints loosen

Asking yourself "What's different today?" and really using your senses and powers of observation can be of great help. The fact that something out of the ordinary happens one time may not mean anything at all, or it may be the first of a series of happenings that will lead to something more serious. Write the "odd thing" in your notes for later reference.

Looking, hearing, touching, smelling, and tasting will give you a lot of information. It is your responsibility to transmit the information to your supervisor or case manager.

Reporting

Some important instructions that you need during your orientation to the agency are how to report information, who to report it to, and when to report it. You have a right to know these "who, what, when, and how" procedures and a responsibility to ask if you aren't told.

In most agencies, one person will be in charge of the care given to the client. This person may be called the "supervisor" or "case manager." This is the person you will probably be instructed to contact when you have information to share about the client.

You will need to exercise judgment in making these reports: Some things need to be reported immediately, even while you are with the client, such as falls. Some things need to be reported as soon as you leave the home. Other things can wait until a regular conference, staffing, or written report. Anything you learn that puts the client in danger should be reported immediately. Such things usually involve physical problems (chest pain, falls, or deep cuts, for example). Other observations may leave you unsure, and you would want to talk them over with the supervisor at your first opportunity. Some observations that leave you unsure might be forgetfulness, decreased appetite, or reduced social contacts. Still other things can wait for regular contact times.

Throughout your career as a home health aide, and especially as a beginner, you should remember that it is **always** better to report something even if you aren't sure how important it is, rather than to risk endangering the client, the agency, and yourself by not reporting it. Good supervisors can help you learn how to sort out the "crisis" from the "unusual," and develop good judgment in reporting. You should never feel or be made to feel that the supervisor is "too busy" or that your information might be "too unimportant." Your supervisor is employed to help you give good client care, and, as you read earlier, a very important part of that care is what you observe and report. When you talk over your observations and your feelings with the supervisor, you can speak freely and voice your opinions and small details. All of these help the supervisor to make decisions; he or she

can help you learn to be more concise and accurate in your oral reports as time goes by.

On the other hand, your supervisor is a busy person, so you won't want to waste time in long, dragged-out stories either. It's a good idea to practice what you're going to say so you can get the story organized in a logical sequence and make it easier for the supervisor to understand.

Documenting

Writing down your observations and actions is a very important part of your job. Your agency will show you the forms they want you to use, and will tell you how often you need to document something in writing, where to do it, and where and when to turn it in.

There's a saying that "The job's not over 'til the paperwork's done." This certainly holds true in home health care. The information you write, which may be called a "narrative," "observation," "notes," or "charting," becomes part of the client's record, or chart. The information contained in client records is of critical importance for these reasons:

1. It is a lasting record of what was done to, for, and by the client. If it is not charted, it is considered not to have been done.
2. It is a record of what was observed about the client.
3. It is a record of how the client reacted to the care that was given.
4. It contains information that can be used by other team members in evaluating the care that was given, and in deciding if changes in the care plan should be made.
5. If the client or family is unhappy with services and decides to complain, or, in the event of legal action, the client record can be used to show that certain things were done on certain dates and times.

When you are writing these reports, it is important that you:

1. **Be factual.** Write only those things that you know to be true, not what someone told you or what you think might be true.

2. **Be objective.** Write what you actually did, saw, heard, smelled, felt, or tasted. Don't try to interpret the cause or the feelings that went along with the observation. If you feel that you really must put something in the record that's your own interpretation, identify it as such.

   Don't diagnose. If the client complains of pains in his chest and arm, don't write, "Mr. Peterson had a heart attack and I called the ambulance." Instead, write, "Mr. Peterson complained of severe grabbing pains in his chest and upper left arm. His face was pale and moist. I called the ambulance. . . ."

   If you observed a large discolored area on the client's arm, write a description of it. Don't write, "Mrs. Jones has a big bruise on her arm where I think her husband grabbed her when he got mad because she wet the bed." However, if the client told you this was what had happened, you could record it as, "Mrs. Jones told me that her husband was angry because she had wet the bed, and he grabbed her by the arm. There is a two-inch discolored, purple area on her left forearm just below the elbow."

3. **Be concise.** Plan your words before you write them. Use enough words to give clear information, but don't "write a book." The important facts should be obvious to another person reading your notes.

4. **Be neat.** Take care that your handwriting or printing is legible. If your writing is very small or very sprawling, try to improve it. If you make a mistake, cross it out with a single line and initial the mistake; this shows you made and corrected the error.

5. **Be accurate.** Be sure the record shows exactly what you did, and if it's appropriate, what the client's reaction was. If you weren't able to carry out some activity that was assigned, give the reason ("I couldn't do the laundry because the washer was broken"). This shows that you didn't forget the activity or purposely fail to do it. Be sure measurements (pulse, temperature, intake and output) are correct.

6. **Sign and date every entry in the record.** Most agencies will want you to sign your name and title (Mary Simmons, HHA) at the end of every entry. It's important to put the date (month, day, and year) and the time the visit began and ended.

7. **Be sure what you write relates to the goals** set for and by the client. Don't let yourself fall in the bad habit of continually writing "No change," "Client was okay today," or other meaningless phrases. If the goal is to have the client learn better housekeeping methods, you might write, "Today Mrs. Kitt washed the dishes immediately after lunch."

8. **Be descriptive.** "The kitchen was a mess" doesn't give as much information as "The sink was piled full of dishes coated with dried-on food. Spilled milk had soured on the floor. Roaches were crawling across the counter."

9. **Use the correct words and abbreviations.** In Unit 4 you can find some lists of the proper words and approved abbreviations to use in describing your observations. Try to use these words properly, instead of using slang, and learn their correct spelling. Your reports will be more respected if you learn to use the right words and correct abbreviations, Figure 3-7.

Confidentiality

Clients in the home setting have many rights to safeguard their well-being. They include the right of confidentiality. **Confidentiality** means that the home health aide's knowledge of all aspects of the client's condition belongs to the client. The home health aide cannot reveal this information without the consent of the client. Put in simple terms, it means **don't gossip about the client.** Don't tell your family, your friends, or anyone else any details about the client; this includes not revealing even the name or address of the client. In small towns or neighborhoods, it's hard to avoid the inquisitive friend or neighbor who wants to know about the people you work with. Sometimes another client asks questions about a friend who also receives home health aide service. You should not even acknowledge that the person is a client. It's a good idea to practice some responses so you won't be caught off guard. Try some comments like "I'd

Complete daily narrative on side 2 of this sheet.

Check if care was given for each box below.	Sat.	Sun.	Mon.	Tues.	Wed.	Thurs.	Fri.
Date:							
PERSONAL CARE Assist with bath							
Comb hair							
Shampoo							
Foot care							
Skin care							
Shave							
Toileting ☐urine ☐BM ☐pericare							
Care of eyeglasses/hearing aids							
Assistance with clothing changes							
Prep for HS							
Linen change							
Other:							
NUTRIT Meal preparation							
Meal service & clean up							
Feeding							
Food/Shopping							
ACTIVITY Turn & position							
Transfer							
Dangle							
Assisted ambulation							
Accompany to medical appointments							
HSKPG Cleaning							
Laundry							
OTHER							

Signature of RN _____ Signature of Supportive Home Health Aide _____

Please report any changes or information concerning client needs to supervising RN.

Progress Notes

Clients Name:

Medical Record No:

Figure 3-7   Sample charting form for the home health aide to complete

DATE	NARRATIVE	AIDE SIGNATURE

DAILY NARRATIVE NOTES

Clients Name:

Medical Record No:

Figure 3-7   *Continued*

rather not discuss my work" or "If you're interested in how Mrs. Chambers is feeling, why don't you call her? I'm sure she'd like to talk to you."

Keeping client information confidential also means that if you're approached by a newspaper, television, or radio reporter and asked to give information or pose for pictures regarding your job or clients, you should refer the reporter to your case manager for approval.

It's just as important to use good judgment in what you say about your coworkers, supervisor, or the agency. If you're unhappy or dissatisfied with working conditions or behaviors, express that discontent to someone in the agency who can do something about it. Don't do your griping to your family and friends. This would only give the agency a bad reputation, and no improvement in conditions would result.

Liability

Liability refers to the degree to which you are held responsible for something that goes wrong on the job. Probably the most important protection from liability that is available to you is to **do only and exactly what your supervisor instructs you to do.** When you follow these instructions, your agency assumes responsibility for your actions. There are some pitfalls that you should recognize and avoid:

1. **Doing more than is assigned.** Practice saying "no" in a nice way, encouraging the client to contact the supervisor if more services are wanted. When you do something that wasn't assigned, you are assuming responsibility (liability) for these acts, and your agency is no longer responsible.
2. **Doing less than is assigned.** This may put the client in danger and lead to a charge of **negligence,** which means "an action or lack of action that leads to an accident or injury."
3. **Doing hasty, careless, or poor-quality work.** You've received training in the proper way to carry out your work activities. It's your responsibility to work carefully. Sometimes, even with the greatest amount of care being taken, accidents happen: a valuable vase

breaks while you're dusting it or a client falls. If you've been carrying out your assigned duties and exercising a normal amount of care, you are not usually held liable for the damage or injury that results; agencies carry liability insurance to cover these kinds of accidents.

4. **Using your car for work activities without notifying your insurance company.** This particularly applies to taking clients out in your car without letting your insurance agency know, even to the doctor's office or clinic appointments. If an accident occurs, you might be heavily liable for injury. It's also a good idea to be sure the agency approves of your taking clients in the car, Figures 3-8 and 3-9.
5. **Failing to do accurate reporting and documentation.** If you see a client doing something wrong, such as failing to take medicine properly, abusing another family member, or being abused by others and you don't include that in your report because you tell yourself, "She doesn't like the taste of that medicine and anyway, it's so expensive" or "He's such a nice man, he couldn't possibly have meant to bruise his wife like that," you're leaving yourself open to charges of negligence.

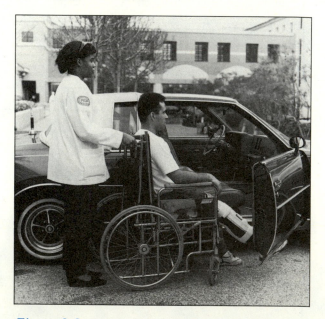

Figure 3-8   Always have the permission of your agency before transporting a client in your own car.

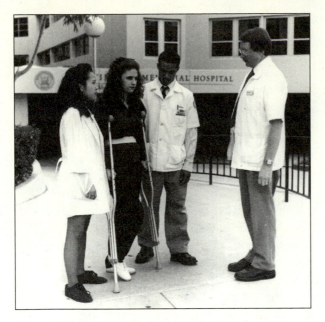

Figure 3-9 Occasionally an aide may need to accompany a client to the outpatient department of a hospital for therapy.

6. **Failing to act in an emergency.** You should know what the emergency plan is for each client you care for, and you should be prepared to follow it. In a life-threatening situation, call for an ambulance before calling the supervisor. But don't try to perform first aid or cardiopulmonary resuscitation (CPR) if you haven't been trained to do so.

7. **Attempting to do things that are beyond your abilities.** It's okay to say, "I don't know how to do that. Let's see if we can get someone who does." You aren't employed as a nurse, a plumber, an electrician, or a counselor . . . don't try to be one.

8. **Injuring yourself or the client** by doing something you aren't assigned or adequately trained to do. If you have been assigned to do something you don't feel comfortable doing, ask for more training. Trying to do something without assignment and adequate training, such as moving a client with a Hoyer lift, can leave you liable for injury that results.

9. **Failing to report** unsafe working conditions that later cause injury to you or another home health aide. Don't take unnecessary risks. Follow the agency procedures for reporting.

Ethics

Ethics is a standard or code of behavior. It is a code concerned with what is "right" and what is "wrong." Doctors and nurses take an oath when they are licensed in which they promise to help and care for clients without causing unnecessary pain or suffering. Although there is no written code for home health aides, there is a definite set of standards they are expected to uphold as they practice their profession.

Ethical Standards

- Be honest in your dealing with clients and coworkers. Stealing involves not only the taking of objects or money, it involves falsifying reports of time and activities.
- Never discuss the financial, emotional, family, medical, or other problems of the client with outsiders.
- Respect the cultural and religious practices of the client and family.
- Never walk out in the middle of an assignment. Some people may be more pleasant to work with than others. If personality conflicts or the work load is impossible to deal with, the aide should try to finish the shift, then call the case manager and explain the problem. If the aide is working a private case or did not get the job through an agency, the problem should be discussed directly with their employer. Having accepted the duties as an employee, a home health aide is ethically bound to give service for the wages paid.
- Refuse tips.
- Report possible cases of abuse.
- Do not have sexual interactions with a client.
- Safeguard the confidential information you acquired from any source concerning the client.
- Do not adjust the client's care plan without permission of the case manager.

Professional Standards

- Maintain high standards of personal health and appearance.
- Be dependable and reliable. When accepting a job, you must be on time and prepared to fulfill all obligations.

- Carry out the responsibilities of the job in the best way you possibly can. This means being sure you understand the assignment and how to do it and asking questions when you are in doubt.
- Show respect for the client's privacy and modesty.
- Recognize and respect the right of clients to determine their life-style, even if it's not one you would choose.
- Keep your professional life separate from your personal life. Personal problems of the home health aide should not be discussed with the client or the client's family. Working hours should be addressed to the needs of the clients.
- Control your normal reactions to chronic disability or the living conditions of the client.
- Maintain safe conditions in the working environment. An aide needs to follow basic rules of safety in caring for the client and when working with equipment and supplies.
- Do not use client's medications for your own health problems.

Ethical Dilemmas

The home health aide may be faced with ethical problems while caring for a client. For example, an aide may be asked in the workplace to perform tasks that are not part of the job description. Instead of getting angry or upset when asked to do such tasks, an aide may say that the agency must give permission before such work can be done. By letting the agency supervisor explain to the client what is or is not allowed, the aide keeps a good relationship with the client and the client's family.

Sometimes home health aides find themselves in a home where the family members are abusive and hit or otherwise harm the client or each other. Aides must report such behavior to their supervisors immediately.

What can a home health aide do if a client or member of the client's family makes a sexual advance? An aide should not tolerate this kind of behavior. A health aide should never become sexually involved with a client. The aide must firmly state that such behavior is not acceptable. If that does not solve the problem, walk away from the client and tell him/her that you are going to report this incident to the supervisor. You must not permit or put up with sexual harassment. Try to handle the situation with diplomacy and tact, but always refuse to participate in any sexual behavior.

Sometimes a client is so grateful for the care provided or the attention given by an aide that he or she will offer extra money or gifts to the aide. Sometimes a client may be confused or under the influence of medication and offer money to the aide. Although it may be tempting, accepting a tip or gift under these circumstances is not ethical practice. If the client continues to offer extra money or gifts, report this to your supervisor.

Sometimes a client may become too attached to one particular aide and may become very dependent on or manipulative of the aide. This could lead to a variety of problems. The aide may feel that it is all right to "let down" on the job because the client likes him/her so much, or the client may avoid asking the aide to perform certain tasks. The client may ask the aide to "break the rules" such as by adding salt to a salt-free diet or sugar to a sugar-free diet.

When a client becomes too dependent on an aide, the client may stop trying to improve his/her own ability to perform the activities of daily living. The aide's job is to help the client achieve the maximum quality of life and become as self-sufficient as possible.

For these reasons, some agencies prefer to rotate home health aides occasionally. A particularly difficult case is another reason for rotation. Such a case would occur if the client requires a great deal of personal service, or if the environment is especially depressing, or if a client is extremely demanding. In these situations the aide may suffer "burn out." This means that the aide loses interest or enthusiasm for the job and becomes less effective or careless. Generally, a home health aide is assigned a client who has an immediate need. For example, such a need would occur if a client had just returned from the hospital or nursing home and had no one at home to help him/her until self-care could be resumed. A home health aide would also be needed during the terminal stages of a client's illness. If the client is resuming self-care, an agency will "wean" the client by slowly cutting the aide's hours to the point where the client realizes there is no longer a need for an aide.

A client may have to make a decision whether to die in a hospital or at home. The client and/or the client's family may ask the aide for advice. The home health aide listens to the family and client but lets them make the decision. Sometimes by just talking to another person, the client or family can make a decision. The aide can then report the request to the supervisor at the agency, who can arrange for counseling for the client and/or family or for referral to an appropriate agency.

Another question is what forms of address to use. A home health aide should introduce herself or himself as "Ms., Mrs., or Mr. Smith." The client should be addressed as "Ms., Mrs., or Mr. Jones." Although our society is very informal today, calling a client by his or her first name is unprofessional and demeaning to the client unless the client requests it.

Applying Ethical Standards at Work

The home health aide who adheres to ethical standards will always be worthy of employment. Home health aide is a challenging and ever-changing career. Every job will be different. Some jobs will be more interesting than others; some will be extremely difficult.

A pleasant, calm manner is the best asset a home health aide can develop. One can be sympathetic and understanding of the client's condition but one should not become emotionally involved with the client or family.

Occasionally, the interpersonal relationships within the family unit are poor. The home health aide must learn to stay out of **intrafamily** disputes. Remaining uninvolved is not always easy. One or more family members may try to get the aide involved through manipulation. **Manipulation** is trying to control another's thoughts or actions for one's own personal gain. A mother, for example, might complain to the aide about how unkind her daughter is. The aide should simply say, "Now, Mrs. Jones, you'll have to talk about that with your daughter. If you like, I'll ask her to stop in so you can clear

this up." In other situations, children may try to manipulate. For example, a child might ask the aide's permission to go out, knowing that the parents would never allow this privilege.

Client's Rights

The home health aide must respect the rights of the clients. The following is a list of common client rights that are mandated by Medicare and Medicaid regulations.

1. Every client shall be treated with consideration, respect, and full recognition of the client's dignity and individuality.
2. Every client shall receive care, treatment, and services that are adequate, appropriate, and in compliance with relevant federal and state law.
3. Every client has the right to be free from mental and physical abuse.
4. Every client shall be informed of these rights in writing.
5. Every client who is responsible for fee for service shall be given a statement of the services available by the agency and related charges.
6. Every client shall participate in the development of the plan of care and discharge plan and be informed of all treatments, when and how services will be provided, and the name and functions of any person and affiliated agency providing care and services.
7. Every client has the right to refuse treatment after being fully informed of and understanding the consequence of such actions.
8. Every client shall be informed on the procedure for submitting complaints to the agency. If the client is not satisfied by the agency response, the client may complain to the State Department of Health and Social Services.
9. Every client shall have the right to recommend changes in policies and services to agency staff, the area office representatives of the department, or any outside representative of the client's choice free from restraints, interference, coercion, discrimination, or reprisal.

10. Every client shall receive respect and privacy, including confidential treatment of client records, and the right to refuse release of records to any individuals outside the agency.
11. Every client has the right to privacy.
12. Every client has the right to request change of caregiver.
13. Every client has the right to be informed of the state consumer hot-line telephone number.

Home Health Aide's Rights

As a employee of an agency or your client, you also have rights. Examples of your rights are:

1. The right to take pride in a job well done
2. The right to make suggestions and complaints within designated channels without fear of retaliation
3. The right not to be abused physically, verbally, or sexually by clients
4. The right to recommend care plan changes designed to facilitate care delivery and reduce caregiver stress
5. The right to be informed when complaints concerning client treatment are alleged against you
6. The right to a fair hearing with your case manager
7. The right to a confidential investigation
8. The right to be informed of the investigation's outcome

Case Study: Client Confidentiality

The following situation is a common one many home health aides meet on an assignment. Remember that information about the client's condition is not to be shared with friends and neighbors. Select the proper responses to the situation. If you select an inappropriate response, discuss the response with your classmates and/or teacher and determine why it is inappropriate:

The situation: For 8 months on this assignment, you have accompanied Mr. J to the neighborhood grocery each Friday morning to assist him in doing his weekly grocery shopping. You've gotten to know the check-out clerk; you, she, and Mr. J have a running joke about his fondness for very ripe bananas. This past month has been different: Mr. J has had some light strokes and is not permitted to leave his apartment, so you have been doing the shopping for him at the same store.

The problem: The clerk has noticed that Mr. J hasn't been with you. You are at the cash register now, and five people are in line behind you. The clerk comments on Mr. J's absence and asks you what's wrong with him.

How would you reply without revealing any confidential information about Mr. J and without hurting the clerk's feelings?

Some possible responses are listed below. Which are acceptable and appropriate?

1. I'm not allowed to talk about my clients.
2. I shouldn't tell you this, but he's been having some strokes, and frankly, he's acting kind of strange, if you ask me.
3. I'll be sure to tell Mr. J you were asking about him. I'm sure he'll be glad to know that you missed him.
4. He had other commitments.
5. It's none of your business.
6. He just didn't come today; I hope he'll be with me next week.

Responses 3, 4, and 6 are all appropriate and reveal nothing about Mr. J while still being polite to the clerk. Response 2 is a definite breach of confidentiality as well as showing disrespect for Mr. J. Response 1 is acceptable, but not very sensitive to the clerk's concern. Response 5 is unacceptable.

9. The right to confidentiality of your work record, except where release of information is required by court order

Client Abuse

Client abuse, neglect, or mistreatment will not be tolerated by your employer or your supervisor. All home health aides are expected to use a professional, caring approach with all clients. There are many forms of abuse. **Abuse** is treatment that reasonably could cause physical pain, physical injury, mental anguish, or fear. Abuse may be verbal, sexual, physical, mental, bodily punishment, involuntary seclusion, mistreatment, or neglect.

- **Verbal abuse** is using depreciative terms or remarks either orally, written, or by gestures to describe someone.
- **Sexual abuse** is making sexual advances to someone or fondling another in inappropriate places.

- **Physical abuse** is hitting, slapping, or pinching another person. Another example is forcing a treatment on a person that the person has requested not to be done.
- **Involuntary seclusion** is placing the client in his or her room without the person's consent or not allowing the individual to visit with others.
- **Mental abuse** is threatening or humiliating an individual.
- **Mistreatment** is using profanity or obscene words, shouting, teasing, or any other method to punish or humiliate another person.
- **Negligence** is failing to follow the established procedures for the care of an individual.

If a home health aide knows that a client is being abused by the client's family or by another caregiver, the aide is obligated by law to report it. If the home health aide does not report it, the aide is just as guilty as the person doing the abusing.

Case Study: Job Ethics and Confidentiality

Sue, a home health aide, travels to work by bus. She is quite friendly with her fellow travelers and very often the conversations are about jobs and daily happenings. Sue has been with her client for several months and without thinking, talks about her job and the nearly blind lady she cares for. She mentions the address and apartment number. She talks about her client's illness and even mentions her case manager and the agency for which she works. In the course of conversation, she tells how her client keeps cash in her desk drawer. These conversations have taken place over several weeks, and Sue didn't realize just how much information she had given.

Sue doesn't work on weekends. One Monday, she arrives to find her client very upset and frightened. It seems that on Satur-

day, the doorbell rang. When the client asked who was there, she was told that it was Kathy, the case manager at Jefferson Health, Inc., Sue's agency. She said Sue had failed to have her time sheet signed and couldn't be paid until it was signed by the client. The client opened the door and let Kathy in. She was given a paper to sign and then Kathy asked if she could use the bathroom. The client gave permission and when Kathy came back from the bathroom she took the signed paper and left. She also took $350 and a diamond ring from the client's desk drawer.

1. What faults were Sue's in this situation?
2. What "rights" did Sue abuse in the above situation?
3. If you were Sue's case manager, how would you handle this situation?

SUMMARY

....

- The person entering the career of home health aide must be flexible about working hours and conditions.
- A home health aide must be capable of working in many different situations and dealing with all age groups and must be well organized in each working environment.
- It is essential that the home health aide adhere to ethical standards of practice and respect the client. As a member of the health team, the home health aide is expected to behave in a suitable manner.
- The needs of the client should be uppermost in the aide's planning, but the other duties must also be completed.
- When necessary, a home health aide should inform the client as to limitations of an aide's duties.
- The home health aide must maintain the confidentiality of the client. Information about the client must not be shared with friends and neighbors of the client or with the family of the aide.
- Accurate observations of the client's physical and emotional states and the details of the client's environment are important components of the overall care of the client. Document all observations thoroughly and accurately as required by the agency.
- The home health aide is required to report information to the supervisor or other personnel at the agency. Know who to report to, how to report, and when to report. Learn the procedures and also know how and when to report emergencies.
- The home health aide can be held liable or responsible for accidents or injury to the client or environment. Perform only those activities you have been trained to do and that have been approved for the client by your supervisor. Follow the care plan for the client. Know and avoid the actions that could result in liability.
- A home health aide should be aware of the client's rights and respect these rights.
- A home health aide also has rights that the client must respect.
- Client abuse, neglect, or mistreatment of any type will not be tolerated. If an aide knows of abuse or mistreatment, the aide must document and report it.

REVIEW

1. Name two career adjustments a home health aide might be expected to make.
2. Define ethics.
3. Name two client care responsibilities of the home health aide.
4. List three home care responsibilities of the home health aide.
5. List six characteristics of the client's physical condition that you would observe.
6. List five actions to avoid that could lead to liability.
7. List two examples of unethical behavior of a home health aide.
8. List four client's rights.
9. List four types of client abuse and give an example of each.
10. Information about a client's diagnosis:
    a. should be kept confidential
    b. can be shared with your coworkers
    c. can be relayed to the client's family
    d. is of no importance to the home health aide caring for the client

11. The case manager asks the aide to do something for a client, but the aide does not know how to do it. The aide should:
    a. ask a family member in the home to do it
    b. call the agency and tell them that the case manager has asked you to do something you do not know how to do
    c. look in your pocket manual and try to find out how to do it
    d. tell the case manager immediately that you do not know how to do it

12. The home health aide will be expected to adapt to:
    a. irregular hours
    b. variety of assignments and settings
    c. variety of different types of equipment
    d. all are correct

13. Which of the following gives the most information?
    a. "The kitchen is a mess."
    b. "No change in skin color."
    c. "Has red open area on left arm below elbow the size of a dime."
    d. "Client okay today."

14. Ethical conduct for a home health aide involves:
    a. doing everything the client asks you to do
    b. discussing your personal problems with the client to relieve the client's boredom
    c. carrying out the responsibilities of your job in the best way you can
    d. all of the above are correct

15. Which of the following is a form of physical abuse?
    a. refusing to give a diabetic client candy
    b. forcing a client to be fed through a stomach tube after the client told the doctor "no" for this method of receiving nourishment
    c. making sexual advancements toward your client
    d. forgetting to give your client a bath

Unit *4* Developing Effective Communication Skills

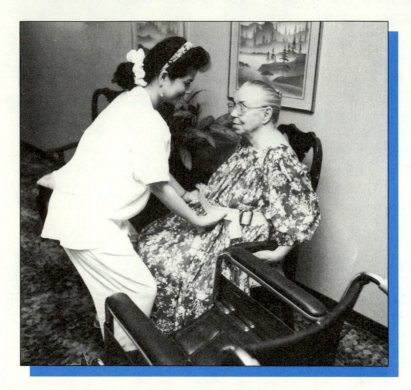

KEY TERMS

....

abbreviations
aphasia
body language
dyslexia

illiterate
listening
medical terminology
nonverbal communication

pitch
therapeutic
tone
verbal

LEARNING OBJECTIVES

....

After studying this unit, you should be able to:

- Identify the sender-message-receiver process.
- Explain the difference between verbal and nonverbal communication.
- List four rules for improving aide/client communication.

- Identify two examples that apply rules of good communication.
- Identify characteristics of speech that affect communication.
- Give an example of a precise way to report an observation.

What do most people think of when they see or hear the word communication? Do they think of what they say and how they say it? Do they think of words written in a book, magazine, or newspaper; or do they think of television, radio, or a telephone? Communication involves all of these and more. What is communication? It is simply the sending and receiving of information.

Humans have developed many methods of communication. Cavemen drew pictures. Early Egyptians developed a complicated system using symbols written on stone. Indians used smoke signals. Homing pigeons carried written messages from one area to another.

Words are one of the tools of communication. From the time a baby puts two syllables together and says "ma ma" or "da da," vocabulary begins to develop. Because vocabulary is an important part of communication, and clear communication is a necessity between the aide, agency, client, and family, home health aides should continue to add new words to their vocabulary both during and after training.

Basic Components of Communication

Communication is a two-way process. It involves a sender and a receiver as well as a message, Figure 4-1. In a conversation, the role of sender and receiver alternates from one to another. In this way there is an exchange of ideas and information. **Listening** is an important part of communication. When the receiver is busy thinking of how to reply to the sender, the meaning of what is being said may be lost.

Meaning and Use of Words

Insights in dealing with others can be gained by understanding the importance of accurate communication and by listening carefully to the

Errors in the Communication Process

Sender uses words that the receiver does not understand.

Sender does not speak loud enough.

Sender speaks too fast.

Sender gives instruction in too many words and too great of detail.

Sender speaks in a language that the receiver does not understand.

Receiver has a problem hearing and only hears half of what the sender is saying.

Receiver is not listening.

Receiver has lost the ability to understand spoken words.

Receiver has tuned the message out.

Receiver has mind on another topic.

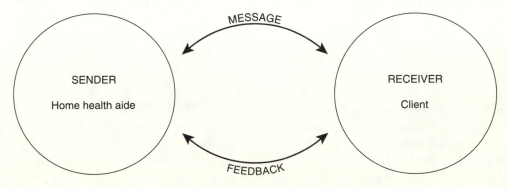

Figure 4-1   Important elements of the communication process

words communicated. Words can be soothing, harsh, cruel, or kind. Some words have a special meaning to certain people. Such words may have a strong effect or an emotional impact because of the past experiences of the listener. For instance, "widow" is a word used to describe a woman whose husband has died. To a recently widowed woman, the word can be frightening. A woman who has been dependent on her husband usually has a strong feeling of loss. She also may feel anger, rejection, worry, and terrible loneliness. To a woman who has not been widowed, the word has less personal meaning and little or no emotional impact.

Words can be simple or complex. The home health aide must make sure that the words used mean exactly what they are intended to say. Words can be used as weapons to hurt or embarrass others. They can also cheer and comfort.

Verbal Communication

Verbal or voice communication is using speech to give a message. When speaking with clients, the home health aide should use words that the client can understand. It is helpful to get feedback from the client to be sure the client is receiving the intended message.

Verbal communication is an important part of the home health aide/client relationship. The aide should be mindful of the effect that voice communication has on clients and their families and work to improve voice quality.

Voice Volume and Tone

Loud voices often sound harsh and can cause anger in the listener. The listener may then respond harshly, causing an argument. When the aide speaks too softly, it may be hard for the listener to understand what has been said. The home health aide must use special care in communicating with clients and their families.

Tone is the expressive quality of the voice that gives meaning. When speaking, tone is a vital part of communication. A home health aide should speak clearly to be understood and pleasantly to avoid upsetting the client. If a client is hard of hearing it is better to speak in

short sentences and form words carefully, sitting or standing, facing the client. This will give the client the chance to read your lips as you speak. Be sure not to talk too fast or use a sentence that is too long. If the client has a hearing aid, encourage the client to wear it after checking the battery. If the client can hear out of one ear better than the other, speak toward the client's good ear. Do not shout or talk to the client while you are in a different room.

Voice Pitch

Speaking voices vary in **pitch.** This quality may be high or low. Some sounds are so low or so high that the human ear cannot perceive them. In speaking, women's voices are normally higher pitched than men's. This is mainly due to a difference in the physical structure of the vocal chords.

Some voices are very unpleasant to listen to. They may be hoarse and harsh sounding, grating to the ear. The middle range of voice is more pleasing than the very high or very low.

Regional Accents and Speech Patterns

Regional accents vary. The southern accent is a soft, slow drawl; an eastern accent is often fast, clipped, and nasal sounding. There are Boston, Chicago, Brooklyn, and Bronx accents, to name a few. Nothing is wrong with any of these accents, and most people are not aware of how they sound to others. However, they are extremely aware of accents different from their own. The speed with which people speak is another difference that may be noticed.

It is possible to change speech habits. For example, "ya know," "yeah," "like," and "um" endlessly repeated during a conversation can be very boring to the listener. During class, listen carefully when another student is speaking. Try to pick out the tone, pitch, speed, and speech patterns that are most pleasant to listen to.

Content of Speech

An aide is expected to avoid crude and vulgar language while on the job. Also, for the sake of the client, the aide's personal life should remain separate from his or her working life. In other words, communication with the client should be

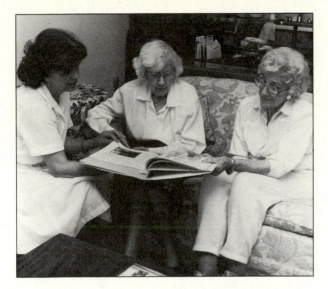

Figure 4-2   An aide, client, and family member looking through client's favorite book together

limited to shared experiences in the work situation. An aide's personal problems should not interfere with the job. The client has enough problems with which to cope without adding the aide's personal problems to them. The aide cannot do proper work if attention is focused on personal problems instead of the client's needs.

It is a good idea for the home health aide to find out the client's current or former hobbies or interests, Figure 4-2. This will give the aide a few ideas on what to discuss with the client. It's a good idea to keep the conversation centered on pleasant and happy topics. It is **therapeutic** (helpful for the healing process) for the aide to encourage clients to express their anger about their illness, disability, or other problems. Generally, it is more therapeutic for the aide to try to focus the conversation on something other than the illness.

Many times a homebound client begins to think only of oneself, and this could lead to depression or mental illness. An aide then needs to try to refocus this person's attention to some other topic. The lives of ill or disabled people are restricted. As they lose a sense of freedom and the ability to move freely, their world shrinks. They may not get out of the house for days or weeks. They may seldom have company, and their children may be unable to visit regularly. It is not unusual for them to talk about themselves and their health and their body

functions. An aide should try to turn the client's attention to more positive topics.

Nonverbal Communication

Communication is not limited to words. It can also involve emotions and body language. Information expressed without the use of words is called **nonverbal communication.** It is possible to communicate without words by using gestures such as hand movements, frowns, and smiles. Use of gestures instead of words is also called **body language.** Body language may be combined with words to reinforce the meaning of the words. This reinforcement helps to make communication clear. Body language could, however, be just the opposite, or contradict, the spoken words.

Touch is a form of nonverbal communication, Figure 4-3. It can be used to relay concern to the client or it can have negative effects if it is used to discipline a client. There are also "safe" places on the client's body that an aide can touch and "unsafe" places. Examples of therapeutic touch is holding an Alzheimer's client's hand while walking her and giving her a hug when you come or go, if permissible. Examples of "unsafe" touch are feeling a woman's breast or hitting her while working with her.

Imagine an elderly client who has no control of the bowels or bladder. Some home health aides tend to be very cold and busi-

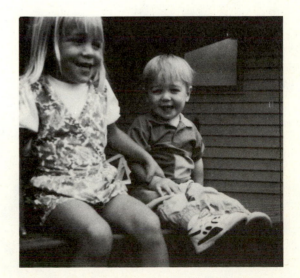

Figure 4-3   Touch is important at any age.

nesslike when cleaning the client and changing the bed. Instead of showing patience and understanding, they may become rude or unkind by making a cruel remark or by holding their nose or making a face while cleaning the client. The home health aide has a responsibility to show compassion and sensitivity to all clients.

Consider the following situation. The mother has just told her child to pick up the toys and clean up the mess in the room. The mother is very angry because the child had not done it earlier. As the mother is walking out of the room with her back to the child, the child says, "Yes, Mama, I'm sorry." The child sticks out her tongue at the departing parent and "makes a face."

What kinds of communication are being used? This is an example of words communicating one thing and body language another. This sort of contradiction would also be seen if a home health aide were cleaning up after a client had soiled the bed and the aide said, "Let me get this cleaned up so you will be more comfortable," and at the same time rolled the eyes and fanned away the bad odor. The aide's body language speaks louder than the words spoken to the client and causes the client to be embarrassed. Sometimes the words lose their meaning and the body language is what is communicated. The home health aide must be careful of the message body language gives as well as the choice of words spoken.

Written Communication

Writing is another form of communication. However, written words have no meaning for the person who is **illiterate** (cannot read) or who cannot see. In some conditions of the elderly, the person might lose the ability to read or to comprehend what is read. In other instances, a person can read one language and not another. An example of this would be a person who speaks and reads Spanish but not English. If this client is given an English form to read, the client will be unable to understand it.

Some people have difficulty communicating because of a learning or physical disability, such as aphasia. **Aphasia** causes a person to use words incorrectly or may totally impair a person's ability to speak. **Dyslexia** is another type of learning disability that makes it difficult for a person to read and understand the words that are seen.

Medical Terminology

The home health aide is usually required to keep a written record of the care given a client and of the client's response to that care. In doing so, the aide may use special medical terminology in describing care procedures or a client's condition.

Medical terminology involves the use of special words and abbreviations that relate to medical subjects. These medical words or terms provide members of the health care team with a precise means of communicating important information about clients under their care, Figure 4-4.

If a client under the care of a home health aide were to suddenly change color—turn pale, or red in the face, or even become blue, how could this be best described? Of course, the home health aide could say, "Mrs. Jones looks as white as a sheet" or "She looks like she's burning up" or "My client looks kind of bluish around

VAGUE REPORT	MENTAL
My client looks bluish around the lips.	Client is cyanotic.
Mrs. Jones looks as white as a sheet.	Mrs. Jones is pale.
Mr. Smith looks very red in the face.	Mr. Smith is flushed.
She feels like she's burning up.	Her temperature is elevated to 102°F.
Susan feels just like ice.	Susan's skin is cold and clammy.

Figure 4-4 Choosing precise words communicates information more clearly.

the lips." However, by using proper medical terminology, the home health aide could communicate more clearly by saying, "My client is cyanotic (blue), the TPR (temperature, pulse, and respiration rate) is as follows," or "The client is flushed, temperature is elevated to 102° . . ." or "The client is chalky, skin is cold and clammy, TPR is. . . ." In this way, the home health aide has stated the problem in a way that communicates more facts. If you report in clear and concise words, you will save your supervisor time.

Abbreviations

The home health aide should become familiar with commonly used **abbreviations** (brief, or shortened, forms of words). Some common ab-

breviations include Dr (doctor), RN (registered nurse), BM (bowel movement), @ (at), and ea (each). Many other abbreviations, such as TPR (temperature, pulse, and respiration rate), will be used throughout this text. Figure 4-5 provides a list of abbreviations that may be frequently encountered. Figure 4-6 is a list of abbreviations used in the diagnosis of a condition or disease of a client. Many times more than one diagnosis will be listed for a client.

Communication with Clients

Interpersonal relationships are developed through communication. Touching, speaking, laughing, and crying are all ways of communicat-

$\bar{a}$ - before	O_2 - oxygen
ad lib - as desired	od - every day
ac - before meals	OT - occupational therapy
ADLs - activities of daily living	oz - ounce
Amb - ambulatory	$\bar{p}$ - after
bid - twice a day	pb - partial bath
BM - bowel movement	pc - after meals
BP - blood pressure	PO - by mouth
BRP - bathroom privileges	prep - prepare for
C - Celsius	prn - when needed or necessary
$\bar{c}$ - with	pt - patient
CBR - complete bedrest	PT - physiotherapy, physical therapy
cc - cubic centimeter	q2h - every 2 hours
c/o - complains of	q3h - every 3 hours
CPR - cardiopulmonary resuscitation	q4h - every 4 hours
dc - discontinue	qd - every day
drg - dressing	qid - four times a day
F - Fahrenheit	qod - every other day
Fe - iron	ROME - range of motion exercises
ff - force fluids	$\bar{s}$ - without
HOB - head of bed	SOB - short of breath
HOH - hard of hearing	Spec - specimen
HS - hour of sleep	SSE - soapsuds enema
Ht - height	stat - immediately
I & O - intake and output	Temp - (T) - temperature
K - potassium	tid - three times a day
Lab - laboratory	TLC - tender loving care
lb - pound	TPR - temperature, pulse, respiration
mL - milliliter	VS - vital signs: TPR and BP
Na - sodium salt	w/c - wheelchair
NPO - nothing by mouth	Wt - weight

Figure 4-5 Standard medical abbreviations must be learned to understand medical orders and to chart correctly.

AIDS - Acquired immunodeficiency syndrome	DM - Diabetes mellitus
Alz - Alzheimer	Fx - Fracture
ARC - AIDS-related complex	MI - Myocardial infarction (major heart condition)
ASHD - Arteriosclerosis (hardening of the arteries)	
CA - Cancer	MS - Multiple sclerosis
CBS - Chronic brain syndrome	PID - Pelvic inflammatory disease
CHF - congestive heart failure	TB - Tuberculosis
COPD - Chronic obstructive pulmonary disease	TIA - Transient ischemic attack (small stroke)
CVA - Cerebral vascular accident (stroke)	URI - Upper respiratory infection
DD - Developmental disabled	UTI - Urinary tract infections
DJD - Degenerative joint disease	VD - Venereal disease

Figure 4-6   Abbreviations used in the diagnosis of a condition or disease. Many times more than one diagnosis will be listed for a client.

DO	DO NOT	EXAMPLES
Show acceptance of the client's feelings first, before explaining what can be done.	Pass judgment, argue with the client, or set blame on the client or others.	After you just finished changing the client sheets, the client spills his orange juice on the clean sheets. Do you yell at him or look on it as a simple accident?
Let the client talk.	Rudely interrupt or give advice.	The client is always talking about something that is very boring and uninteresting to you. Do you change conversation to something you like to talk about?
Show interest in what is said.	Pretend to be busy or change the subject abruptly.	
Show concern for your client's condition. Ask if the client is comfortable or if you can help in any way.	Give false encouragement as to a client's prognosis.	You know your client's husband knows that his wife has a terminal illness. You keep telling him that she is getting better every day and will soon be well.
Allow the supervisor to answer when a client wants to know about his or her medical condition.	Tell your own medical history.	You have read the client's medical history, which states she has heart problems. You interpret the doctor's notes about the client's medications and their effects on the client.
Tell the client what you are going to do before you do it. Also, explain procedures as you are doing them.	Assume the client understands the steps or the purpose of a procedure.	You transfer the client using the mechanical lift the first time without explaining the procedure to her. The aide must remember that the client is the employer, and if he or she prefers something done a certain way, the aide must comply if it is a reasonable request. Everyone has different ideas on how routine personal care should be done. Many times there are several ways of doing things correctly. If you are supportive of the family unit and work with them as fellow team members, the client will receive better care as a result.

Figure 4-7   Following these guidelines helps make communication more meaningful.

ing. The home health aide should keep in mind a few simple rules for setting up lines of communication in the work situation, Figure 4-7.

Humor has been found to be so effective in healing that some health care professionals are making it a regular part of the care plan. A home health aide might ask a client what makes him or her laugh. Sometimes it might be a funny joke or a rerun of a comedy TV show such as "Cheers." Shared laughter can improve communication between a client and home health aide. However, use humor carefully and appropriately so it is not misunderstood as mocking or ignoring the seriousness of a situa-

tion. Humor can make people feel good about themselves and ease stress. Some therapists prescribe "humor breaks" for families of terminally ill clients. The theory is that if you can laugh for a few moments, you may be better able to cope with illness or death.

Communicating with the Client's Family

The more people involved in a home health care situation, the more a possibility exists for miscommunication and misunderstanding. If an aide is assigned to a home where a husband is the client and the wife is well and not receiv-

Case Study: Communication

The following is a typical situation that may arise when caring for a client. As you read the description of the situation, consider appropriate responses. Then compare your responses with those provided and make a selection of the most appropriate ones. If inappropriate choices are made, determine why they are inappropriate.

The situation: You are the home health aide assigned to work with Mrs. T from 10:00 AM until 12:30 PM on Monday through Friday. One of your assigned duties is to prepare Mrs. T's noon meal, with enough planned leftovers for Mrs. T to prepare a light supper for herself. Your supervisor has told you that Mrs. T has very limited money available for food purchases, so you must be careful to not waste food or plan expensive menus.

The problem: Ever since Mrs. T was a child, she has been accustomed to offering food to anyone working at her home at a mealtime. When you prepare a meal, she asks you to sit down at the table and share the meal with her. When you say that the leftovers are for her supper, she says she'll just eat cold cereal then. It looks like she's getting angry because you won't eat with her.

What are some of the responses you might make that will encourage Mrs. T to eat,

but allow you to refrain from eating her food? Some possible responses are:

1. Thank you, but I'm going to eat lunch with a friend as soon as I leave here.
2. Thank you, but I have to go home and fix a meal for my family, so I'll eat with them.
3. I couldn't possibly eat your food!
4. I'm allergic to this kind of meat so I can't eat it.
5. Thank you for asking. I don't believe I'll eat a full meal right now, but if it's all right with you, I'll sit down and have a cup of tea while you eat.
6. I brought my lunch today, so I'll get it out of your refrigerator and sit with you while we both eat.
7. If I were to eat with you and then eat with my family when I get home, pretty soon I'd be too fat to fit through your door!

Responses 1, 2, 5, 6, and 7 are acceptable. If you plan to use 5 or 6, be sure your supervisor has approved your taking lunch time while in a client's home. Responses 3 and 4 won't leave Mrs. T feeling very good about herself. Can you think of some other possible responses?

SITUATION	POOR RESPONSE	BETTER RESPONSE
Client is in pain.	"Stop complaining; take an aspirin and you'll feel better."	"I see that you are in pain. Tell me more about where it hurts."
Client tells you all the details of her operation.	"I had a friend who had the same thing. She never got well and was in terrible pain."	"My, you've really had a rough time; you must be happy to be back home."
Client asks your advice about a personal matter.	"Well, if I were you I'd stop talking to that person. . . she's no good."	"I know that you are upset. What are some possible solutions?"
Client complains that you did something the wrong way.	"Nobody could please you. It's no wonder you have no friends."	"The way you're used to may also be correct, but this is the way I was taught in class. I'll check with the supervisor the next time I call."
Client is restless and cranky—should be napping.	"It's your nap time and I am due for a coffee break."	"You don't seem sleepy. Would you like to talk for a while before you take your rest?"
Client on salt-free diet says food tastes terrible.	"That's what you're to eat, so stop complaining."	"It must be hard to get used to eating your food without salt. Perhaps using the salt substitute the dietitian recommended would help."
Client on sugar-free diet pleads with you to put "just a little" sugar in her tea.	"Well, just a half spoon of sugar couldn't hurt."	"I know it's not easy to give up sugar, but your health comes first. Try the sugar substitute your dietitian ordered."
Client claims she needs bedpan even though she used it only 20 minutes earlier.	"It's your imagination. You know you don't need it again."	"You must be uncomfortable. I'll get it for you."
Client has soiled bed the second time in one day and is very upset.	"Why didn't you tell me you needed the bedpan? What an awful mess."	"It's hard not to feel embarrassed, but it takes just a few minutes to change the linens."
It's time for lunch but the client states she is not hungry.	"Eat the soup before it gets cold."	"I can warm it up and serve it later when you feel hungry. Just try one teaspoon and then I will put it back in the refrigerator for later."
Aide wants to give client a bath. Client says she is too tired.	"How could you be tired? You just woke up. Anyway I have to bathe you now."	"Yes, you must be tired but I have to give you a bath before I leave this morning."

Figure 4-8   Situations assuming client is able to communicate and is not mentally impaired

ing any attention, friction may arise when an aide comes on the scene. The wife may show signs of jealousy over the special attention given by a female aide to her husband. The aide may feel caught in the middle and be getting instructions or orders from all sides. The aide must keep calm and listen to the requests, questions, and advice offered. Then the aide must state that he/she is only permitted to take orders from the supervisor. If conflicting requests are made by the family, the aide must remain friendly and appear interested while going ahead with the job as assigned.

Another example would be a family that is affected by the illness of a parent. The aide should try to get the family involved in making the client comfortable. Ask family member(s) to name the client's favorite foods and to state what the client likes to talk about. Try to learn more about the client from them and then put that information to good use when caring for the client. You can be supportive of the family members by being sympathetic, by being understanding, and by listening. If you are supportive of the family, they will be able to give more support to the ailing family member.

Sometimes family members will ask an aide to do personal work for them. This is not acceptable. The aide can say that he/she will have to get permission from the agency or suggest that the family member call the agency to see if such a request is appropriate. It is wrong to talk back to the client or to the client's family. If an aide should find it impossible to cope with a particular client or the client's family, the agency supervisor should be advised immediately.

HEARING IMPAIRMENT
1. Always be sure to get the listener's attention, verbally or by touch.
2. Position yourself so that the listener can view your face clearly.
3. Speak slowly and clearly at a full, but not excessively loud level. Form words carefully and keep sentences relatively short. Avoid unnecessary chatter that may confuse the hearing-impaired client.
4. Use facial expressions or gestures appropriately to help express yourself. Visual clues are important in helping the hearing-impaired client to understand what you say.
5. Check to make sure your client has understood what you said. If not, rephrase the message, trying to give more clues. (Example: *Message:* "The nurse will be dropping by this afternoon to check on you." *Rephrased:* "Your nurse, Ms. Anderson, will be coming here at 3:00 to check the dressing on your leg.")
6. Try to reduce distractions in the immediate environment.
7. Avoid chewing gum or placing your hands at your mouth when you speak.
8. Demonstrate your willingness to take the time and energy to communicate with your client, without losing your patience.

SPEECH IMPAIRMENT
1. Position yourself close to the client in a quiet setting to avoid unnecessary strain or frustration.
2. Speak to the client in a normal fashion.
3. Try to phrase questions so that they may be answered either yes or no.
4. Watch the lips of the speaker to help you pick up additional clues as to the message being communicated.
5. If you do not understand a portion of your client's message, repeat the portion of it you did understand and request clarification of the remainder. (Example: "I understand that you are hungry, but I do not understand what you would like to eat.")
6. Limit the time of your conversations so as not to tire your client.
7. Keep paper and pencil within your client's reach, if necessary.
8. Demonstrate your willingness to take the time and make the effort to communicate, without losing your patience. Provide encouragement for your client to speak.

Figure 4-9   Guidelines for communicating with hearing- and speech-impaired clients

Stop to think about the guidelines in Figure 4-7. Are they not based on common sense? Clients and their families are to be spoken to and treated in the same way that the home health aide would want to be spoken to and treated. Remember, too, that communication does not always need words. Sometimes a gentle pat on the arm or a smile can communicate more than any choice of words.

Communication is a combination of many skills. A home health aide must develop these skills in order to become successful. Figure 4-8 shows several examples of aide/client communications. Note how the choice of words can affect interpersonal relationships. The better responses are based on the rules shown in Figure 4-7.

Guidelines for communicating with hearing- and speech-impaired clients are shown in Figure 4-9.

SUMMARY

- One of the skills a home health aide must develop is the art of communication.
- It is always wise to think before speaking. The tone of voice and the pitch, as well as the content of what is said, are all part of verbal communication.
- Nonverbal communication includes body language such as gestures, touching, and facial expressions.
- Communications can only be delivered when there is a sender and a receiver. This means that part of the art of communication is learning to be a good listener.
- Written communications must be very clear. This requires properly spelling words and writing clearly so that the message can be read.
- Many times a home health aide will be asked to keep a chart of the client's responses or to record certain information about the client, such as temperature, pulse, and respiration rate. Special terminology or abbreviations may be used for this purpose. Use short and concise terms when reporting to your supervisor.
- Accuracy is an absolute must when making a client's record.
- When communicating with an elderly or disabled person, the home health aide should be patient and gentle.
- The aide should keep in mind that illness affects the emotions. Some clients may whine and cry. Others may appear to be angry and short-tempered.
- It is the duty of the home health aide to keep the lines of communication open. Clients and their families must be spoken to and treated in the same way that the home health aide would want to be spoken to and treated.

REVIEW

1. Give two examples each of verbal and nonverbal communication.
2. How can the home health aide give a precise report of observations made?
3. List four rules for improving communications with clients.
4. What four elements are involved in communication?
5. List two techniques to remember when communicating with a client who is hard of hearing or has a speech impairment.

6. Mrs. Lindsay is blind. You should:
   a. touch her to get her attention
   b. move furniture and items around to provide for variety
   c. provide step-by-step explanation of what you are doing
   d. have her walk in front of you as you guide her from behind

7. Match Column I with Column II (abbreviations of diseases)

   Column I

   ___1. AIDS
   ___2. CHF
   ___3. DM
   ___4. DJD
   ___5. Fx
   ___6. Alz
   ___7. TIA

   Column II

   a. Alzheimer
   b. Acquired immunodeficiency syndrome
   c. Congestive heart failure
   d. Diabetes mellitus
   e. Transient ischemic attacks
   f. Fracture
   g. Degenerative joint disease

8. You are talking to a client with a hearing loss. You should do all of the following except:
   a. speak clearly and slowly
   b. speak in front of the client so the client can read your lips
   c. shout
   d. use short sentences and simple words

9. Body language is:
   a. use of gestures instead of words
   b. a form of verbal communication
   c. of no concern to the home health aide
   d. used only when a client is unable to hear

10. Match Column I with Column II

    Column I

    ___1. ADLs
    ___2. TLC
    ___3. qod
    ___4. stat
    ___5. HOH
    ___6. c/o
    ___7. qid

    Column II

    a. complains of
    b. activities of daily living
    c. four times a day
    d. tender loving care
    e. immediately
    f. every other day
    g. hard of hearing

Unit 5 Understanding Differences: Individuals, Families, and Cultures

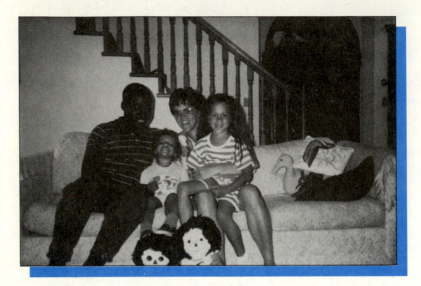

KEY TERMS

blended families

children with special needs

culture

divorce

environment

extended family

family unit

interracial family

life-style choices

living style

psychosocial

separation

single-parent families

two-career families

vegetarians

LEARNING OBJECTIVES

After studying this unit, you should be able to:

- List three ways in which families may differ.
- Identify one way illness might affect a family.
- Discuss racial and religious prejudice.
- Identify what is meant by a family unit.
- Define environment and culture.
- List three main minority groups in the United States.

- Explain three different types of family unit.
- Describe two typical differences between a family today and a family in the early part of this century.
- List two customs regarding health care that are different in a minority culture.

Home is a word with a great deal of emotional impact. It has a special meaning for most people. It recalls mental images of shared family experiences and geographical locations or even of anger or sadness. One may speak of one's home as the country, state, or town of birth. It may be thought of as the house where one lives. It can be a small room in a boarding house or a spacious place in the suburbs; but to the people living there, it is home. A home health aide may be assigned to many different types of homes, from modest to wealthy. The care standards provided by the home health aide are the same in all types of homes. Standards of cleanliness are to be maintained, using whatever equipment is available. An aide is expected to work with individuals and within **family units** and develop good interpersonal relationships.

The home health aide must recognize that each client is an individual unique in many ways from any other person. Each client has different needs, and each reacts to illness or disability in different ways. The aide must be prepared to adapt to the changing and unique needs of the client and the client's family and to work with the client without criticizing the client's or family's life-style.

The Family Unit—Past and Present

What is a family unit? By many laws, a family unit is made up of a married couple and their natural or adopted children. A family may also include relatives such as aunts, uncles, cousins, grandparents, or in-laws, Figure 5-1. In today's society, however, a family may also be made up of nonrelated members who live together under one roof. As a large or small group, they usually share some common interests and financial duties.

Historical Perspective

Early in this century, a majority of the population lived in rural areas. Home and family were the center of life. Farming or agriculture was the main industry or source of income.

The family unit was often an **extended family.** Different generations—grandparents, par-

ents, and children—lived together and shared responsibilities. They were self-sufficient for their own needs of food, clothing, and shelter. The average income per family was often less than $900 a year. Babies were cared for by older women in the family. As the children grew up, they were given chores suited to their age. They were expected to feed the farm animals or milk the cows. Each member of the family worked to help the family survive as a whole. The families at that time were large, which was necessary to help do all the farm work. The average life span was less than 50 years in the early 1900s.

Because of lack of transportation and limited phone service, social life was limited to the local neighborhood. It usually was centered around the relatives, close neighbors, school, and the church. Close family and community ties provided stability and strength to the family unit. Rarely did children move far away from their parents.

Technological advances creating employment and military service eventually led chil-

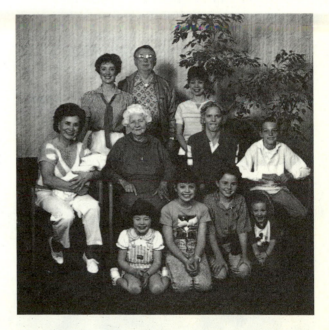

Figure 5-1   Continuum of life. The characteristics of the different age groups are reflected in this group picture. This is an example of a traditional extended family. (From Hegner and Caldwell, *Nursing Assistant, A Nursing Process Approach,* 6E, copyright 1992 by Delmar Publishers Inc.)

dren away from their parents' homes. Travel became easier and industrial jobs drew families away from their rural environment. Family members became more mobile and more educated and found employment in a variety of jobs and places.

Current Perspectives

We have moved from being an industrial society to being a computer society. The year 2000 is fast approaching, and individual and family life is continuously changing. Technology has improved the lives of family members in many ways, but it has also created new problems. Families are smaller—the average number of children per family is two. Many children now are being raised not by an extended family, but by a single parent, Figure 5-2. Single families are all different. A well-known TV star with one child has very different options and opportunities than a young, unskilled, divorced mother of two preschoolers. However, a recent study has shown that single parents spend approximately the same amount of time with their children as parents from two-parent families. Another study recently done showed that children from single-parent families do as well as children from two-

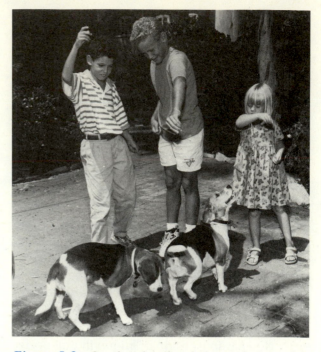

Figure 5-3   Stepbrothers and sister playing with the family dogs

parent families in both intellectual and academic achievement in school.

Another type of family that is emerging in our society is called a **blended family.** An example of this type of family is when parents of children remarry. Children in this type of family do far better economically than those from a single-parent family, but may have more emotional problems adjusting to their new parent, stepbrothers, and stepsisters, Figure 5-3. **Interracial family** units are also increasing in our society and are more accepted than in prior years, Figure 5-4. Part of this acceptance arises from a better understanding and knowledge of different races by individuals and society. Color of skin is not the important issue in marriage, but rather the ability to relate to one another and share similar values.

Divorce and separation are never acceptable, just more common and therefore, more routine; there is also less stigma attached to divorce and separation than in prior generations. Divorce has been shown to adversely affect children both physically and emotionally. The standard of living for a woman usually declines after a divorce. It is quite common for women after a

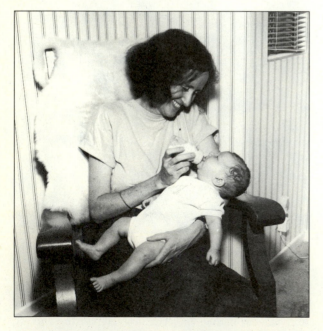

Figure 5-2   Single-parent family—mother with her new baby

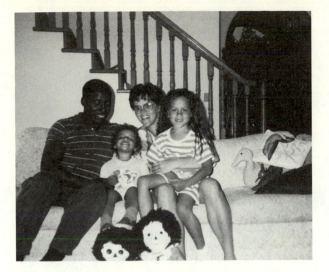

Figure 5-4   Interracial family—the blending of two cultures

divorce not to have health insurance, which in many instances, will stop her from seeking medical care unless it is an emergency.

Two-career families are becoming very evident in our society. Women are continuing their education and seek jobs with higher pay and more satisfaction. Over 60% of families with children under 18 have parents that both work. Many women work to help pay the bills, others work for personal satisfaction. Studies have shown that women who work outside of the home have less physical and emotional problems than their counterparts who stay at home. Their common problem is not having adequate time to do everything they want to do. Husbands in today's families are expected to do some household chores and also help with raising the children.

Younger children from these various types of families are often cared for in day-care centers. If a parent's income is below a certain amount, the government will assist in paying their weekly fee for the day care. The number of day-care centers has grown tremendously in the last decade. Studies have shown that children benefit in many ways by attending a well-run day-care facility.

Young **children with special needs,** whether physical or emotional, may be cared for by a home health aide often in the child's own home. The aide may be sent into the home on a regular basis to care for the child while the par-

ents work, or to assist the parent in doing personal care for the child. Another reason for assisting with care for the child with special needs is to relieve the parent for a few hours to prevent "burnout." Children with special needs do need more care than normal healthy children. Some families are very willing and able to give this special care required, whereas other families may have difficulty dealing with the disability and giving the necessary care. In some cases, finances are often strained due to the extra expense involved in caring for children with special needs. Extra expenses can be incurred due to more physician visits and medications, or when needing to purchase special equipment such as wheelchairs, mechanical lifts, etc.

Another type of **living style** becoming more common is two people of the same sex setting up a household together. It might be two women living together or two men. If you are assigned to care for clients in this household, you must not comment on this living style. Another type of living style that is becoming more common is a man and woman who are not married living together. When you are working in this household, you must not comment on this arrangement. You are there to care for the client and not to judge the life-style.

A life-style choice of an increasing number of individuals is to remain single; others may fall into this category because of divorce or death. There is a difference in the age, number, and quality of lives of these individuals. Single individuals may be either 18 or 99 years of age. Some single individuals will have a limited income to live on, whereas other will live in poverty. A few will live with relatives mainly because of financial reasons, others have their own household. Many have built up a network of friends who care for one another, whereas others live a lonely life. If a single individual does get ill and this person has no friends to assist with routine personal care, a home health aide will be employed to do the necessary care. The aide must be aware of not only the physical needs of this individual, but also the psychosocial needs such as talking and relating to other people.

Changes in life-style have altered social and moral attitudes. In many cases, these changes have weakened and made family units less stable. Also, family members are living longer and require more assistance than in prior generations. It is not uncommon for children to be in their seventies and parents in their nineties. Because family members cannot always rely on one another for care, they must seek help from outside the family. This outside source might be respite care, adult day care, or a home health aide coming directly into their parent's home.

General Background About Contrasts Creating Family Differences

In less than 20 years, roughly 14% of United States residents will be over age 65. One of the fastest growing age groups today is the 100+ age group. Total population groups are changing. African Americans make up 12% of the United States population and are the largest minority group. Hispanics constitute about 8% of the total population. Hispanic culture is the predominant culture in California. The Asian and Pacific Islander Americans number over 11 million, the third largest minority group. Speaking over 30 different languages and bringing with them 30 different cultures, the Native Americans are a minority group with about 1.6 million people.

From reading the above statistics it is easy to recognize the diversity of our population. This diversity should strengthen the country, but first the nation must recognize a few problems. It is difficult to make generalizations about cultures and problems within each culture. One common problem among the minorities is adequate access to proper health care. There is a higher incidence of infant deaths and acquired immunodeficiency syndrome (AIDS) in these groups. Beside having poor access to proper health care, their income and quality of housing is lower than those of most white Americans.

Customs of Minority Cultures

The Native American diet is high in carbohydrates and fats and low in protein, vitamins, and minerals. Indian medicine and religion cannot be separated. Native Americans do not separate emotional illness from physical illness. If modern Western medicine does not work for an ill Native American, the person will use the traditional healing practices or alternate between the two.

Puerto Ricans and Haitians believe in the "hot-cold" theory, in which illnesses are classified as hot or cold. If a disease is a hot disease, it must be treated with a cold remedy. An example is if a person is anemic (low in iron) and pregnant (a hot condition), then a wise doctor would order the woman to take her iron pills with cold water.

In some Hispanic homes all medicines are taken before breakfast and are usually done nine times in a row. Hispanic people also believe that potatoes have many medicinal uses. They also have strong family ties.

Each culture has unique characteristics and customs derived from its ancestors. When you are assigned to care for clients from a different culture than your own, obtain additional information about the particular culture. You will then be better prepared to understand the client's life-style and to offer better quality care.

It is estimated that 59.3% of the population are members of churches, synagogues, or temples. The *major* religions in the United States are:

Protestant denominations (Christian, Baptist, Methodist, Episcopalian, Presbyterians, etc.). In addition, there are various *sects,* groups that are too small to be considered a denomination.
Catholic (Roman Catholic, Old Catholic, Polish National Catholic, Russian Orthodox, and American Catholic).
Jewish (Reform, Conservative, and Orthodox).

There are also Muslims who follow the writings of Mohammed; Buddhists who believe in the teachings of Buddha; and atheists, who do not believe in God, to name only a few.

From reading these statistics, it is quite clear that in America people are free to practice (or not practice) religion. This is a nation that prides itself on offering the gift of freedom to all people. Freedom, however, does not mean that a person can do whatever he or she may choose. There are laws that all must follow so that we will not live in chaos.

What does all this mean to a home health aide? Prejudice grows out of ignorance and lack of knowledge about others. Prejudice is forming an opinion without knowing all the facts. Those who hold preconceived, irrational opinions often feel hatred or strong dislike for a particular group, race, or religion. Some people feel threatened by those whose skin color is different or fear practices that are unfamiliar to them. It is clear that the average individual cannot be knowledgeable about all of the differences among people. However, each individual should keep an open mind and be sensitive to the religious, cultural, or ethnic practices of others.

As home health aides go from client to client, they will meet persons of other cultures, religions, color, or nationality from their own, Figure 5-5. This can be viewed as an opportunity to discover interesting and informative facts about others. The more a person knows, the less likely a person is to be prejudiced. An aide must always remember that there are unpleasant individuals in the world. Being unpleasant has nothing to do with one's race, color, language, or religion.

Religious practices, traditions, types of food, and manner in which food is prepared are very often determined by the culture and religion of the individual. The home health aide must (1) accept the practices of others, (2) be sensitive to the client's needs, and (3) follow the instructions given by the case manager in meeting the needs of the client regardless of religion, color, or creed. An aide must not judge clients, but must allow them the freedom to follow their own practices and beliefs while the aide provides safe and proper care.

Families differ in size, ages of members, likes and dislikes, customs, and habits. They differ in political beliefs, financial resources, and ethnic background. Each family has its own living standards, religious practices, and standards within the community. Many normal contrasts exist. However, health or social problems can also create contrasts. Some families include children with special needs. Members of other families may have suffered emotional breakdowns. Alcoholism, **psychosocial** problems, and addiction to drugs or gambling may cause family

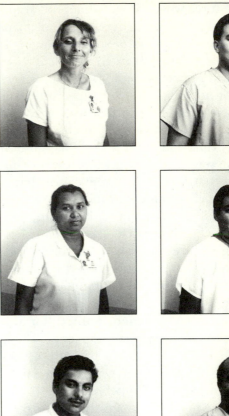

Figure 5-5   Home health aides and clients represent many cultures.

problems. The home health aide should be aware of these problems. They may determine how the aide plans work schedules and what work must be done.

Language Differences

How can an English-speaking aide communicate with a client who only speaks Spanish, French, Chinese, or any other language?

1. Be sure that the case manager explains in detail the home and nursing procedures to be given in each case. If a home health aide knows exactly what is expected, he or she can follow a plan of action.
2. Maintain a pleasant and friendly manner, smile and touch the client, and try to show

with gestures what you are doing or would like to do. For instance, it is lunchtime; pantomime holding a fork or spoon, bringing it to your mouth and back to the plate. Nod your head up and down for yes or back and forth for no. Hold up toilet paper and ask if the client needs to go to the bathroom. Hold up a glass to see if the client might want a drink. Although it may take time to establish ways to communicate, it is very important that the client understand what is being done. An aide can take the time to find special ways to communicate. One possibility might be to make a little scrapbook showing pictures of food, drink, bed, chair, bathroom, telephone, towels and shampoo, or other everyday items. The client could point to a picture and you would know immediately what the client wanted. Or, the aide could point to a picture to let the client know that it is time to have a bath, for instance. Try to make certain that the client understands what is happening!

3. If there is a family member who speaks both languages, let him or her act as an interpreter to help establish lines of communication. Another suggestion would be to have the family member write down common words that the client uses, with English interpretations. If a client does not speak English, an aide should face the client, speak softly, not make sudden jerking movements, and look pleasant. Yelling does not make communication any clearer and may upset the client as well. Speak clearly in short sentences, using gestures to help get the message across.

4. Recognize that there are differences in what is acceptable and unacceptable to persons of other cultures. In some societies, people do not look directly at a person who is talking to them. Some people do not like to be touched, even in a friendly and nonthreatening way, by a stranger or nonfamily member.

Cultural Differences

Culture is the way of life passed down to children from generation to generation. Cultural influences include language, moral codes, customs, and laws. Culture is a learned behavior. A child at birth speaks no language. A Chinese baby raised by a German family would grow up speaking German, not Chinese. Culture is the result of the social surroundings that affect the growth of an individual. The sum total of the conditions surrounding an individual is called the **environment.** Examples of cultural customs that might be seen by a home health aide include:

- *When and what a family eats.* Farm families often have their main meal at noon. Those who live in cities most often have their largest meal at night when all the family members are at home. The spices and seasonings preferred by a family are often culturally determined. Greek and Italian families may use heavy garlic seasonings. Some Texans prefer hot, spicy foods because they have acquired part of the Hispanic culture.

- *The accepted response to pain or grief.* Native Americans have been considered a stoic people. They are taught from infancy to show no response to pain and not to cry. Other cultures may encourage outward expression such as screaming, crying, or tearing their clothes to show grief.

- *How children are disciplined.* In Japan, children are taught from infancy not to make unnecessary noise. When a baby cries, it is picked up at once and soothed so that the cries will not disturb others. In general, American parents are more permissive than English parents. Most people discipline a child in the way they were disciplined by their own parents.

Religious Practices

Whether or not one follows a religion is an individual decision. However, that personal decision is greatly influenced by one's culture. When working in a home where there are strong religious practices, the home health aide must respect the customs and practices of that family.

Most religions set aside Sunday as a day of worship and rest; exceptions to this are Judaism and Seventh Day Adventists, which celebrate the Sabbath on Saturday. Special dietary laws are often observed. Some religious groups do not eat meat, limit the types of meat eaten, or restrict meat on certain days. Many nonreligious groups also do not eat meat or animal products and are referred to as **vegetarians.** Fast day (no food or drink are consumed for a certain period of time) may also be observed in varying degrees. Orthodox Jewish families may have two or more sets of dishes and utensils for cooking and eating: one set is used only for dairy foods, another set for meat dishes, and a third set is used only during the Passover celebration. Observing Jewish law in this manner is part of keeping a Kosher home. Families that practice special dietary customs will usually instruct the home health aide as to the family's special requirements. The aide must carry out such special instructions without passing judgment.

Among some religious groups, it is customary for the minister, priest, or rabbi to make regular visits to the homebound members of their congregations. A telephone number of the clergy is usually given to the aide. This number should be kept near the phone so the aide can call if the need arises. To a deeply religious family, the minister, priest, or rabbi is a vital member of the health team; they give spiritual and psychological support to the client. The home health aide has a duty to respect the religious beliefs and practices of the client and family.

Racial Prejudice and Discrimination

What is the role of the home health aide in homes where life-style, racial, educational, and economic background and cultural differences are present? Home health aides are expected to provide the services for which they have been trained, to the best of their ability.

But how does one function in an environment that is very different from what one is used to? It is important to recognize and accept the fact that no two people are alike. It is the individual and cultural differences that make up the fabric of our society. Just because a group

believes in "supernatural healing" or does not eat certain foods, doesn't make them "wrong"; it just makes them different. An aide must be aware of and allow the client to follow special dietary or ritualistic rules practiced within a household.

Many individuals are frightened or wary of people who are different from themselves. Sometimes color of skin, language, or religious practices get in the way of understanding each other. Although it is not always easy to accept individual or cultural differences, a health care professional must avoid hurting the feelings of the client.

One home health aide went to a new client's home and asked the elderly lady if she were Jewish. The client said that she wasn't Jewish, but that her name was of German origin. The aide replied that the name sure sounded Jewish, and went on to say that she didn't like Jews. The client was very upset. She called the case manager and reported the incident. She said she didn't think the aide should have brought the subject up. She also said that she was very angry at being called Jewish!

This was an actual example of two prejudiced individuals. The aide didn't like Jews. The client showed her own prejudice by implying that she, too, didn't like Jews.

Unfortunately, some older persons are set in their ways and find it hard to adapt to the changes that have taken place in our society over the past 20 or more years. There is little one can do to bring them into this century! Probably the best thing to do is just try to ignore any prejudicial remarks and try to say a few things positive about the culture.

On the other hand, it is totally inappropriate for an aide to make prejudiced remarks or be judgmental about the client or the client's life-style. Of course, there are times when an aide and client simply cannot adjust to each other. In such a situation, the aide should talk to the case manager and may be reassigned to another client.

SUMMARY

· · · · · · · · · · · · · · · · · ·

- Rich or poor, the home is usually the focus of family life. Within a home, the family unit lives by its own rules and standards.
- One of the responsibilities of the home health aide is to respect the rights of the client and the family within the home.
- The roles and responsibilities of parents today are not as rigid as in prior generations; more fathers help with household tasks and child rearing and mothers have jobs outside of the home. Single-parent families and blended families are becoming more common and more accepted in our society.
- As a home health aide, you will be exposed to many different cultures and customs.

- When working with a client who cannot speak the same language the aide does, the aide may need to find ways to communicate with the clients other than with words.
- The home health aide comes into a home as a stranger to give personal care to the client and provide home care. The aide can ease some of the problems caused by illness.
- A home health aide should take pride in doing a job well.
- When helping a family in trouble, the aide should always show respect for the customs and life-styles of that family.

REVIEW

1. Name three ways in which families may differ.

2. What is meant by an extended family?

3. Define culture.

4. Give two examples of prejudice.

5. List three major minority groups in the United States.

6. Explain three different family groups.

7. List two customs regarding health care that may be different in a minority culture.

8. Clients sometimes have culture beliefs with which the home health aide does not agree. Which understanding would be the best guide for the home health aide?
   a. pretend to have the same beliefs
   b. explain your own beliefs in detail
   c. understand that each person has a right to their own beliefs and should be respected
   d. explain why you do not agree with the client's beliefs

9. One of the most common problems that minorities have in our society is access to adequate health care.
   a. true
   b. false

10. The Spanish culture is the largest minority group in the United States.
    a. true
    b. false

11.   A common problem of two-career families is having adequate time to do the things they want to accomplish.
  a. true
  b. false

12.   It is inappropriate for an aide to make prejudicial remarks or be judgmental about the client's life-style.
  a. true
  b. false

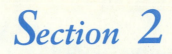

Section 2

Basic Anatomy and Physiology

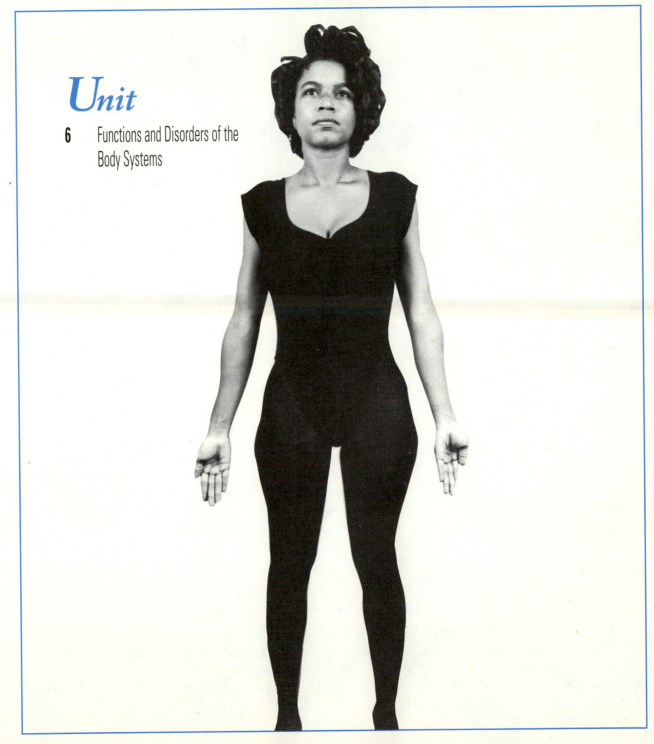

Unit

6 Functions and Disorders of the
Body Systems

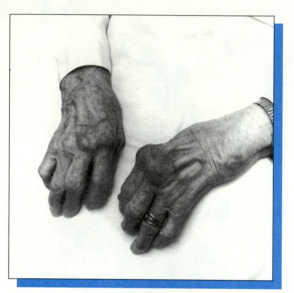

KEY TERMS
. . . .

anemia
atherosclerosis
arthritis
auditory
bony prominences
contracture
cystitis
dermis
ducts
emphysema

epidermis
epilepsy
fracture
gangrene
hemiplegia
hemophiliac
hypertension
hypotension
impacted

incontinent
ligaments
otosclerosis
paraplegia
peristalsis
phlebitis
pressure areas
quadriplegia
sensory deficits

LEARNING OBJECTIVES
. . . .

After studying this unit, you should be able to:

- Identify one function of each body system.
- Name the five senses.
- Identify one disorder in each body system.
- Identify the relationship among cells, tissues, organs, and systems.

- Identify the difference between hereditary and environmental factors.
- List two factors that influence body development.

Human beings have often been compared to machines. When functioning perfectly, the body operates as smoothly as a well-oiled machine. The human body, however, is much more efficient than any machine. Unlike a machine, the human body can often repair itself, e.g., new skin can grow over a wound. When the body functions at its peak efficiency with all of its parts working like a finely tuned engine, it is in a state of wellness.

The body is a complex organism. It is made up of millions of cells, which are the smallest structural units of the body. Many cells make up a tissue and tissues make up organs, Figure 6-1. Organs act together in making the total body function. All of these separate units interact

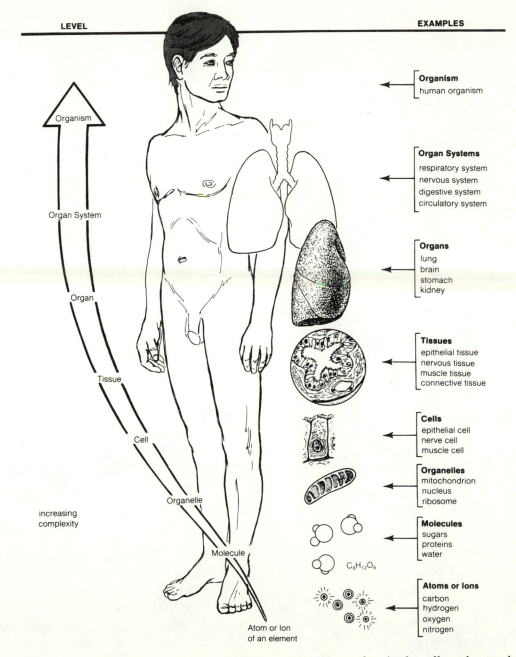

Figure 6-1   The human body is highly organized from the single cell to the total organism. (From Fong, Ferris, and Skelley, *Body Structures and Functions,* copyright 1989 by Delmar Publishers Inc.)

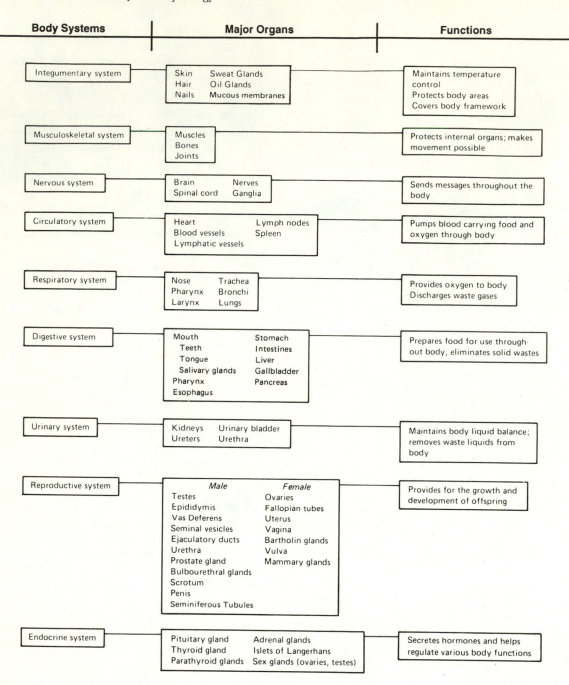

Body Systems	Major Organs		Functions
Integumentary system	Skin Sweat Glands Hair Oil Glands Nails Mucous membranes		Maintains temperature control Protects body areas Covers body framework
Musculoskeletal system	Muscles Bones Joints		Protects internal organs; makes movement possible
Nervous system	Brain Nerves Spinal cord Ganglia		Sends messages throughout the body
Circulatory system	Heart Lymph nodes Blood vessels Spleen Lymphatic vessels		Pumps blood carrying food and oxygen through body
Respiratory system	Nose Trachea Pharynx Bronchi Larynx Lungs		Provides oxygen to body Discharges waste gases
Digestive system	Mouth Stomach Teeth Intestines Tongue Liver Salivary glands Gallbladder Pharynx Pancreas Esophagus		Prepares food for use throughout body, eliminates solid wastes
Urinary system	Kidneys Urinary bladder Ureters Urethra		Maintains body liquid balance; removes waste liquids from body
Reproductive system	*Male* *Female* Testes Ovaries Epididymis Fallopian tubes Vas Deferens Uterus Seminal vesicles Vagina Ejaculatory ducts Bartholin glands Urethra Vulva Prostate gland Mammary glands Bulbourethral glands Scrotum Penis Seminiferous Tubules		Provides for the growth and development of offspring
Endocrine system	Pituitary gland Adrenal glands Thyroid gland Islets of Langerhans Parathyroid glands Sex glands (ovaries, testes)		Secretes hormones and helps regulate various body functions

Figure 6-2   The body systems and their major organs and functions

within the body in systems. There are nine body systems, each one performing a necessary function in the body, Figure 6-2.

Integumentary System

The skin, which is the largest component of the integumentary system, is the body's first means of defense against germs. The skin is the largest organ of the body. It covers the entire outer surface and the inside surfaces of all the body's openings (nose, mouth, ears, vagina, etc.). Skin is made up of two layers of tissue. The outer layer is the **epidermis** and the inner layer is the **dermis,** Figure 6-3. Other parts of the integumentary system are the nails, hair, oil and sweat glands, and mucous membranes.

The integumentary system protects the

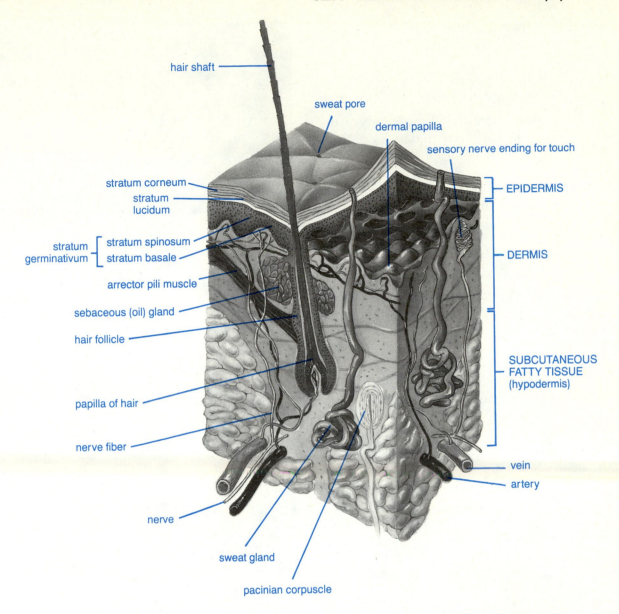

hair shaft

sweat pore

dermal papilla

sensory nerve ending for touch

stratum corneum

stratum lucidum

EPIDERMIS

stratum germinativum

stratum spinosum

stratum basale

DERMIS

arrector pili muscle

sebaceous (oil) gland

hair follicle

SUBCUTANEOUS FATTY TISSUE (hypodermis)

papilla of hair

nerve fiber

vein

artery

nerve

sweat gland

pacinian corpuscle

Figure 6-3 Cross section of the skin (From Anatomy and Physiology insert, copyright 1992 by Delmar Publishers Inc.)

body but also has other functions. It regulates body temperature and works with the nervous system to sense touch, pressure, pain, heat, and cold.

The pores or natural openings in the skin surface are protected by oil glands and sweat glands. As the body perspires (sweats) through the skin pores, the air evaporates the perspiration and the body feels cooler. Secretions from these glands are helpful in keeping germs from entering the pores. When the skin is cut or there is an open sore, germs can enter the body easily. Once germs get beyond the skin, the other body defenses start to work. White blood cells surround the germs and try to stop them from going deeper into the body. The pus that forms on a skin wound is made up of dead white blood cells that have fought off the germs.

Hair protects the body in several ways. The eyebrows keep sweat from falling into the eyes. The tiny hairs inside the nose and ears stop small particles from entering and causing damage. The eyelashes keep small objects from getting into the eye. These hairs all act very much like a screen door on a house in keeping out unwanted organisms. The skin itself screens out harmful rays from the sun which may cause burns and harm the body.

Common Disorders of the Integumentary System

Pressure Areas (bedsores). The care given to the skin of a person confined to bed or a wheelchair is extremely important. When the body gets little exercise, the skin is one of the first areas to break down. Breakdown most often occurs where the skin covers the bones. These places are called **bony prominences,** Figure 6-4.

The back of the head, elbow, knees, and heels are common places to watch for signs of skin breakdown. A pressure sore is a breakdown in the skin that covers a bony area. Some common causes of pressure sore development are injury to the skin due to friction and shearing when turning or repositioning a client, leaving a client in one position too long, poor skin cleansing, and poor nutrition. The first sign is a

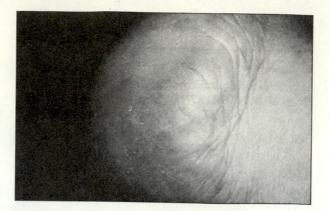

Figure 6-5A First indication of tissue ischemia (stage one) is redness and heat over a pressure point such as this heel. (Photo courtesy of Emory University Hospital, Atlanta, GA; from Hegner and Caldwell, *Nursing Assistant, A Nursing Process Approach,* 6E, copyright 1992 by Delmar Publishers Inc.)

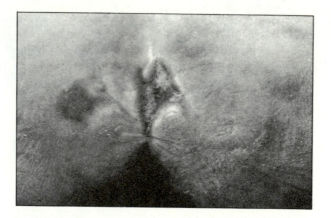

Figure 6-5B Stage two is marked by destruction of the epidermis and partial destruction of the dermis. NOTE: Photo shows coccygeal (sacrum) area. (Photo courtesy of Emory University Hospital, Atlanta, GA; from Hegner and Caldwell, *Nursing Assistant, A Nursing Process Approach,* 6E, copyright 1992 by Delmar Publishers Inc.)

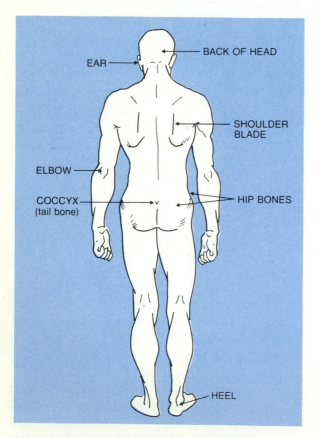

Figure 6-4 Pressure sores most often form over bony prominences.

warm looking reddened area. Within 18 to 24 hours the reddened area can become an open sore. The client's bed linens should be kept clean and dry at all times. If the client is left in a urine-saturated bed, the skin may begin to break down quickly. The client should be turned at least every 2 hours.

The first sign or stage of a pressure sore development is a reddened area as stated above,

Figure 6-5A. If not treated it will soon develop into stage two, Figure 6-5B. In this stage a blister will form and there will be small breaks visible on the client's skin. If not treated, it can rapidly progress to stage three where the blister breaks open and there is a well defined sore visible, Figure 6-6A. The fourth stage occurs when the open area extends to the muscle, bones, and other underlying structures, Figure 6-6B. These sores can vary greatly in size and are places where infections can set in readily.

The home health aide role is mainly in the prevention of the development of pressure sores. If a client develops a reddened area, the aide should gently rub lotion around this area. The aide will need to reposition the client every 2 hours. The client's bed linens should be kept clean and dry at all times. The client should be exercised as condition allows. The aide can assist the client with these exercises. When bathing a client be sure to use soap sparingly because soap dries the skin and makes the skin susceptible to skin breakdown. Many special devices are available to place on the bed or on the specific part of the body to aid in the preven-

tion of pressure sores. Examples of these are air mattress, water mattress, gel foam pad, egg crate mattress or cushion; lamb's wool or sheepskin pads; elbow and heel pads, Figures 6-7, 6-8, and 6-9. These special devices can prevent the skin from rubbing against the bed clothes but do not take the place of good skin care. The type of clients most susceptible to pressure sores are bedbound or chairbound or persons with impaired ability to reposition themselves. As a home health aide you need to check these types of clients on an ongoing basis for any signs of skin breakdown. Prevention is the first goal of the home health aide. Once a pressure sore develops, it may take weeks or months to heal.

Some other common skin disorders and their treatments are described in Figure 6-10.

Musculoskeletal System

The musculoskeletal system is made up of bones and muscles. It protects the internal body organs and makes body movement possible. The skull, for instance, forms a protective cover-

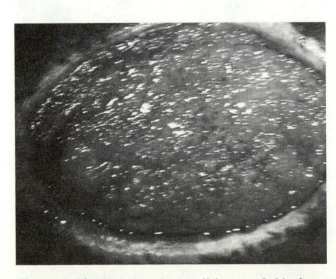

Figure 6-6A   In stage three, all layers of skin have been destroyed. A deep crater has been formed. NOTE: Photo shows right hip. (Photo courtesy of Emory University Hospital, Atlanta, GA; from Hegner and Caldwell, *Nursing Assistant, A Nursing Process Approach*, 6E, copyright 1992 by Delmar Publishers Inc.)

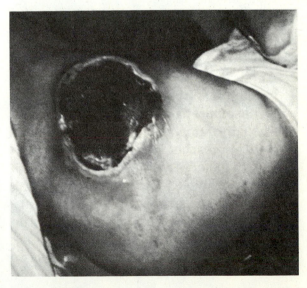

Figure 6-6B   In stage four, tissue destruction can involve muscle, bone, and other vital structures. (Photo courtesy of Emory University Hospital, Atlanta, GA; from Hegner and Caldwell, *Nursing Assistant, A Nursing Process Approach*, 6E, copyright 1992 by Delmar Publishers Inc.)

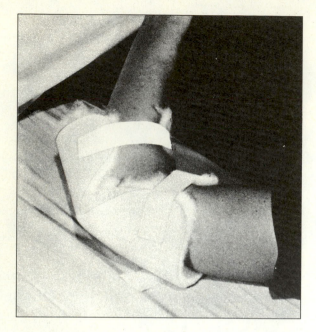

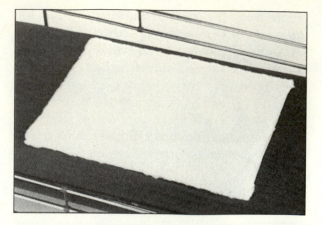

Figure 6-8A Pad of synthetic sheepskin (Photo courtesy of J.T. Posey Company, Arcadia, CA; from Hegner and Caldwell, *Nursing Assistant, A Nursing Process Approach,* 6E, copyright 1992 by Delmar Publishers Inc.)

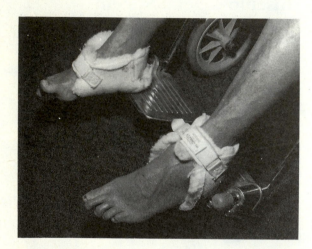

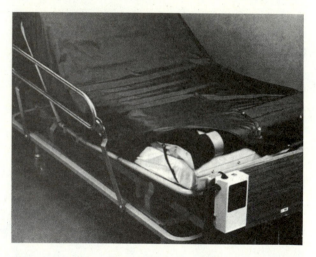

Figure 6-8B Alternating low airloss mattress overlay. Alternating air pressure in mattress cells constantly changes pressure points against the client's skin and gently massages the skin. (Photo courtesy of National Patient Care Systems; from Hegner and Caldwell, *Nursing Assistant, A Nursing Process Approach,* 6E, copyright 1992 by Delmar Publishers Inc.)

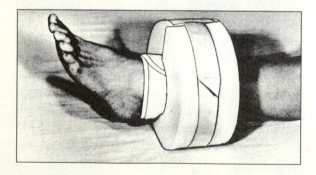

Figure 6-7 Pads reduce skin irritation and help prevent pressure sores. (Courtesy of the J.T. Posey Company, Arcadia, CA)

ing for the brain. The spinal column surrounds the spinal nerves leading from the brain. There are over 200 bones in the body, Figure 6-11. Bones are joined together by tough elastic fibers called **ligaments.**

Joints allow the bones to be moved in certain ways, Figure 6-12. The elbows and knees have hinge joints, which move in only two directions like hinges on a door. The joints at the shoulder and pelvis are ball and socket joints. They provide circular movements. The wrist, ankles, and spinal column have gliding joints connecting the various bones. These allow only a limited sliding movement.

Skeletal muscles are attached to the bones and are stretched over joints. Certain muscles produce motion by pulling on the bone when they receive messages from the nervous system. These muscles are called voluntary muscles because their movement is controlled by the brain. For example, the eye sees a $5.00 bill on the floor. The picture is relayed to the brain. The brain, through the nervous system, tells the body to bend over and pick up the bill. This is an example of voluntary muscle action or one which the body chooses to perform.

Other muscles, called involuntary muscles, form the walls of organs. They, too, receive messages through the nervous system but they work automatically, or without any conscious effort by the individual. The heart is an example of an involuntary muscle as it pumps blood throughout the body without any conscious effort.

The musculoskeletal system constantly interacts with other systems. The interior of the bone produces new blood cells for the circulatory system. Muscles move in response to mes-

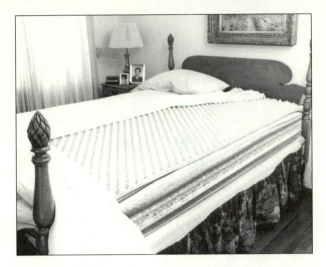

Figure 6-9 Egg crate mattress provides cushioning and mild redistribution of pressure beneath the client.

DISORDER	DESCRIPTION	TREATMENT
Acne	Chronic inflammatory disease of the sebaceous (oil) glands and hair follicles. Characterized by eruptions, cysts, nodules, or pustules that may lead to scarring and pitting of the skin. Often appears at puberty when major body changes commence. Usually appears on the face, neck, and shoulders.	Diet modification Topical medication Cleansing of the skin Surgical skin peeling or removal
Psoriasis	Scaly, itchy skin eruptions that appear at any age.	No cure, but can be controlled by topical medication to relieve itching
Dermatitis	Skin inflammation that causes itching, redness, and skin lesions (sores). May be caused by skin irritants such as poison ivy, allergies, sunburn, or adverse reaction to heat or cold.	Topical medication and avoidance of causal factors
Scabies	Skin lesions caused by mites that burrow into the skin. Transmitted by direct contact, clothing, and linen. Itching may persist several days after treatment. Noticed around fingers, wrists, axilla, waist, under the breasts, abdomen, buttocks, and genitalia. Infection of the lesions is common.	(ordered by physician) Topical medication Antibiotics if infection occurs Antihistamines to relieve the itching

Figure 6-10 Common skin disorders and their treatments

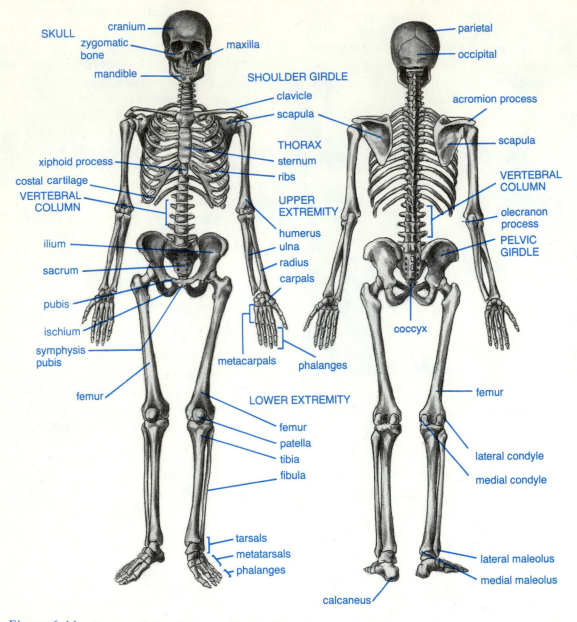

Figure 6-11   Bones of the skeleton (From Anatomy and Physiology insert, copyright 1992 by Delmar Publishers Inc.)

sages from the nervous system. It is not necessary to understand these complex interrelationships. However, it is interesting to note how one system depends on another.

Common Disorders of the Musculoskeletal System

The musculoskeletal system can be invaded by disease-causing microorganisms. However, the most common problems are fractures which are caused by falls.

Fractures.   A **fracture** is a break in a bone. Fractures are treated by immobilizing the bone or fixing it into position. Healing of bones may take several weeks; older people require a longer healing period.

Arthritis.   A musculoskeletal problem the home health aide will probably encounter is arthritis. Although arthritis affects people of all ages, it more commonly occurs in the elderly. **Arthritis** is an inflammation of the

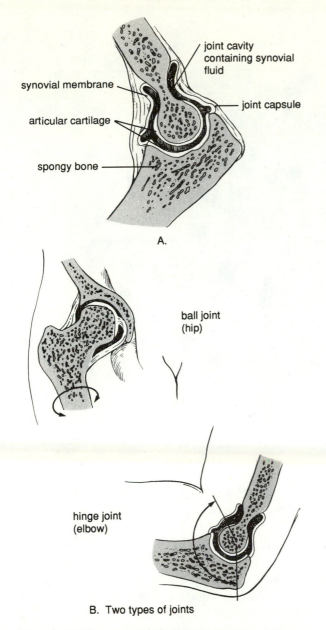

A.

ball joint
(hip)

hinge joint
(elbow)

B. Two types of joints

Figure 6-12 Diarthrotic joints (From Hegner and Caldwell, *Nursing Assistant, A Nursing Process Approach*, 6E, copyright 1992 by Delmar Publishers Inc.)

joints. It is usually painful and causes the joints to swell and become enlarged. Sometimes the bones of the hands and feet curl inward and become deformed.

There is no specific cure for arthritis but there are treatments to relieve some of the symptoms. Pain, muscle spasms and cramps can be relieved by heat from hot baths, heat lamps, paraffin baths, or hot packs. Aspirin, or aspirin substitutes, are considered the safest medication for long-term use. However, the doctor should determine the amount of aspirin the client is allowed to take. Other drugs are also used in the treatment of arthritis but these drugs must be prescribed by the physician. A client with arthritis may need physical therapy or may be treated with a special diet. Unit 18 will go into more detail on the types of arthritis and treatment.

Nervous System

The brain, spinal cord, nerves and ganglia make up the nervous system. This system is the communication center which sends messages to all parts of the body. It is the system that enables the body to see, hear, smell, taste, and touch. Sight, sound, taste, smell, and touch are known as the five body senses. The brain, Figure 6-13, is the master control or main switch of the nervous system. Messages are relayed to the brain from all parts of the body. The brain decides how to respond to each stimulus or message sent by the nerves. Each area of the brain performs a specialized duty. The brain alerts other control centers in the body so that the body correctly responds to a message.

The spinal cord can be compared to the electrical wiring system in a house. All the major nerves of the body are bound together in the spinal cord and lead into the brain. The spinal cord is protected by the spinal column. If the spinal column is damaged or diseased, the spinal nerves may be affected. For example, if one suffers a broken back and the spinal cord is cut or damaged, the nerves below the cut could no longer send messages up to the brain. The parts of the body below the cut could no longer feel pain and the muscles would no longer move.

Paraplegia refers to paralysis of the lower part of the body and both legs. **Quadriplegia** refers to paralysis of both arms and both legs. Both paraplegia and quadriplegia are the results of tumors or injury to the spinal cord. **Hemiplegia** is a paralysis of one side of the body. It is frequently the result of a cerebrovascular accident (CVA or "stroke").

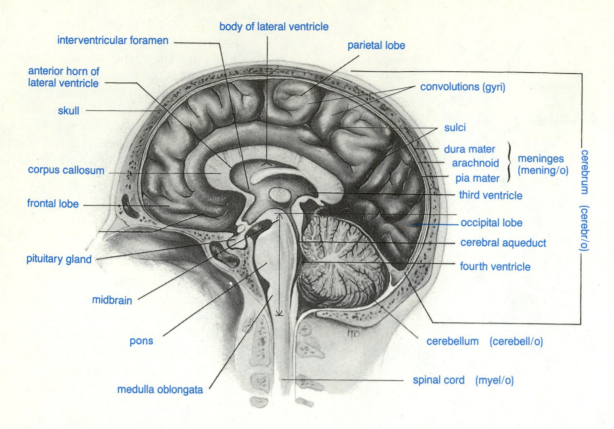

Figure 6-13   The central nervous system—brain and spinal cord (From Anatomy and Physiology insert, copyright 1992 by Delmar Publishers Inc.)

The nerves radiate from the spinal cord to all parts of the body forming a network. The nerve endings might be compared to the electrical outlets in the house. In the body, the nerves are usually ready to receive stimuli. For instance, the hand touches a hot surface, the nerve sends the message to the spinal cord, and it goes to the brain. The brain sends back the message to move the hand. This entire process takes place in an instant so that one is only aware of the result. The time it takes to respond to a stimulus is known as reaction time. As the human body ages, reaction time often slows down a great deal. It also is affected when part of the brain has been damaged as with a stroke.

Common Disorders of the Nervous System

Epilepsy.   **Epilepsy** is a condition that is characterized by various forms of recurrent seizures. These seizures range in severity from momentary losses of consciousness to violent, patterned movements. Clients who have epileptic seizures

are often treated with medication to control the severity and/or frequency of those episodes.

Spinal Cord Injuries.   When a person has an injury to the spinal cord, loss of sensation and function in body parts below the level of that injury often results. Clients who are paralyzed as a result of a spinal cord injury are often prone to the development of pressure areas and **contractures.**

Sensory Deficits.   **Sensory deficits** (decreases in sensory ability such as hearing or vision) commonly affect elderly people, but may also affect others as a result of disease. The home health aide is likely to encounter clients whose vision or hearing is impaired. Such conditions as glaucoma (an eye disorder caused by increased pressure of the fluid within the eye) and cataracts (a cloudy area in the lens of the eye) may severely limit the vision of a client. Elderly persons who are hard of hearing (HOH) may have nerve damage affecting the **auditory** (hearing) nerve, or a disorder called **otosclerosis.** This condition occurs when the bones of the inner ear, Figure 6-14, harden and sound waves are no longer carried in the usual fashion. Hearing ability gradually diminishes. Aged persons also may experience a loss of taste sensation, which may have a negative effect on their appetite. The home health aide should be aware of any sensory deficits a client might have and accordingly adjust the care given.

Circulatory System

The circulatory system delivers food, oxygen, and liquids to every cell of the body. It can best be described as a series of soft, flexible tubes of different sizes. These tubes are blood vessels, which are located in every part of the body. Blood is carried through the vessels bringing nourishment and removing waste products, Figure 6-15.

The organ that provides power to the system is the heart. The heart is a muscular organ about the size of a closed fist, Figure 6-16. Although it is one of the most important organs in the body, it has only one job. That job is to pump blood throughout the body. From the

time the fetus is 3½ months old until death, the heart continues to pump.

The heart has four chambers. Leading into and out of these chambers are the largest blood vessels making up the circulatory system. There are three kinds of blood vessels. The arteries carry blood away from the heart to the body cells. The arteries join the tiny blood vessels called capillaries. The capillaries meet the veins. The veins carry the blood back to the heart. This blood, poor in oxygen, is then pumped into the lungs where carbon dioxide is exchanged for oxygen. From the lungs, the oxygenated blood returns to the heart. The arteries carry the blood away from the heart to all parts of the body. It takes one minute for blood to leave the heart, travel through the arteries, capillaries, and veins and return to the heart. This is a cycle that continues each minute of the day.

As the heart contracts (squeezes together) and expands (relaxes) it pushes the blood into the arteries. The arteries contract and expand in the same rhythm as the heart. The pulse measured at the wrist is the expansion of the radial artery. The blood carried in the arteries is a rich, bright red color. Venous blood is a darker red because it is low in oxygen.

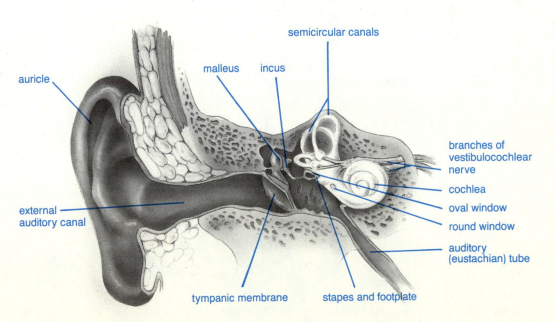

Figure 6-14   Internal view of the ear (From Anatomy and Physiology insert, copyright 1992 by Delmar Publishers Inc.)

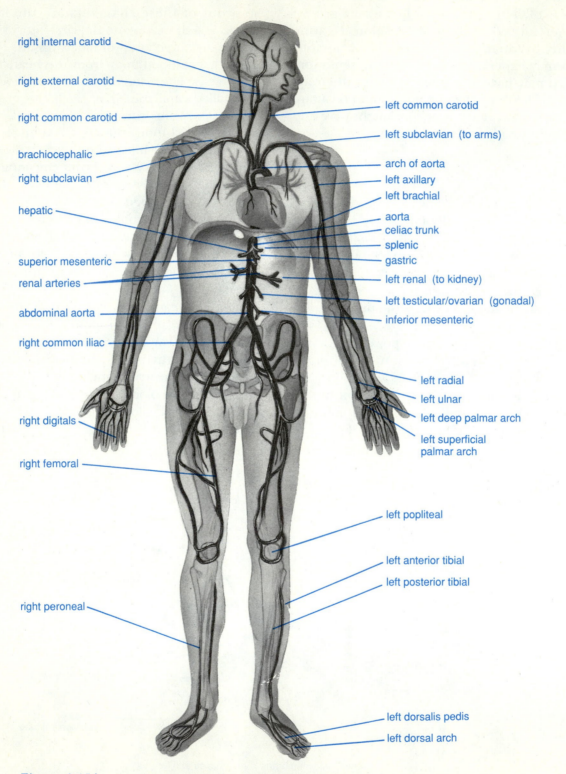

Figure 6-15A   Arterial system carries blood to all parts of the body (From Anatomy and Physiology insert, copyright 1992 by Delmar Publishers Inc.)

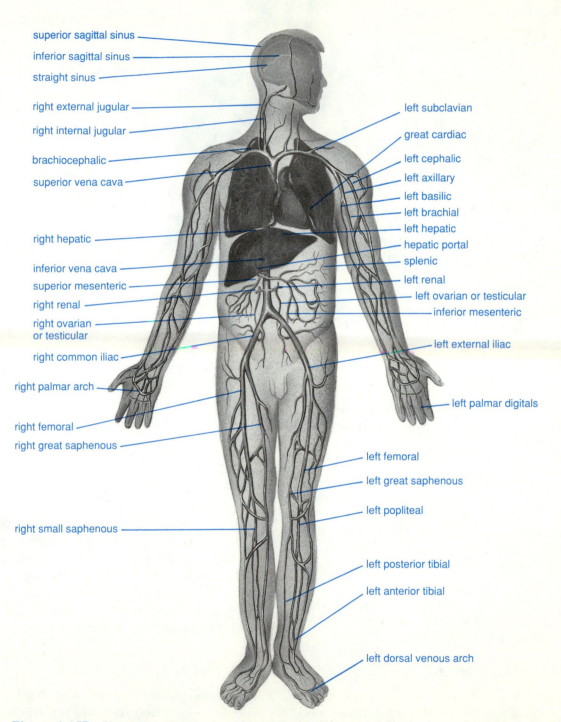

superior sagittal sinus
inferior sagittal sinus
straight sinus
right external jugular
right internal jugular
brachiocephalic
superior vena cava
right hepatic
inferior vena cava
superior mesenteric
right renal
right ovarian or testicular
right common iliac
right palmar arch
right femoral
right great saphenous
right small saphenous

left subclavian
great cardiac
left cephalic
left axillary
left basilic
left brachial
left hepatic
hepatic portal
splenic
left renal
left ovarian or testicular
inferior mesenteric
left external iliac
left palmar digitals
left femoral
left great saphenous
left popliteal
left posterior tibial
left anterior tibial
left dorsal venous arch

Figure 6-15B   Venous system returns blood from all parts of the body to the heart and lungs (From Anatomy and Physiology insert, copyright 1992 by Delmar Publishers Inc.)

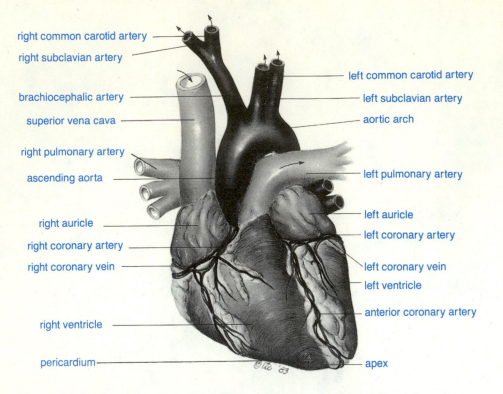

right common carotid artery

right subclavian artery

left common carotid artery

brachiocephalic artery

left subclavian artery

superior vena cava

aortic arch

right pulmonary artery

ascending aorta

left pulmonary artery

right auricle

left auricle

right coronary artery

left coronary artery

right coronary vein

left coronary vein

left ventricle

anterior coronary artery

right ventricle

pericardium

apex

Figure 6-16   External view of the heart (From Anatomy and Physiology insert, copyright 1992 by Delmar Publishers Inc.)

Common Disorders of the Circulatory System

Circulatory disorders are very common in people over the age of 50. These disorders may affect either the heart or the blood vessels. Circulatory conditions are the leading causes of long-term illness and death after the age of 50. The symptoms may be so mild as to be unnoticeable. Damage may have taken place before a victim knows anything is wrong. Cardiac disorders are those that affect the heart itself. Circulatory disorders are those affecting the blood vessels carrying blood throughout the body. The parts of the body most often affected by circulatory disorders are the brain and the lower extremities (feet and legs).

Disorders of the Heart

Angina Pectoris.   Angina pectoris is a mild pain in the chest that radiates to the shoulder, neck, and left arm. It usually results from a lack of oxygen in the heart muscle. It occurs most commonly in middle-aged men after exercising.

Acute Coronary Occlusion (Myocardial Infarction). Acute coronary occlusion (myocardial infarction) is commonly known as a heart attack. It occurs when a blood vessel within the heart muscle closes or is blocked by a blood clot. The seriousness of this condition depends on the size and location of the blockage. The heart may be permanently damaged.

Congestive Heart Failure.   Congestive heart failure occurs when the heart cannot pump enough blood to meet body demands, causing fluid build-up in the lungs and other tissues. Damage to the heart muscle is the usual cause. Acute attacks of congestive heart failure may lead to a chronic condition.

Disorders of the Blood Vessels

Arteriosclerosis.   Arteriosclerosis is hardening of the arteries. **Atherosclerosis** is a type of arteriosclerosis that often occurs in the larger arteries, especially those of the heart, kidneys, and brain. This condition could be compared to a piece of garden hose left lying outdoors. Dirt clogs the insides and the weather changes cause it to become hard and stiff. In the arteries, fatty deposits stop the blood from flowing through and cause loss of elasticity, Figure 6-17. Lack of blood flow causes less oxygen to reach the body cells. The body cells starve as a result.

Gangrene.   **Gangrene** is the death of body tissue caused by lack of adequate blood supply. It may be caused by a lack of blood supply to a body part. The lower extremities are most often affected. The first sign may be a small black spot on the client's large toe.

Phlebitis.   **Phlebitis** occurs when the lining of a vein becomes inflamed, causing a clot to form in the vein. This usually occurs in one leg, which may become swollen and painful to touch. The area may feel warm. The physician may order antiembolism stockings or elastic bandages (such as Ace bandages) to be applied to the affected leg or to both legs.

Cerebral Vascular Accidents.   A cerebral vascular accident (CVA) is also known as a stroke. There are three main causes of a CVA.

- A small blood clot, or plaque called a thrombus, may block a blood vessel in the brain. This prevents oxygen from reaching the brain cells.

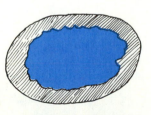

CROSS SECTION OF NORMAL ARTERY

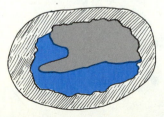

CROSS SECTION OF AN ABNORMAL ARTERY
ATHEROSCLEROTIC PLAQUE FORMATION-
INNER LINING OF THE VESSEL

Figure 6-17   Cross sections of a normal and an abnormal artery

- Arteriosclerosis (hardening of the arteries) may develop in the blood vessels of the brain, blocking the flow of blood.
- A blood vessel in the brain may burst, spilling blood directly into the brain tissues. This is often caused by high blood pressure (**hypertension**).

Disorders of the Blood

Anemia.   **Anemia** occurs when there are fewer than adequate red blood cells. It may result from an excessive loss of blood, from malformation of blood cells, or from a lack of essential nutrients. If blood loss is excessive, hypotension (low blood pressure) may occur.

Sickle Cell Anemia.   In this disorder, seen in African Americans, the client's red blood cells are crescent shaped, like a sickle. The cells do not carry enough oxygen in them, causing anemia. This is an inherited disease for which there is no cure, but new drugs are helping clients. Infections, stressful situations, excessive exercise, and other situations that increase the client's need for oxygen should be avoided. In the United States, this disease is usually found only in African Americans.

Leukemia.   Leukemia is a condition in which too many white blood cells are produced. These excess white blood cells block the normal transport of oxygen to the body's tissues. They may also affect production of new red blood cells. It may also be called cancer of the blood.

Hemophilia.   Hemophilia is a hereditary disease characterized by spontaneous hemorrhages due to a deficiency of a clotting factor in the blood. The classic form of the disease affects males only. If an individual starts to bleed, a special preparation can be given to stop the bleeding.

Respiratory System

The respiratory system consists of the nose, pharynx, larynx, trachea, bronchi, and lungs, Figure 6-18. It is closely linked to the circulatory system. Blood is supplied with fresh oxygen by means of the respiratory system. Fresh air is inhaled into the body and carried to the lungs. The oxygen from the air is carried to all parts of the body by the circulatory system. As oxygen is delivered to the cells of the body, waste gases are picked up and carried back to the lungs where they are exhaled from the body. The most plentiful waste gas is carbon dioxide. In short, oxygen is inhaled and carbon dioxide is exhaled.

Common Disorders of the Respiratory System

Diseases of the respiratory system have now been classified together as chronic obstructive pulmonary diseases (COPD).

Pneumonia.   Pneumonia is an infection of the lung. It is usually caused by bacteria, but there may be other causes such as a virus. It is treated with antibiotics.

Chronic Bronchitis.   Chronic bronchitis often occurs in middle-aged or elderly persons. It can result from a number of acute conditions, asthma, bronchitis, cigarette smoking, air pollution.

Asthma.   Asthma is a condition caused by an allergic reaction, although there are other causes. Often the specific substance causing the asthma cannot be determined. Symptoms may include

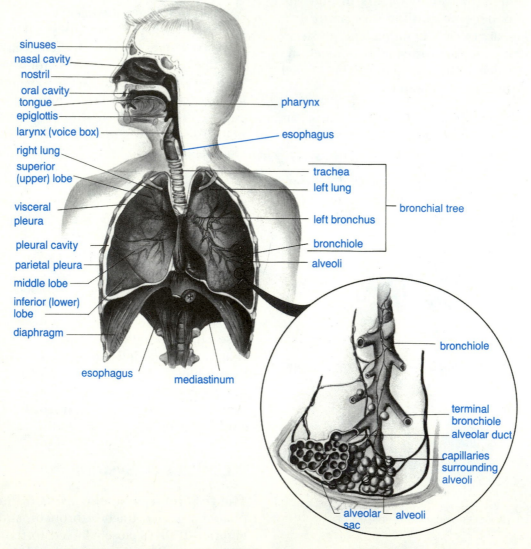

Figure 6-18   The respiratory system (From Anatomy and Physiology insert, copyright 1992 by Delmar Publishers Inc.)

coughing, difficult breathing, wheezing, and a feeling of tightness in the chest.

Emphysema.   **Emphysema** is a lung condition in which the air sacs within the lung lose their elasticity. Breathing is difficult for the person affected by this disease. Medications can relieve the symptoms of emphysema, but there is no cure.

Digestive System

The digestive system changes food into a form that can be used by all the cells of the body. Those parts of food that cannot be used by the body are expelled as waste products.

Food is the fuel burned by the digestive system to provide energy for the entire body. This use of food can be compared to gasoline in a car which burns to give power to the car, or oil in a furnace which produces heat. In the body, the fuel is food; the process of burning this fuel is called metabolism.

Metabolism depends on the proper functioning of each organ of digestion, Figure 6-19. The digestive process begins the moment food is taken into the mouth. The teeth and tongue tear the food into small pieces and mix it with saliva so that it can be swallowed easily. In the saliva, chemical substances called enzymes start to break down the foods into products that can be used by the rest of the body. From the mouth the partially processed food is swallowed, moving into the esophagus. An involuntary wavelike muscle action called **peristalsis** moves food through the esophagus and then into the stomach. Sometimes the body rejects or refuses food during the digestive process. When this occurs, the voluntary and involuntary muscles work together to force the food backward. This is called vomiting or emesis.

The stomach is an elastic, muscular organ that holds the food while gastric enzymes and a strong acid turn food into a semi-liquid state. From the stomach, the food passes into the small intestine. Enzymes in the intestinal juice are especially important in the digestive process. The liver produces bile, which is necessary to absorb fat. Bile is produced in the liver but is stored in the gallbladder. Bile enters the small intestine and breaks up fats in the duodenum so they can be digested and absorbed. The duodenum is the first 10 inches of the 19- to 20-foot small intestine. The jejunum is the second portion of the small intestine. It is about 9 feet long. The ileum is the third portion and is about 9 feet. The pancreas also releases a digestive pancreatic juice into the duodenum. Insulin, which controls sugar metabolism, is also released into the bloodstream from a specific area within the pancreas.

The digestive juices work together to break food down into a simpler form. The usable products of this breakdown are called nutrients. The nutrients are absorbed through the walls of the small intestine. The nutrients are then carried by the bloodstream to all parts of the body. Some portion of food remains in the small intestine because it cannot be broken down or absorbed. This remaining material moves into the large intestine in a semiliquid state. The large intestine, also called the colon, is about five feet long. In this area, much of the liquid from the food is absorbed into the body. This helps maintain the balance of fluids in the body. Peristalsis moves the remaining solid material into the lower part of the colon. When enough waste has collected, the voluntary muscles expel it through the anus. This is a normal bowel movement.

Common Disorders of the Digestive System

Constipation.   A common problem with the bowels is constipation. This is a condition in which bowel movements are hard and difficult. Prevention might include exercise, an increase in fluids, and eating more bulky foods such as whole grain cereals, fruits, and vegetables. Prolonged or long-lasting constipation can cause feces (the technical name for the waste material of the body) to become lodged in the rectum **(impacted).** It may then be necessary for the person to receive an enema or a laxative, or disimpaction by the nurse.

Stools may have blood on the outside surface, which may be the result of bleeding hemorrhoids or rectal cancer. If the stool looks dark, black, or tarry, internal bleeding in the gastroin-

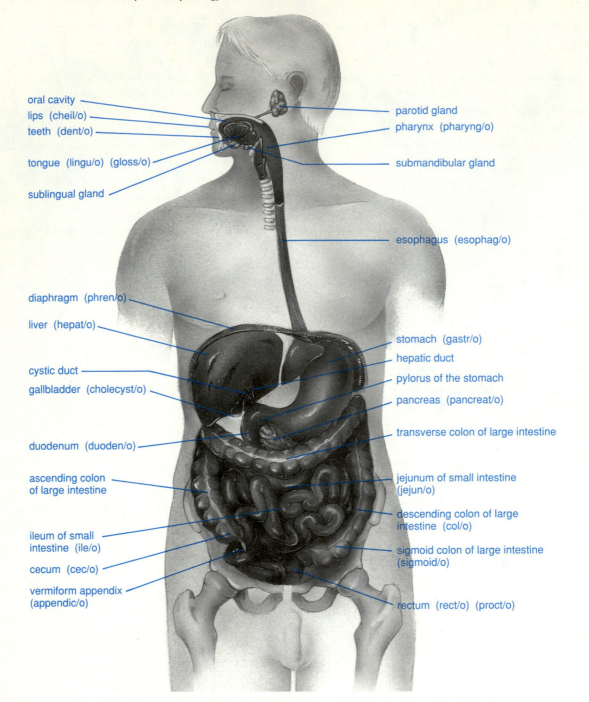

oral cavity
lips (cheil/o)
teeth (dent/o)
tongue (lingu/o) (gloss/o)
sublingual gland

parotid gland
pharynx (pharyng/o)
submandibular gland

esophagus (esophag/o)

diaphragm (phren/o)
liver (hepat/o)
cystic duct
gallbladder (cholecyst/o)
duodenum (duoden/o)
ascending colon of large intestine
ileum of small intestine (ile/o)
cecum (cec/o)
vermiform appendix (appendic/o)

stomach (gastr/o)
hepatic duct
pylorus of the stomach
pancreas (pancreat/o)
transverse colon of large intestine
jejunum of small intestine (jejun/o)
descending colon of large intestine (col/o)
sigmoid colon of large intestine (sigmoid/o)
rectum (rect/o) (proct/o)

Figure 6-19   The digestive system (From Anatomy and Physiology insert, copyright 1992 by Delmar Publishers Inc.)

testinal system may be the cause. Brighter colored blood in the stool may result from bleeding in the lower part of the intestinal tract.

Diarrhea.   Diarrhea is a condition in which feces are watery and frequent. Constipation and diarrhea may result from a number of causes. Proper diet, adequate exercise, and regular elimination of wastes help prevent both constipation and diarrhea.

Heartburn.   So-called "heartburn" results from a backflow of the digestive juices into the lower portion of the esophagus. These juices, because of their high acid content, cause irritation of the lining of the esophagus. Those affected experience a burning sensation.

Urinary System

The urinary system consists of the kidneys, ureters, bladder, and urethra, Figure 6-20. The kidneys are the primary organs of this system. Their function is to filter waste material from the bloodstream. As the blood passes through the kidneys, it undergoes a purifying and recycling process; waste material and excess water are filtered from it. As the blood continues through the kidneys, much of the filtered water and some minerals are reabsorbed into the bloodstream. This reabsorption is necessary to maintain the body's liquid balance. The waste material and excess water (now called urine)

pass from the kidneys into the bladder by way of ducts called ureters. The bladder is a muscular organ for storing urine. When the bladder has accumulated about a pint of urine, nerves sense discomfort. Involuntary muscle contractions of the bladder then empty the urine into the urethra, from which it is expelled. These muscular contractions can be controlled and do become voluntary to a large extent. The normal daily output of urine is between 1500 to 2000 mL (1½–2 qt).

Common Disorders of the Urinary System

Incontinence. Some individuals have no voluntary control of their bladder muscles. This causes them to be **incontinent;** they wet themselves. Incontinence occurs in babies prior to toilet training because they have not yet developed control over the muscles in the urethra.

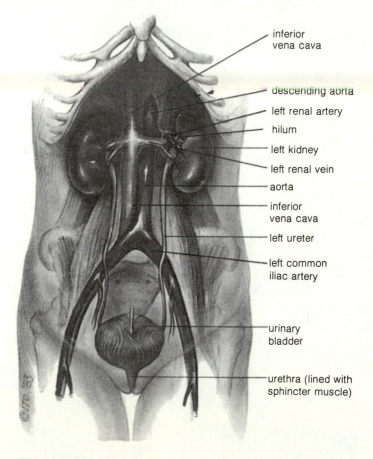

Figure 6-20   The urinary system (From Fong, Ferris, and Skelley, *Body Structures and Functions,* copyright 1989 by Delmar Publishers Inc.)

Cystitis. **Cystitis** occurs when the membrane lining of the urinary bladder becomes inflamed. It can be caused by bacterial infection or a kidney inflammation that has spread to the bladder. This condition usually results in painful urination. It is generally treated with urinary antiseptic medication.

Kidney Stones. Kidney stones are usually caused by an excess of calcium. The urine becomes crystallized and stones may block the ureters and cause painful urination. There is a new technique available now for some clients, whereby the stones can be destroyed by sound waves rather than by surgery.

Reproductive System

The reproductive system consists of organs that are needed to produce a new life, Figures 6-21, 6-22 and 6-23. The male reproductive system manufactures sperm that fertilize the ovum (egg) produced by the female reproductive sys-tem. Sperm are released into the female vagina during sexual intercourse. When a sperm comes together with the female egg, usually in the upper part of the fallopian tube, the egg is said to be fertilized. The fertilized egg travels to the female uterus and begins to develop into a new individual. In this way the human race continues from generation to generation.

It normally takes 280 days from conception (when egg and sperm meet) until an infant is born. The menstrual cycle is interrupted for 9 months of pregnancy. It may be 6 weeks after delivery before the cycle begins again. The menstrual cycle continues until menopause occurs later in life when eggs are no longer released.

Common Disorders of the Reproductive System

The incidence of cancer affecting the reproductive system in both males and females is quite significant. Two common cancers of the reproductive system are breast cancer in women and

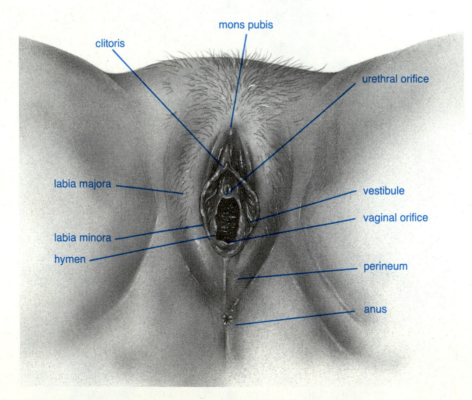

Figure 6-21 Female external reproductive organs (From Anatomy and Physiology insert, copyright 1992 by Delmar Publishers Inc.)

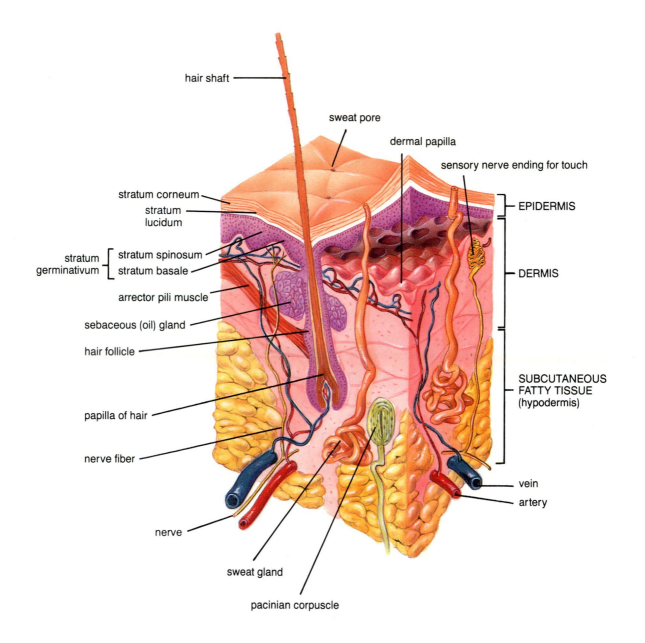

hair shaft

sweat pore

dermal papilla

sensory nerve ending for touch

EPIDERMIS

stratum corneum

stratum lucidum

DERMIS

stratum germinativum — stratum spinosum / stratum basale

arrector pili muscle

sebaceous (oil) gland

hair follicle

SUBCUTANEOUS FATTY TISSUE (hypodermis)

papilla of hair

nerve fiber

vein

artery

nerve

sweat gland

pacinian corpuscle

Plate 1 Cross Section of Skin

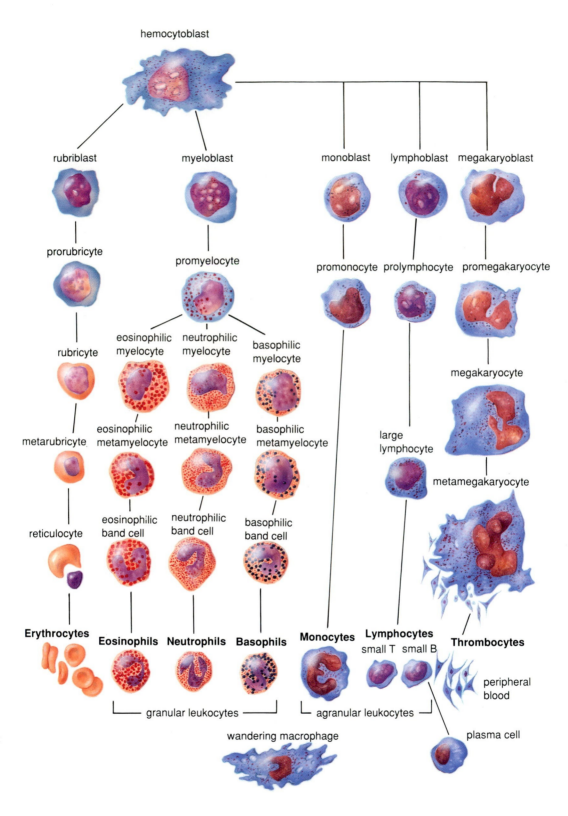

hemocytoblast

rubriblast

myeloblast

monoblast

lymphoblast

megakaryoblast

prorubricyte

promyelocyte

promonocyte

prolymphocyte

promegakaryocyte

rubricyte

eosinophilic
myelocyte

neutrophilic
myelocyte

basophilic
myelocyte

megakaryocyte

metarubricyte

eosinophilic
metamyelocyte

neutrophilic
metamyelocyte

basophilic
metamyelocyte

large
lymphocyte

metamegakaryocyte

reticulocyte

eosinophilic
band cell

neutrophilic
band cell

basophilic
band cell

Erythrocytes

Eosinophils

Neutrophils

Basophils

Monocytes

Lymphocytes

small T small B

Thrombocytes

peripheral
blood

└─── granular leukocytes ───┘

└─ agranular leukocytes ─┘

plasma cell

wandering macrophage

Plate 2 Blood Cells and Platelets

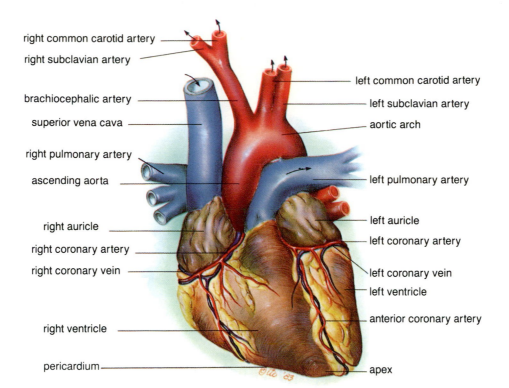

right common carotid artery
right subclavian artery
brachiocephalic artery
superior vena cava
right pulmonary artery
ascending aorta
right auricle
right coronary artery
right coronary vein
right ventricle
pericardium

left common carotid artery
left subclavian artery
aortic arch
left pulmonary artery
left auricle
left coronary artery
left coronary vein
left ventricle
anterior coronary artery
apex

Plate 3 Front View of Heart

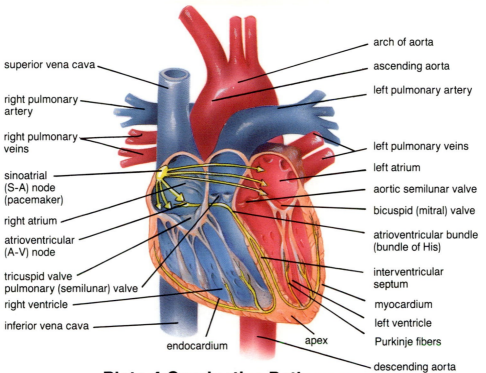

superior vena cava
right pulmonary artery
right pulmonary veins
sinoatrial (S-A) node (pacemaker)
right atrium
atrioventricular (A-V) node
tricuspid valve
pulmonary (semilunar) valve
right ventricle
inferior vena cava
endocardium

arch of aorta
ascending aorta
left pulmonary artery
left pulmonary veins
left atrium
aortic semilunar valve
bicuspid (mitral) valve
atrioventricular bundle (bundle of His)
interventricular septum
myocardium
left ventricle
Purkinje fibers
apex
descending aorta

Plate 4 Conductive Pathways

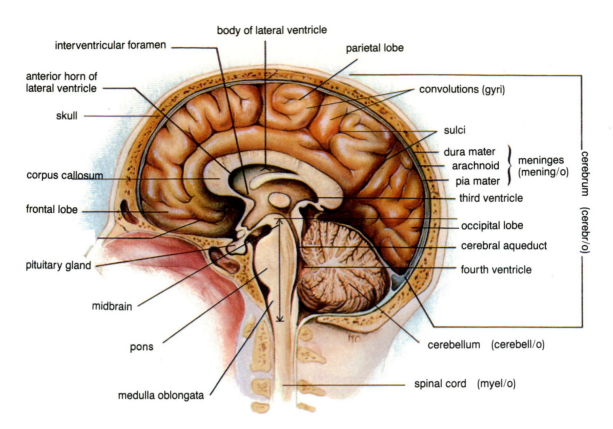

interventricular foramen

body of lateral ventricle

parietal lobe

anterior horn of lateral ventricle

convolutions (gyri)

skull

sulci

dura mater
arachnoid } **meninges (mening/o)**
pia mater

corpus callosum

third ventricle

frontal lobe

occipital lobe

cerebral aqueduct

pituitary gland

fourth ventricle

midbrain

cerebrum (cerebr/o)

pons

cerebellum (cerebell/o)

spinal cord (myel/o)

medulla oblongata

Plate 5A Section of Brain

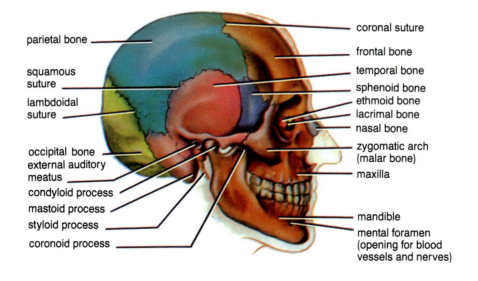

parietal bone

coronal suture

frontal bone

squamous suture

temporal bone

sphenoid bone

lambdoidal suture

ethmoid bone

lacrimal bone

nasal bone

occipital bone
external auditory meatus

zygomatic arch (malar bone)

condyloid process

maxilla

mastoid process

styloid process

mandible

coronoid process

mental foramen (opening for blood vessels and nerves)

Plate 5B Lateral View of Cranium

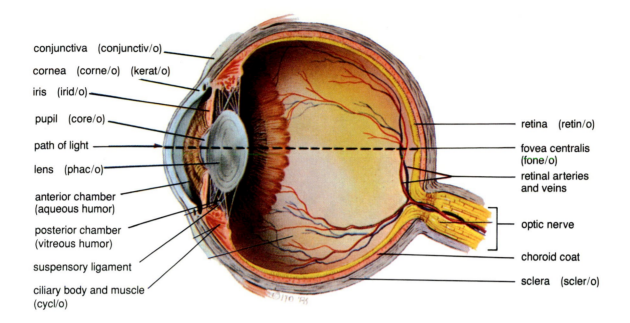

conjunctiva (conjunctiv/o)

cornea (corne/o) (kerat/o)

iris (irid/o)

pupil (core/o)

path of light

lens (phac/o)

anterior chamber
(aqueous humor)

posterior chamber
(vitreous humor)

suspensory ligament

ciliary body and muscle
(cycl/o)

retina (retin/o)

fovea centralis
(fone/o)

retinal arteries
and veins

optic nerve

choroid coat

sclera (scler/o)

Plate 6A Eye Structure

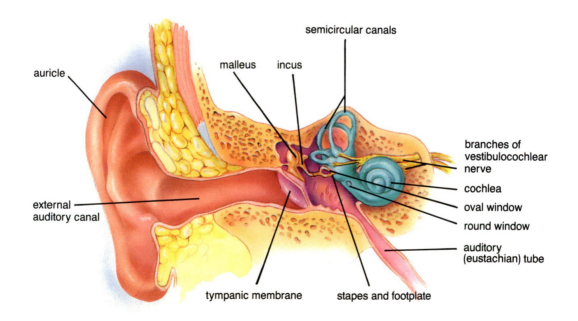

auricle

malleus

incus

semicircular canals

branches of
vestibulocochlear
nerve

cochlea

oval window

round window

auditory
(eustachian) tube

external
auditory canal

tympanic membrane

stapes and footplate

Plate 6B Ear Structure

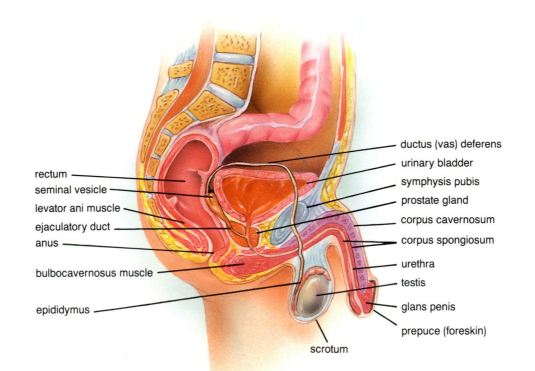

rectum
seminal vesicle
levator ani muscle
ejaculatory duct
anus
bulbocavernosus muscle
epididymus

ductus (vas) deferens
urinary bladder
symphysis pubis
prostate gland
corpus cavernosum
corpus spongiosum
urethra
testis
glans penis
prepuce (foreskin)
scrotum

Plate 7A Male Reproductive

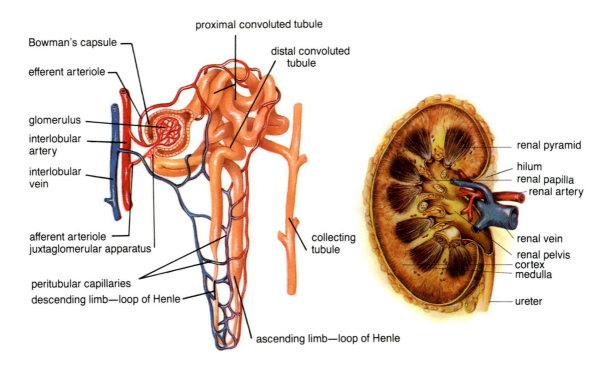

Bowman's capsule
efferent arteriole
glomerulus
interlobular artery
interlobular vein
afferent arteriole
juxtaglomerular apparatus
peritubular capillaries
descending limb—loop of Henle

proximal convoluted tubule
distal convoluted tubule
collecting tubule
ascending limb—loop of Henle

renal pyramid
hilum
renal papilla
renal artery
renal vein
renal pelvis
cortex
medulla
ureter

Plate 7B Nephron and Cross Section of Kidney

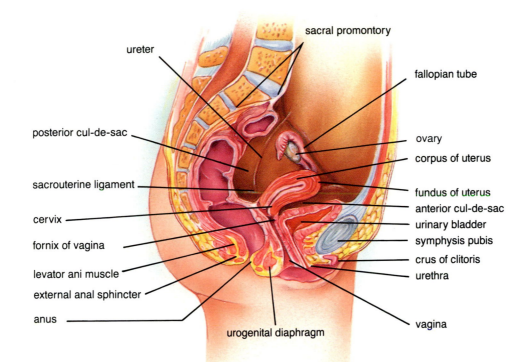

ureter

sacral promontory

fallopian tube

posterior cul-de-sac

ovary

corpus of uterus

sacrouterine ligament

fundus of uterus

anterior cul-de-sac

cervix

urinary bladder

fornix of vagina

symphysis pubis

levator ani muscle

crus of clitoris

external anal sphincter

urethra

anus

vagina

urogenital diaphragm

Plate 8A Female Reproductive

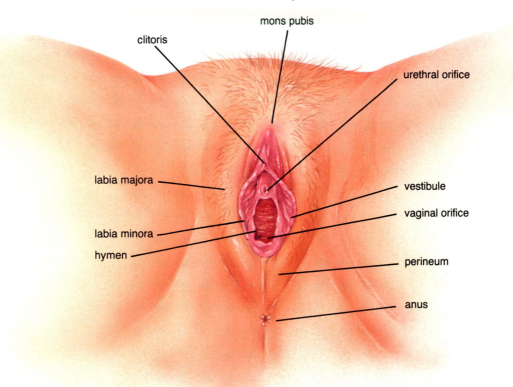

mons pubis

clitoris

urethral orifice

labia majora

vestibule

vaginal orifice

labia minora

hymen

perineum

anus

Plate 8B Female External Genitalia

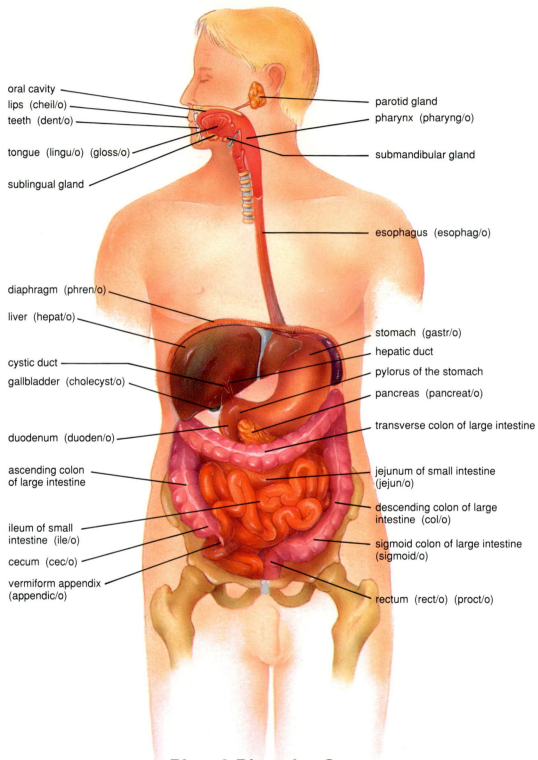

oral cavity

lips (cheil/o)

teeth (dent/o)

tongue (lingu/o) (gloss/o)

sublingual gland

parotid gland

pharynx (pharyng/o)

submandibular gland

esophagus (esophag/o)

diaphragm (phren/o)

liver (hepat/o)

cystic duct

gallbladder (cholecyst/o)

duodenum (duoden/o)

ascending colon
of large intestine

ileum of small
intestine (ile/o)

cecum (cec/o)

vermiform appendix
(appendic/o)

stomach (gastr/o)

hepatic duct

pylorus of the stomach

pancreas (pancreat/o)

transverse colon of large intestine

jejunum of small intestine
(jejun/o)

descending colon of large
intestine (col/o)

sigmoid colon of large intestine
(sigmoid/o)

rectum (rect/o) (proct/o)

Plate 9 Digestive System

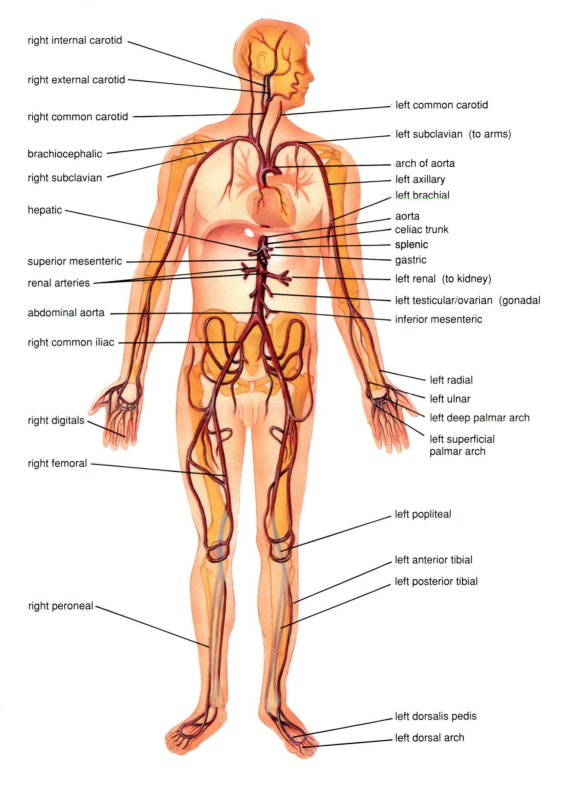

right internal carotid

right external carotid

right common carotid

brachiocephalic

right subclavian

hepatic

superior mesenteric

renal arteries

abdominal aorta

right common iliac

right digitals

right femoral

right peroneal

left common carotid

left subclavian (to arms)

arch of aorta

left axillary

left brachial

aorta

celiac trunk

splenic

gastric

left renal (to kidney)

left testicular/ovarian (gonadal

inferior mesenteric

left radial

left ulnar

left deep palmar arch

left superficial
palmar arch

left popliteal

left anterior tibial

left posterior tibial

left dorsalis pedis

left dorsal arch

Plate 10A Arterial Distribution

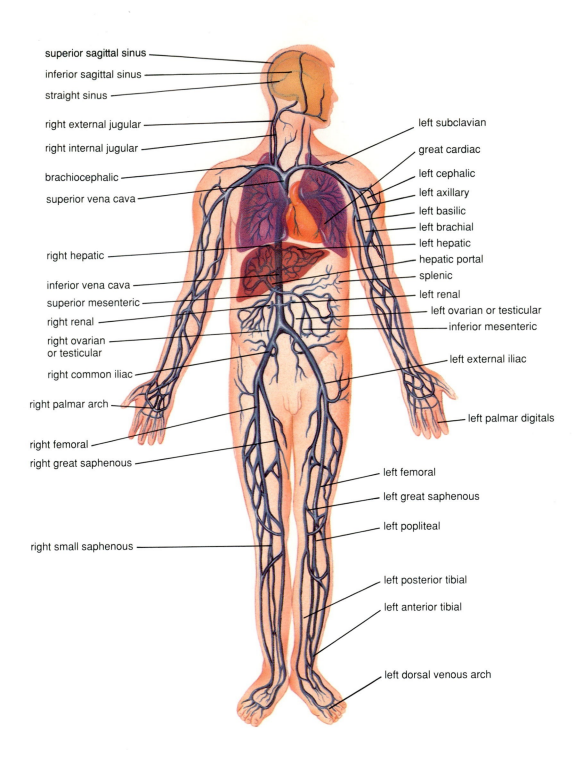

superior sagittal sinus

inferior sagittal sinus

straight sinus

right external jugular

right internal jugular

brachiocephalic

superior vena cava

right hepatic

inferior vena cava

superior mesenteric

right renal

right ovarian
or testicular

right common iliac

right palmar arch

right femoral

right great saphenous

right small saphenous

left subclavian

great cardiac

left cephalic

left axillary

left basilic

left brachial

left hepatic

hepatic portal

splenic

left renal

left ovarian or testicular

inferior mesenteric

left external iliac

left palmar digitals

left femoral

left great saphenous

left popliteal

left posterior tibial

left anterior tibial

left dorsal venous arch

Plate 10B Venous Distribution

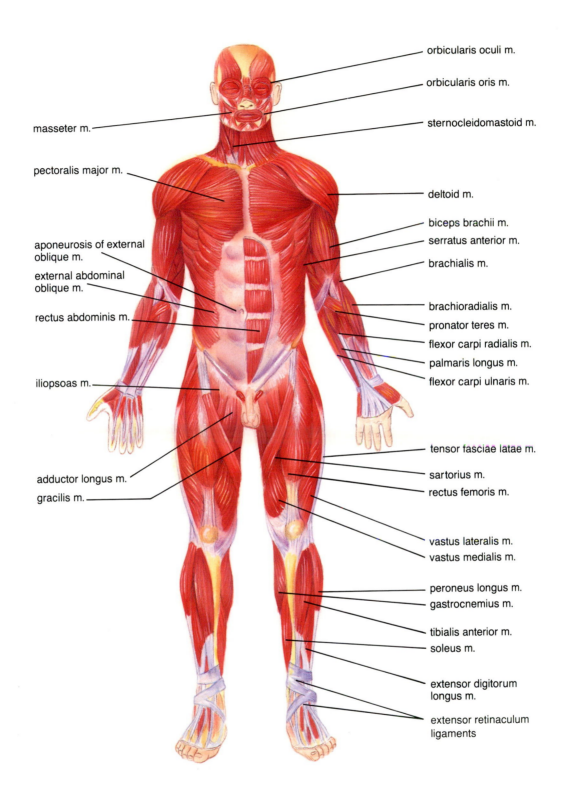

orbicularis oculi m.

orbicularis oris m.

sternocleidomastoid m.

masseter m.

pectoralis major m.

deltoid m.

biceps brachii m.

serratus anterior m.

brachialis m.

aponeurosis of external
oblique m.

external abdominal
oblique m.

brachioradialis m.

pronator teres m.

rectus abdominis m.

flexor carpi radialis m.

palmaris longus m.

flexor carpi ulnaris m.

iliopsoas m.

tensor fasciae latae m.

sartorius m.

adductor longus m.

rectus femoris m.

gracilis m.

vastus lateralis m.

vastus medialis m.

peroneus longus m.

gastrocnemius m.

tibialis anterior m.

soleus m.

extensor digitorum
longus m.

extensor retinaculum
ligaments

Plate 11A Muscular System, Anterior

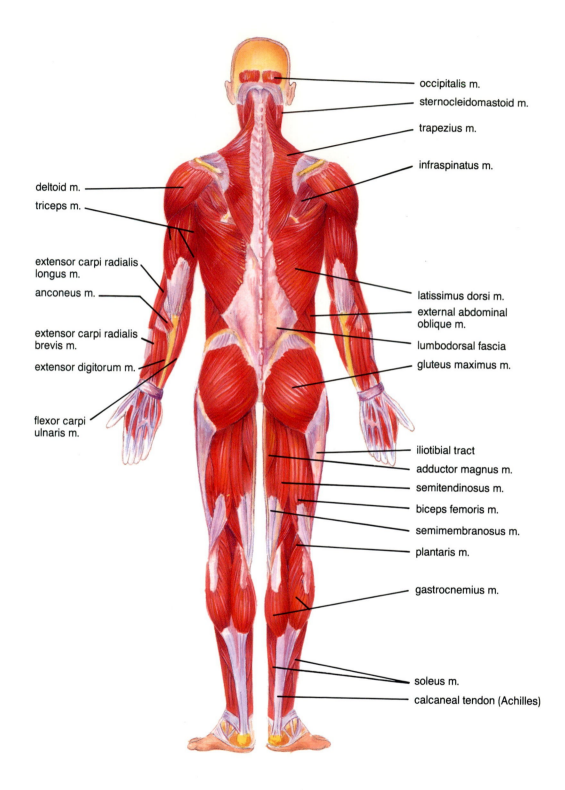

occipitalis m.

sternocleidomastoid m.

trapezius m.

infraspinatus m.

deltoid m.

triceps m.

extensor carpi radialis longus m.

anconeus m.

extensor carpi radialis brevis m.

extensor digitorum m.

flexor carpi ulnaris m.

latissimus dorsi m.

external abdominal oblique m.

lumbodorsal fascia

gluteus maximus m.

iliotibial tract

adductor magnus m.

semitendinosus m.

biceps femoris m.

semimembranosus m.

plantaris m.

gastrocnemius m.

soleus m.

calcaneal tendon (Achilles)

Plate 11B Muscular System, Posterior

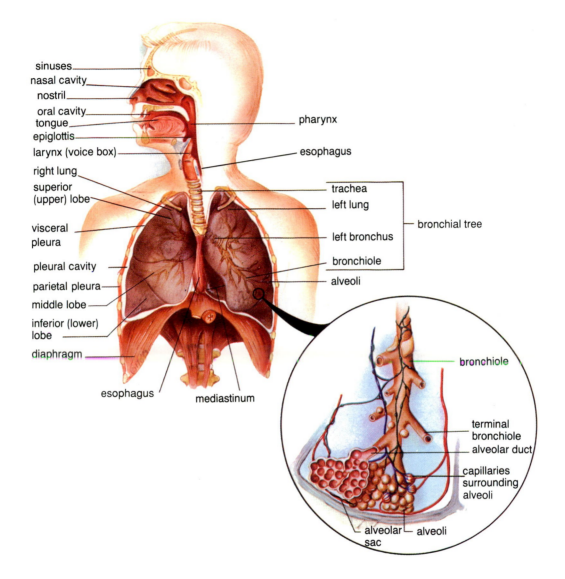

sinuses
nasal cavity
nostril
oral cavity
tongue
epiglottis
larynx (voice box)
right lung
superior (upper) lobe
visceral pleura
pleural cavity
parietal pleura
middle lobe
inferior (lower) lobe
diaphragm

pharynx
esophagus
trachea
left lung
bronchial tree
left bronchus
bronchiole
alveoli

esophagus
mediastinum

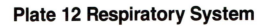

bronchiole
terminal bronchiole
alveolar duct
capillaries surrounding alveoli
alveolar sac
alveoli

Plate 12 Respiratory System

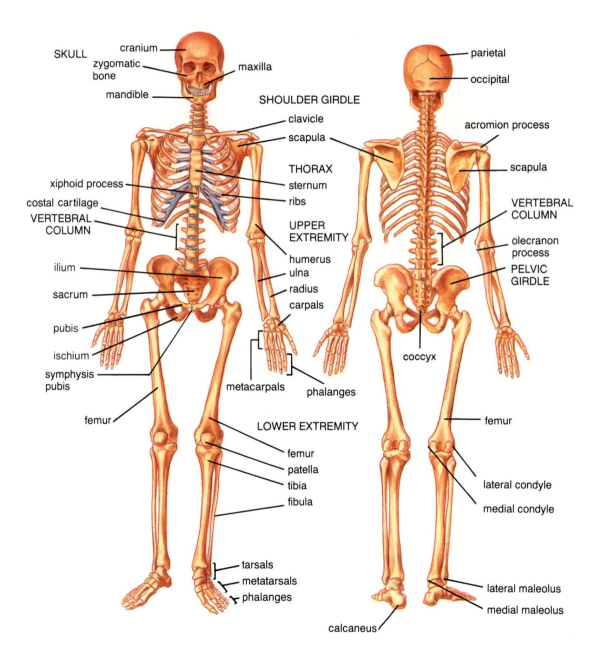

SKULL

cranium

zygomatic bone

maxilla

mandible

parietal

occipital

SHOULDER GIRDLE

clavicle

scapula

acromion process

scapula

THORAX

sternum

ribs

xiphoid process

costal cartilage

VERTEBRAL COLUMN

VERTEBRAL COLUMN

UPPER EXTREMITY

humerus

ulna

radius

carpals

olecranon process

PELVIC GIRDLE

ilium

sacrum

pubis

ischium

symphysis pubis

coccyx

metacarpals

phalanges

femur

femur

LOWER EXTREMITY

femur

patella

tibia

fibula

lateral condyle

medial condyle

tarsals

metatarsals

phalanges

lateral maleolus

medial maleolus

calcaneus

Plate 13 Skeletal System

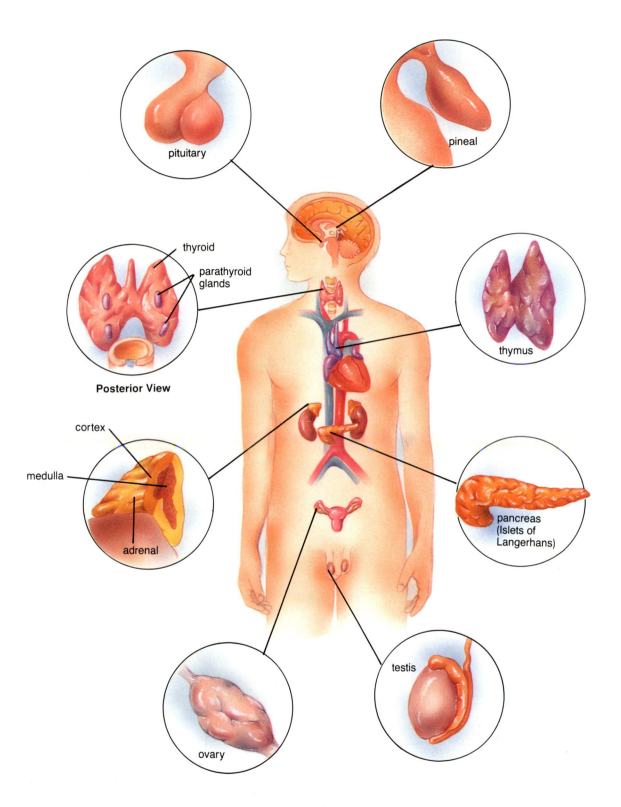

Plate 14 Endocrine System

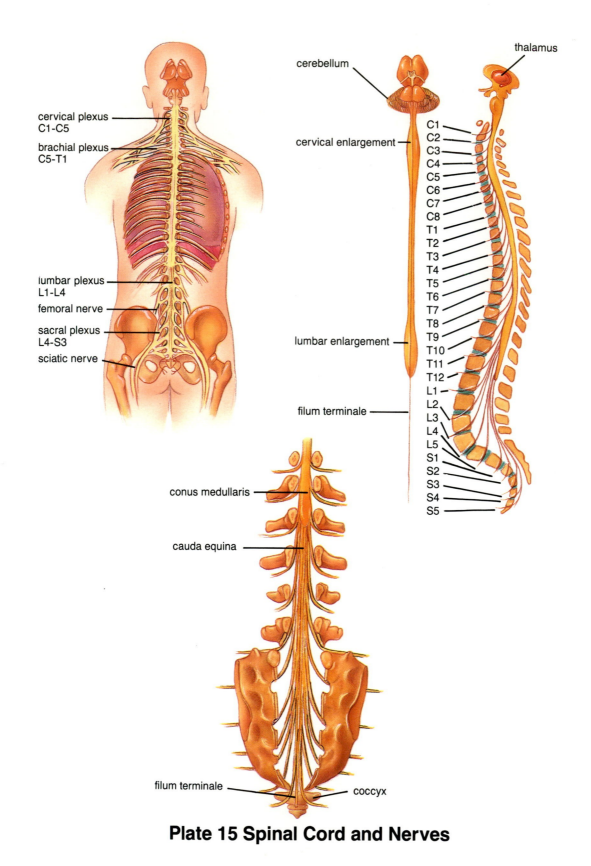

cervical plexus
C1-C5

brachial plexus
C5-T1

lumbar plexus
L1-L4

femoral nerve

sacral plexus
L4-S3

sciatic nerve

cerebellum

thalamus

cervical enlargement

lumbar enlargement

filum terminale

C1
C2
C3
C4
C5
C6
C7
C8
T1
T2
T3
T4
T5
T6
T7
T8
T9
T10
T11
T12
L1
L2
L3
L4
L5
S1
S2
S3
S4
S5

conus medullaris

cauda equina

filum terminale

coccyx

Plate 15 Spinal Cord and Nerves

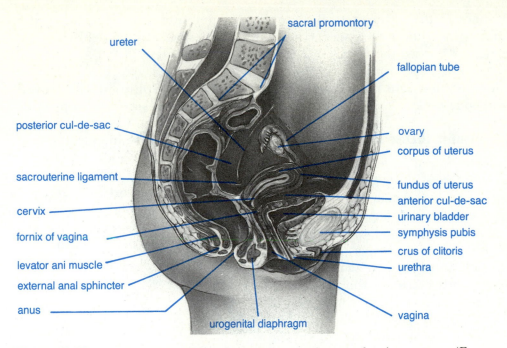

Figure 6-22   Lateral view of the female internal reproductive organs (From Anatomy and Physiology insert, copyright 1992 by Delmar Publishers Inc.)

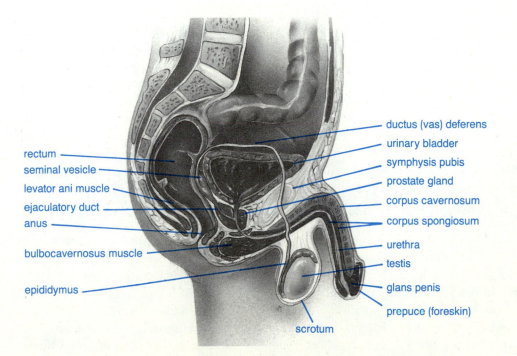

Figure 6-23   The male reproductive system (From Anatomy and Physiology insert, copyright 1992 by Delmar Publishers Inc.)

prostate cancer in the older man. Both are treatable if caught in the early stages. Care of cancer clients is discussed more fully in a later unit. In addition, sterility or infertility (inability to have children) often is the result of an abnormality of this body system.

Sexually Transmitted Diseases (STD)

Gonorrhea, syphilis, and other infections transmitted through sexual contact are called venereal diseases (VD), or sexually transmitted diseases (STD). Over the past several years there has been an alarming increase in sexually transmitted diseases. In today's society, it is not unusual for people to be sexually active with several partners. This increases the chance for contact and incidence of VD. In some areas of the country, VD has reached epidemic proportions. The germs can be passed on to anyone who has sexual intercourse with an infected person. Direct sexual contact with an infected person is the most common way in which gonorrhea is spread.

Gonorrhea.   Gonorrhea can develop within 48 hours after contact. Usually the first sign of the infection in males is painful burning during urination. The next stage is a yellowish green discharge from the penis. The female's symptoms include a burning sensation and painful urination; the vaginal area may become red and tender, with a discharge present. It is common for the female to have no symptoms at all. This absence of symptoms is dangerous since the woman will not know that she needs treatment. The symptoms may go away within a few days, but the microorganisms may move into the reproductive system and do further damage. Untreated gonorrhea can cause permanent damage to the reproductive organs (pelvic inflammatory disease or PID) and even cause sterility. A person who suspects exposure to gonorrhea should have an examination at once. To detect the gonorrhea germ, a laboratory test is done on the discharge. Penicillin and tetracycline are both used to treat gonorrhea.

Babies born to mothers infected with gonorrhea may become blind as a result of contact with the germs causing gonorrhea in the vagina during birth. The eyedrops given to the newborn in the delivery room help to prevent blindness.

Syphilis.   Syphilis shows up very quickly in males. Open sores develop on the penis very early in the course of syphilis. If the germs are not killed early in the illness, they spread throughout the body. Secondary skin lesions (sores) may appear on the face. From contact with these open sores, the germs can be passed from person to person. Untreated syphilis can lead to severe brain damage, mental illness, heart disease, and death. In the female, syphilis is not as easy to detect; the germs continue to invade the body while the female is unaware of it. Women who have syphilis and become pregnant can pass syphilis to the fetus. Children born with active syphilis may be born with birth defects. Blindness is a frequent syphilitic complication at birth. Penicillin or tetracycline are drugs of choice for treatment of syphilis. The earlier the treatment, the more effective it is.

Care of the client with acquired immunodeficiency disease (AIDS) is discussed in Unit 15.

Herpes.   Herpes is a viral infection that is spread by direct contact from the site of infection to the site of contact. There are two types of viruses that can cause herpes—herpes type 1 (HSV-1) and herpes type 2 (HSV-2). These viruses can infect the mouth or genitals. Generally HSV-1 occurs above the waist, and HSV-2 below the waist. It is estimated that 30 million Americans now have genital herpes. There is no cure for herpes but a new drug called acyclovir has been effective in reducing the frequency and duration of herpes outbreaks. This drug can only be obtained through a prescription.

Symptoms of the disease vary from one person to the next. The first symptoms may be a tingling or itching sensation. Blisters may appear within 2 to 20 days after infection. The first episode lasts on the average of 3 weeks. Subsequent attacks usually last around 5 days. The blisters may be accompanied by swollen glands, headache, muscle aches, or fever.

Endocrine System

The endocrine system is made up of ductless glands that secrete substances within the body called hormones, Figure 6-24. The glands in this system do not have **ducts** (little tubes) and are, therefore, unlike tear and sweat glands. Hormones are chemicals that are secreted directly into the blood or lymph. They are carried throughout the body to regulate and control specific body functions. They are very powerful substances and direct the functions of other systems. Each hormone has a special job to do, Figure 6-25. It only takes a small amount of hormone to trigger a body reaction. Most scientists agree that the brain sends messages to the endocrine glands. These messages cause the gland to secrete the hormone needed by the body. For instance, in a time of physical danger the adrenal gland secretes a hormone called adrenalin. The adrenalin causes the heart rate to increase. This forces more blood through the body, which increases the nourishment to the muscles. Sugar is released into the body giving it quick energy. The adrenalin also speeds up the body's reflexes. All of these changes occur rapidly, making the body able to react and save itself or others from harm.

The thyroid gland regulates the metabolic rate of the body. This determines the speed that food is turned into energy.

Common Disorders of the Endocrine System

Hyperthyroidism and Hypothyroidism.   The activity level of the thyroid has a direct influence on the body's metabolism. Some people are able to eat large quantities of food without gaining weight. They have an overactive thyroid gland and their food metabolizes (burns up) quickly. These people tend to be restless and irritable. When the thyroid gland is underactive, food is not used fast enough and is converted into fat. The person with an underactive thyroid gland becomes sluggish and slow moving and tired. One of the excuses used by many overweight people is that they "have a thyroid condition."

However, most people who are overweight have normal thyroid function.

Diabetes.   The endocrine gland of most interest to the home health aide is the pancreas. The endocrine part is known as the islets of Langerhans and is involved in the condition called diabetes.

The islets of Langerhans secrete insulin and glucagon. They control the use and distribution of sugar in the body. When insulin is not produced, the body metabolism is thrown off balance. A condition called diabetes may develop. Diabetes is a chronic disorder that can be controlled by medication, and/or proper diet and regular exercise. Diabetes is described more completely in Unit 16.

The Remarkable Body

Imagine how hard it would be if, each second of the day, you had to consciously perform every body function. Most people take their bodies for granted as long as everything seems to be in good working order. Think of all the activities constantly taking place and all of the things that could go wrong. Maintaining a state of wellness seems miraculous.

The human body is remarkable because it can continue to work when some of its parts break down. Damaged brain cells cannot be "repaired," but there are so many brain cells that new ones can be trained to take over. Many of the body structures are in "pairs." A body has two arms, two legs, two kidneys, two eyes. In the well body all of the parts work together.

What happens when one of a pair becomes diseased? In the case of kidneys, one can be removed surgically and the other will take over the work. The person with only one kidney must be more careful with diet and generally take more health precautions than the average person. A person can return to a state of wellness with even one kidney. The human body and mind are able to adapt. The home health aide's efforts are important in helping a client adapt physically, mentally, and emotionally, Figure 6-26.

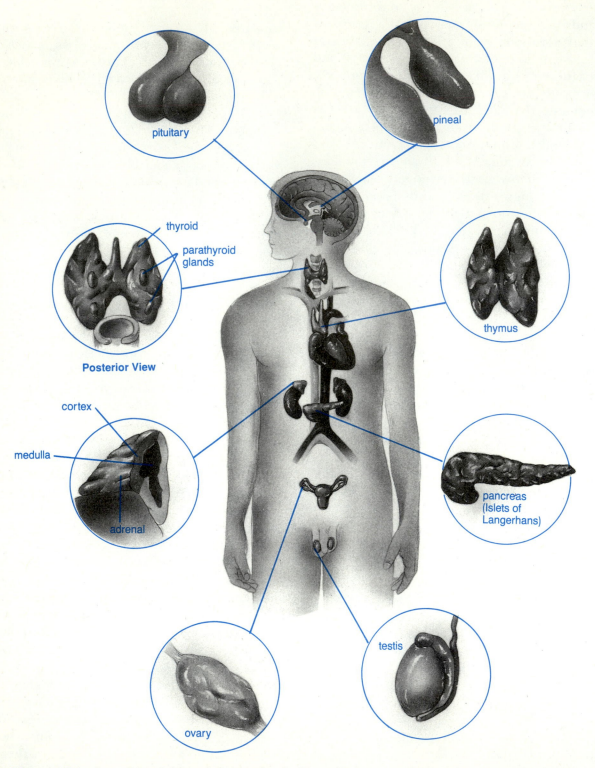

Figure 6-24 Location of the endocrine glands (From Anatomy and Physiology insert, copyright 1992 by Delmar Publishers Inc.)

Pituitary gland	Once called "master gland" of the body; secretes a number of hormones which regulate many bodily processes. The pituitary is completely controlled by the hypothalamus, a part of the brain.
Thyroid gland	Helps to regulate the metabolic rate and growth process.
Parathyroid glands	Regulate metabolism of calcium and phosphorous.
Thymus gland	Regulates immunity to infectious diseases during infancy and early childhood; becomes smaller as body ages.
Adrenal glands	Adjust body to crisis and stress; increase blood pressure; speed reactions; metabolize carbohydrates and proteins.
Islets of Langerhans	Produce insulin needed to burn sugar in body. (Too little insulin causes diabetes; too much insulin causes hyperglycemia.) Also produce glucagon to raise blood sugar.
Ovaries	Produce ovum (egg) for reproduction; secrete estrogen and progesterone which develop and maintain secondary sexual characteristics (breasts, pubic and underarm hair, etc.).
Testes	Produce sperm to fertilize ovum; secrete male hormones called testosterone.

Figure 6-25   Functions of the glands of the endocrine system

Factors that Influence Body Development

Bodies come in all shapes and sizes. There are records of men who have been as tall as 9 feet and as short as 26½ inches. These statistics are interesting because they show the tremendous

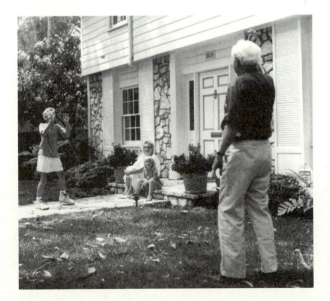

Figure 6-26   Exercise increases the efficiency of all body systems.

contrasts possible within the human body. Just as there are contrasts in size, there are other individual differences. Heredity is the passing of traits from parents to their children. Heredity can determine height, weight, general appearance, skin color, talents and abilities, basic physical wellness, and many other things. All children get half of their heredity from each parent. However, some traits are more dominant than others. This explains why some children are more like one parent than another.

Another factor that helps determine body size, shape, and wellness is environment. Environment is the sum total of the circumstances, conditions, and surroundings affecting the development of an organism. Some environmental factors that may affect growth are nutrition, financial conditions, climate, number of children in the family, and the parents' ages and occupations. The child who is born healthy with good hereditary characteristics is likely to start life as a well person. If the child grows up in a healthy environment where it is well fed, clothed, sheltered, respected, and loved, the child will continue to be well physically and mentally. An identical twin with the same heredity would not be as likely to develop into a well person if the twin was raised in an unhealthy environment. Many argue about which is more important, heredity or environment. One side believes that good heredity can overcome poor environment. The other side claims that good environment can rescue a child with poor heredity. It is clear, however, that both contribute to a person's development. Ways to control heredity are limited; however, environment can, to some extent, be controlled. The role of the home health aide is involved in improving environmental conditions for the client.

SUMMARY

· As one begins to understand the way the body works when it is well, the effects of illness are easier to grasp.
· Good mental outlook, healthy body cells, proper nutrition, rest, exercise, and good relationships with others are all part of wellness.

· The body systems work together and depend on one another to make the body function harmoniously.
· The body functions and development are affected by both heredity and environment. Changes in the environment can affect the health of individuals.

REVIEW

1. Name the nine body systems.
2. Name one function of each body system.
3. List one disorder for each of the nine body systems.
4. What is the largest organ of the body?
5. What might be suspected if a red, warm-looking spot appears on a bony prominence?
6. What is the difference between hereditary and environmental factors?
7. List two factors that may influence body development.
8. List four changes that can occur in the elderly due to the aging process.
9. Which of the following respiratory disorders is not correctly described?
   a. Pneumonia—an infection of the lung, often caused by a bacteria or virus
   b. Emphysema—a lung condition in which the air sacs within the lung lose their elasticity
   c. Asthma—narrowing of the air passages, often due to an allergic reaction
   d. Chronic obstructive pulmonary disease (COPD)—general term that may include asthma, chronic bronchitis, and emphysema
   e. All of the above are correct
10. A condition caused by loss of calcium in the bones is:
    a. osteoporosis   c. leukemia
    b. arthritis   d. anemia
11. Glaucoma and cataracts may result in:
    a. decreased mental function   c. aphasia
    b. loss of vision   d. paralysis

12.   Match Column I with Column II

Column I
___1. cystitis
___2. peristalsis
___3. incontinence
___4. phlebitis

Column II
a. no voluntary control of the bladder
b. involuntary wavelike muscle action
c. inflammation of the bladder
d. inflammation of a vein

13.   Match Column I with Column II

Column I
___1. anemia
___2. paraplegia
___3. gangrene
___4. quadriplegia
___5. leukemia

Column II
a. paralyzed from waist down
b. unable to move arms and legs
c. death of tissue
d. lack of iron in the blood
e. cancer of the blood

Section 3

Understanding Human Development and Age-Related Health Problems

Units

7 Infancy to Adolescence

8 Early and Middle Adulthood

9 Late Adulthood

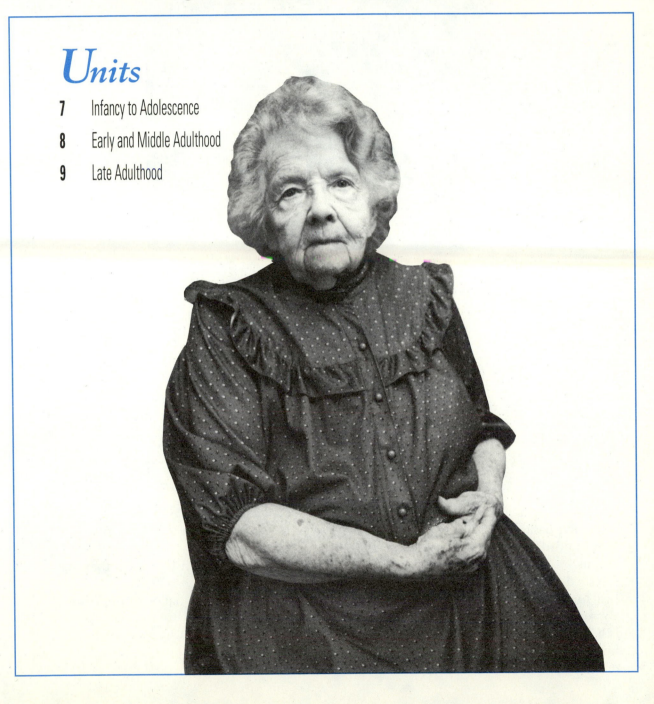

Unit *7* Infancy to Adolescence

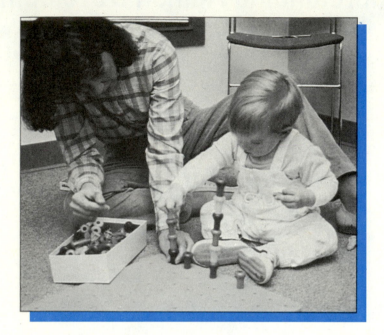

KEY TERMS

adolescence
bonding
cerebral palsy
cesarean section
child abuse

conception
cystic fibrosis
fetal alcohol syndrome
gestation period
immunity

low-birth-weight
premature
puberty
sibling rivalry
sudden infant death syndrome

LEARNING OBJECTIVES

After studying this unit, you should be able to:

- Name five basic needs of the newborn infant.
- Identify three immunizations necessary for infants.
- List six disorders of the newborn.
- List four behavior patterns associated with abused children.
- List four conditions that can occur in an infant if the mother drinks alcohol during pregnancy.

- Recognize definitions for five of the key terms listed.
- Name two health problems that may affect adolescents.
- Identify changes that occur at puberty.

An aide who is assigned to care for a newborn infant and the mother is usually going into a happy environment. If it is a first child, both parents may be very attentive toward the baby and watch its every move. Of course, the newness wears off, and suddenly they are faced with a demanding, helpless human being for whom they are entirely responsible. Even so, this is usually a positive assignment.

Pregnancy

Conception is the fertilization of the female egg by male sperm. This union forms the beginning of a new individual. The time from conception to birth is called the **gestation period.** When a woman is pregnant, it is essential that she receive prenatal care either from a physician or a midwife. Many complications of pregnancy and birth disorders may be prevented by good prenatal care. It is an important duty as a home health aide to encourage your client to seek prenatal care. If the client is pregnant, the aide should encourage the client to eat a balanced diet.

Labor and Delivery

Infants are most often delivered by a doctor in the hospital. However, in some areas, this situation is changing. Normally, a woman goes into labor and delivers the baby with assistance of an obstetrician. The baby moves from the uterus into the vagina and passes out of the body. This normal process is eased, however, by use of medications, health facilities, and trained personnel.

In some cases it may be necessary to deliver the baby by **cesarean section.** This is a surgical technique in which an abdominal incision is made into the uterus and the infant is lifted out. After a cesarean section, the mother needs extra time to recover. The incision site must be kept clean to prevent infection. The aide may be instructed to assist the mother to clean the incision and apply clean dressings.

Bonding is a process of attachment of mother, father, and infant happening immediately after birth. The newborn infant is placed on the mother's abdomen nude so that both parents can make eye contact with the child and feel and cuddle the infant. This initial contact is very important as it assists in creating positive emotional ties between the parent and child and the child and the parents. Cuddling and fondling are important in the first few months of the newborn's life. The home health aide needs to encourage a new mother and father to hold, talk, and play with the baby often. The newborn needs to develop a sense of trust and security to develop into a trusting and secure adult.

Normal Infant Growth and Development

As an infant grows, both physical and mental abilities develop. In the first month, infants are quite helpless. They totally depend on others to meet their basic needs, Figure 7-1. Infants need to be kept warm and dry and they need to be fed and allowed to sleep. Giving love to the infant also fulfills a basic need. Infants need to be held, cuddled, and crooned to as much as possible.

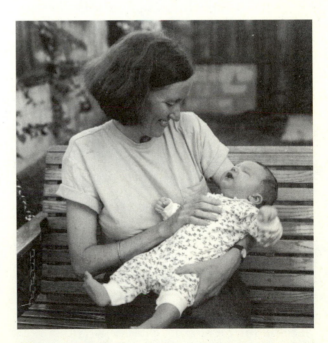

Figure 7-1   Mother holding and talking to her new baby

By age 2 months, babies can raise their heads and cry when they want to be picked up. They notice lights and sounds and begin to babble. They get used to certain patterns, especially the time to eat and time to sleep. Usually by the fourth month an infant sleeps 8 to 12 hours at night and naps during the day. Regular schedules of meals, activity, and sleep are needed.

Normal Weight Gain

Normally, infants weigh between 5 and 8 lb (2.3 to 3.6 kg) at birth. During the first 5 days, a weight loss of several ounces is expected. Until birth, all the baby's needs are supplied within the uterus through the umbilical cord. Birth is a shock to the baby's system and it takes a few days for the infant's body to adjust. When the body starts to function, a weight gain of 6 to 8 oz (0.17 to 0.23 kg) a week is normal. Birth weight is usually tripled by age 1 year. In the second year, the weight increases at a rate of 0.5 lb (0.23 kg) per month.

Nutritionists believe that a child's weight should be controlled. The formation of too many fat cells in childhood can lead to obesity in adulthood. It is important for children to eat a well-balanced diet. All of the body's systems need the right foods so that they will develop in a strong and healthy way.

Immunizations

Babies are born with natural **immunities.** This means that they have some built-in resistance to germs for 1 to 3 months. However, once born, a child's body is exposed to many new germs. To protect infants from common childhood diseases they are given vaccines, Figure 7-2. At 2, 4, and 6 months, an infant should be given vaccines against diphtheria, pertussis (whooping cough), and tetanus. These three vaccines are combined, and given in one injection called a DPT shot. An oral vaccine for poliomyelitis is also given at 2, 4, and 15 months. Vaccines for measles, mumps, and rubella are given after a child is 1 year old. HbCV, a new vaccine for meningitis caused by Hib is now recommended to be given at 2, 4, 6, and 15 months. A test for tuberculosis is given at 1 year

Infant	2 months	DTP*, OPV■, HbCV♦
	4 months	DTP, OPV, HbCV
	6 months	DTP, HbCV
	15 months	HbCV, MMR+
	15–18 months	DTP, OPV
	4–6 years	DTP, OPV, MMR
Adult	14–16 years and every 10 years thereafter	Td•

* DTP means Diphtheria, Tetanus and Pertussis
\+ MMR means Measles, Mumps and Rubella
■ OPV means Oral Polio Vaccine
♦ HbCV is vaccine for meningitis caused by Hib disease
• Td means Tetanus and Diphtheria

Figure 7-2   Infant and child immunization schedule

in addition to the vaccines. Boosters of DPT and polio vaccines are given two more times before the child enters school. Many states do not permit children to begin school until they are properly immunized. Parents should keep records of their children's immunizations. They should also record the childhood diseases contracted by their children and the age of the child when they occurred.

Common Health Problems in Infancy

One common problem with newborns is premature birth. An infant born before full term (before 37 weeks of **gestation**) is considered **premature.** Some also judge prematurity by low birth weight. A newborn weighing less than five pounds may be premature. However, some babies are full term yet weigh less than five pounds. A newborn in this condition is called a **low-birth-weight** baby.

Some infants are born with diseases, injuries, or malformations. These abnormalities may be inherited through the parents' genes. Conditions also may result from diseases or drugs present in the mother's body during pregnancy. Common abnormal infant conditions are described in Figure 7-3. Children with one of these conditions need special medical

CONDITION	DESCRIPTION	TREATMENT
PKU (phenylke-tonuria)	Body is unable to break down a certain amino acid. Mental retardation, convulsions, and eczema are common.	Specific diet begun early in infancy prevents symptoms. Test for PKU at birth.
Cerebral palsy	Defect, injury, or disease of the brain tissue which causes lack of muscle coordination and possible paralysis; person has shaking and muscle spasms with poor balance.	No cure but treatment varies and may include muscle relaxants, orthopedic surgery, use of casts or braces, exercises.
Congenital heart disease	Malformation of vessels, valves, or chambers in the heart; results in faulty circulation and usually cyanosis.	Surgery is often successful in restoring normal functioning.
Down syndrome	Chromosome abnormality causing retardation and typical physical malformation.	No treatment but many persons can be taught to live with some independence.
Hydrocephalus	Defect in the absorption of cerebrospinal fluid; fluid builds up and increases the size of the head.	Common treatment is with surgery. Shunts are commonly used to divert fluid away from brain and into the abdomen.
Sickle cell anemia (thalassemia)	Abnormal sickle-shaped red blood cells break down easily and cannot transport oxygen efficiently; fever, blackouts, and pain. (African American population)	Blood transfusions. No cure.
Leukemia	Overproduction of immature white blood cells; anemia, internal bleeding. Person has increased risk of infection, fever, pain in the joints and swelling of the lymph nodes, spleen, and liver.	Chemotherapy
Tay-Sachs	Degeneration of the central nervous system; infant does not develop mentally; disease affects those of Jewish ancestry.	No cure; infant usually does not live beyond age 1 year.
Cystic fibrosis	Inherited malfunction of the pancreas, intestinal, and sweat glands, and the respiratory system	No cure; special diet and respiratory care prolongs life.
Cleft lip/cleft palate	Fetal growth incomplete. Infant may have problems feeding. Cleft palate may alter tooth formation and cause speech problems.	Surgical repair, special feeding nipples and special therapy.
Fetal alcohol syndrome	Set of signs and symptoms and problems that newborn babies have if their mother drinks during pregnancy: (1) smaller baby; (2) small head; (3) weak heart or kidney problems; (4) failure to thrive; (5) peculiar appearing flat face with narrow eyes and drooping lips.	No cure—supportive care. The child may experience some degree of mental retardation for the rest of his/her life.
Sudden infant death syndrome	Baby stopped breathing while asleep.	Place monitor on babies with suspected breathing problems.

Figure 7-3 Abnormal conditions that exist in infants may require medical attention and sometimes long-term adjustments for the infant and family.

and emotional care. The aide may need to help the mother and family members adjust to meeting the child's special needs.

Responsibilities of the Home Health Aide

Often a mother must leave one or more children at home while she is at the hospital. The aide may be assigned to attend to the children then or after the mother has returned home with the newborn. The children are likely to want to be near the mother and may want to play with the baby. Sometimes older children are too rough with the baby even though they do not intend to be. The children also may be jealous of the new member of the family. This jealousy is called **sibling rivalry.** At these times, the home health aide should give the children extra attention. The aide can make the children feel important by giving them chores to do for the baby or mother. They should be praised for being helpful. Children may need help adjusting to the role of being a big brother or sister. The aide should be sure that the older children wash their hands before touching the baby. If they have colds they should be kept away from the baby until they are no longer contagious.

Besides the older children, the aide cares for the mother and the newborn. These duties include:

• bathing the infant
• diapering
• feeding the infant
• preparing the formula
• doing added laundry such as diapers and crib sheets
• caring for the mother
• assisting the mother if she is breast-feeding
• accident prevention

Handling Visitors

Many visitors will likely come to see a newborn infant. One of the aide's duties is to make sure that the mother does not get over-tired. A new mother should rest for a period in the morning and afternoon. Most mothers are happy to show off their newborn infant. However, it is a good idea to plan ahead with the mother as to how to handle visitors. Visitors should not stay too long and should not come in great numbers. The home health aide must encourage the mother to set the standards as to who can and cannot hold the baby. Visitors who have colds or similar infections should be discouraged from going near the baby. The mother and home health aide should wear a disposable mask if they are coughing or have a cold. Babies are born with some natural immunity to germs. However, it is unwise to expose them to disease when it can be avoided.

Toddlers and Preschoolers

Ages 1 and 2 are known as the toddler stage. The toddler approaches life with a great deal of interest, Figure 7-4. A favorite activity is exploring the immediate environment, creating a need for safety precautions. As the infant grows into a toddler, muscle coordination increases, and physical skills expand and improve greatly. Toddlers learn to walk and to feed themselves. Social skills and language become more meaningful.

Ages 3 through 5 are considered the preschool age group. The preschool years are a time of slower physical growth but a time of increased motor skill development and an increase in language and social skills. By age 3, the child plays alongside other children of the same age, Figure 7-5. Toilet training is usually mastered by the time the child is 5 and ready to start school. The preschooler is learning to be less dependent.

School-age Children

A child beginning school often needs time to adjust to the new situation. Some children find it difficult to leave the familiarity of home. However, most children enjoy being with other children. A school-aged child generally can follow simple instructions. It is important that children be given small jobs so that they feel a sense of responsibility. Praise for achievements is better than punishments for mistakes, Figure 7-6.

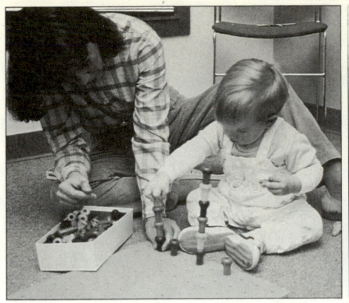

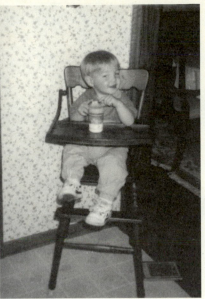

Figure 7-4A   The toddler begins to develop gross manual skills. (Photo courtesy of Henrietta Egleston Hospital for Children, Atlanta, GA. Photograph by Ginger Lovering; from Hegner and Caldwell, *Nursing Assistant, A Nursing Process Approach,* 6E, copyright 1992 by Delmar Publishers Inc.)

Figure 7-4B   The toddler begins to use a plastic drinking glass.

Adolescence

Adolescence is the age period between 13 and 18 years of age. During adolescence, youngsters become much more private about their lives. The move toward privacy begins around **puberty,** which marks the beginning of the time when the body is capable of reproduction. The teenager begins to realize that no one else knows what he or she is thinking. And because the teenage world is new and fragile, the youngster is very concerned about maintaining that privacy for all his or her thoughts. At the same time the teenage body is changing rapidly; physical and emotional needs are demanding. As a home health aide, you will rarely be assigned to care for an adolescent unless there is a physical problem with the youth's health, such as an accident (body in a cast) or childhood cancer. Open communication between parents and children is healthy and important. If teenagers have a previous history of comfortable verbal give and take with their parents, they will be willing to share unpleasant news with them.

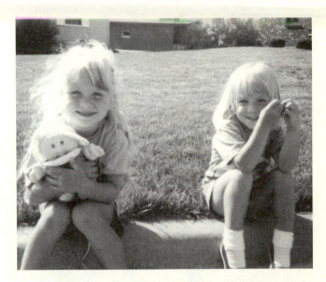

Figure 7-5   Learning to play with peers is important for preschoolers.

An adolescent wants to feel independent, but needs to know that the family can be depended on, Figure 7-7. This is a time when parental guidance and love are extremely important. During adolescence, a child is strongly

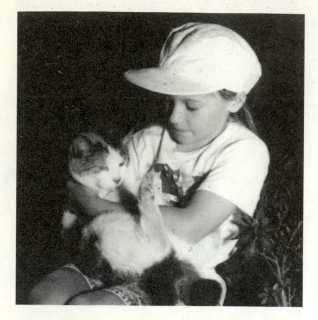

Figure 7-6A   The young person develops motor skills and learns to reach out with concern for other living things. (From Hegner and Caldwell, *Nursing Assistant, A Nursing Process Approach,* 6E, copyright 1992 by Delmar Publishers Inc.)

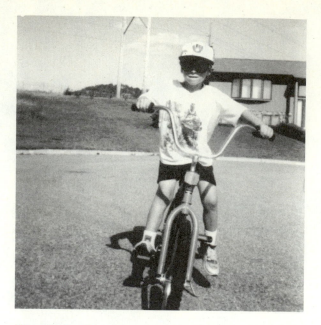

Figure 7-6B   The younger person develops motor skills by riding a bicycle.

influenced by the peer group (those of the same age), Figure 7-8. Parents should be aware of who their children are with. Showing support, reassurance, and concern for the teenager's well-being is essential.

Physical Changes in Puberty

Puberty beings sometime between the ages of 10 and 15 when the endocrine system releases hormones in both males and females. At this time, the secondary sexual characteristics begin to mature. In boys, the beard, underarm and pubic hair starts to grow and the voice deepens. There is usually a marked growth rate of both height and weight. At puberty, the male is able to produce sperm and have an orgasm to deposit the sperm in the female.

In young females, the breasts develop and pubic and underarm hair grows. A 28- to 35-day menstrual cycle also begins at puberty. About every 28 days the mature female reproductive system releases one or more eggs (ova). During sexual intercourse the ovum may come in contact with the sperm. If the sperm fertilizes the ovum, a fetus begins to grow.

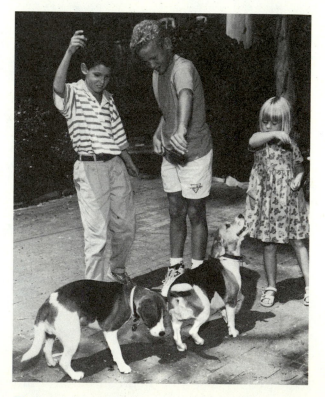

Figure 7-7   Adolescent playing with younger members of his family

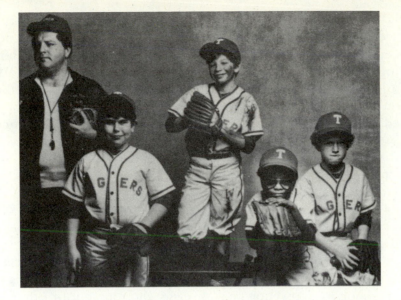

Figure 7-8   Peer relationships are important to the preadolescent who is developing awareness of himself as a sex-identified individual. (Photo courtesy of Hollister Incorporated, Libertyville, IL; from Hegner and Caldwell, *Nursing Assistant, A Nursing Process Approach*, 6E, copyright 1992 by Delmar Publishers Inc.)

Common Health Problems in Adolescence

Adolescents are at an age of experimentation. They often express their independence by trying new things. For some adolescents, this experimentation leads to abuse of drugs or alcohol. Many adolescents also become curious about their sexuality.

Sex-related health problems are especially common with adolescents. An active sex life may pose emotional problems. Diseases passed through sexual contact also may bring about additional problems. The female, in particular, must consider the possibility of becoming pregnant. Sex-related health problems often result from the adolescent having insufficient and inaccurate information.

Teenage Pregnancy.   In addition to an increase in sexually transmitted diseases among adolescents, an increase in teenage pregnancies has also occurred. It is currently estimated that two of every five girls now 14 years old will become pregnant before they are 20 and that one of those five will bear a child. It is now estimated that 42% of teenagers are sexually active. Many teenagers have sex without contraceptives, and when they do go to family planning services, it is often too late.

Few teenagers are ready to handle the responsibilities that accompany pregnancy and parenthood. The decision to raise a child, place the child for adoption, or have an abortion is usually a difficult decision for a teenage girl.

Teenage girls are still growing themselves, both emotionally and physically. Even a healthy, well-adjusted teenager will feel the stress that pregnancy puts on her body. A teenage father may feel emotional stress. The financial and practical aspects of parenthood are usually too much for a teenager to handle.

Pregnancy can be prevented through use of planned birth control methods as well as abstinence from sexual intercourse. Teenagers who desire to be sexually active should be made aware of the methods available. The common methods are the oral contraceptive pill, the diaphragm, the condom, and foam spermaticides. The rhythm method is also practiced by some but is not very reliable. Condoms are recommended for the male to use to prevent transmission of sexually transmitted diseases.

Religious practices may determine the type of birth control used. In any case, it is wise for the teenager to consult a medical doctor, family planning clinic, or school nurse. The only advice a home health aide should offer is to mention that one of the persons should be consulted.

Substance Abuse.   Drug use among adolescents has been on the increase over the past 20 years. It is recognized that "pot" smoking, "pill popping," and the use of hard drugs have increased the crime rate and caused serious health problems, both physical and mental. Many families have been destroyed because of the aftermath of drug abuse by its members. Drug awareness programs are run in schools to alert young people to the dangers involved. Legislation has been passed in an effort to stop drug abuse. Television and radio programs continue to tell of the harmful effects of drug abuse.

Parents should see that their children are well informed about the dangers and effects of drug abuse. A loving home environment where the child feels accepted and is able to talk about concerns and feelings helps to deter drug abuse. If a parent sees physical or emotional signs—extreme mood swings, lethargy, overactivity, nervousness, red eyes, sniffling, needle marks, or other unaccountable signals—professional help should be sought.

In America today there is another "drug" being used more and more by young people. Alcohol abuse has become a major problem. Children as young as 6 and 7 years of age are abusing alcohol. In fact, according to one recent report, among youth the average drinking age nationwide is 11.5 years. Parents often are not as concerned about drinking as they are about other drugs. They seem to feel that alcohol is less harmful than drug abuse. Unfortunately, the truth is that youthful drinking is a serious and dangerous problem. Drinking can lead to cirrhosis of the liver, which is irreversible. It can also lead to permanent brain damage. Moreover, drinking is a major cause of death on the highway due to driving while intoxicated (DWI). The fact that it is illegal to drink below the age of 21 has not slowed down the consumption of alcohol by minors.

Alcohol is an accepted part of our adult society, but all too often its negative influence reaches the younger generation. Organizations such as Al-Anon and Alateen are educating drinkers and helping them to stop drinking for at least "one day at a time." DARE or Drug Awareness Resistance Education is a group organized to stop young people from getting started on illegal drugs.

Child Abuse, Maltreatment, and Neglect

According to Social Services law, Sec. 412, an abused child is one who is under 18 years of age whose parent or other legally responsible for his or her care or any person in a caregiver's situation:

- inflicts or allows to be inflicted on such child physical injury by other than accidental means, or
- creates or allows to be created a risk of physical injury to such a child by other than accidental means which might cause death or serious disfigurement, impairment of function of any bodily organ
- commits or allows to be committed, a sex offense against such a child
- allows, permits, or encourages such a child to engage in prostitution
- allows such a child to engage in acts or conduct of a sexual nature, i.e., videotaping sexual acts

Examples of maltreatment and neglect of children are:

- improperly fed, clothed, or deprived of any emotional support
- allowed to drink alcohol or given illegal drugs
- chained or locked in a closet
- kept in an environment where mice, rats, cockroaches, or other pests can harm the child
- left alone in an apartment or house or locked in a room while the legally responsible adult is away

• exposed to lead poison from painted walls or furniture

The "legally responsible person" would include a parent, guardian, or custodian. A home health aide working in the household where such conduct as abuse, neglect, or maltreatment occurs is considered a "legally responsible person." Such behavior is not acceptable on the part of an aide or any other legally responsible person. If an aide becomes aware of such abusive treatment, it should be immediately reported to the agency. If the aide does not report the abuse, the aide is as guilty as the person doing the abuse. Child abuse can take place in a wealthy client's home or in a poor client's home. It can come in many forms such as beating a child with a strap to withholding feeding a baby for days because the baby cries. Figure 7-9 lists typical behavior for abused/mistreated children.

Abusive parents or caretakers may have been raised by abusive families themselves. The husband or wife may abuse the spouse. Life crises such as loss of job, debt, or housing problems and substance abuse of alcohol or drugs or gambling losses can lead to abusive behavior; physical or mental health problems may cause a parent to become abusive; or parents who are too young themselves may lack self-discipline to deal with their own children. Many of these parents are not aware of the damage they are doing to their children and may need help themselves to develop better parenting skills. Parents of mentally or developmentally disabled children may be unable to cope with their children's problems. These parents should be encouraged to join support groups with parents with similar problems.

Avoid contact with parents or other adults
Become upset when other children cry
Be extremely aggressive
Be extremely withdrawn
Suffer mood swings
Fear going into home—run away from home
Be overly demonstrative and loving to abusive parent
Blame themselves for being "clumsy" or "bad"
Wear long sleeves to conceal injuries
Appear to have low self-esteem
Attempt suicide

Figure 7-9 Observable behavior patterns of abused/mistreated children

SUMMARY

• Life begins with the uniting of a sperm and an ovum.
• An infant is born and continues to develop through adolescence.
• A home health aide's job in caring for children is to help the family meet the difficult or everyday problems. By understanding the needs of each age group, the aide can prepare for possible problems.
• It is of utmost importance that a woman receive good prenatal care during pregnancy.
• It is very important that "bonding" occur shortly after birth between the parents and the new baby.
• A home health aide needs to be aware of and report signs of child abuse, maltreatment, or neglect.
• Adolescence is a time of rapid physical, sexual, and emotional growth and change. It is important that the parents maintain open lines of communication with their child at this time.

REVIEW

1. What are the five basic needs of a newborn?

2. List three immunizations recommended for infants.

3. Name two health problems that affect adolescents.

4. What physical changes occur at puberty?

5. List three signs of child abuse and three examples of child maltreatment.

6. What is an aide's responsibility if child abuse is suspected?

7. Why is it important for the aide to allow the mother to assume as much care of the newborn baby as possible? What would you look for and document relating to the mother's "bonding" with her infant?

8. What kind of observations would you be likely to make in caring for a newborn infant? An older baby? A toddler?

9. An infant needs to be:
    a. toilet trained immediately
    b. weaned to a cup by 6 months
    c. kept awake during the day so it will sleep at night
    d. loved, held, and fed regularly

10. Typical characteristics of the adolescent phase of development are:
    a. likes to maintain privacy of his/her thoughts
    b. sex-related problems are especially common
    c. alcohol abuse can become a major problem
    d. all of the above are true

11. Match Column I with Column II (childhood conditions)

    Column I
    ___1. PKU
    ___2. Hydrocephalus
    ___3. Down syndrome
    ___4. Cystic fibrosis
    ___5. Sickle cell anemia

    Column II
    a. inherited malfunction of the pancreas
    b. defect or injury of the brain tissues
    c. unable to break down a certain amino acid
    d. defect in the absorption of brain fluid and head is enlarged
    e. abnormal sickle-shape red blood cells that are very fragile

12. Signs and symptoms of fetal alcohol syndrome are:
    a. small head
    b. weak heart
    c. flat face with drooping lips
    d. all of the above are correct

Unit *8* Early and Middle Adulthood

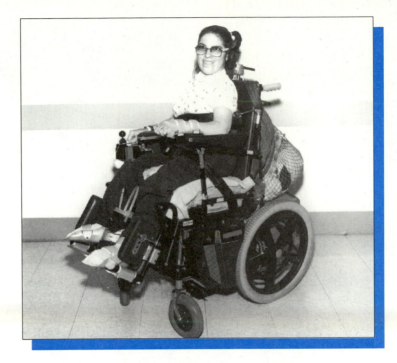

KEY TERMS

• • • • • • • • • • • • • • • • • • • •

early and middle adulthood
empty nest syndrome
mammogram
menopause

multiple sclerosis
Pap smear
preventive health measure
prognosis

rheumatoid arthritis
self-esteem
sigmoidoscopy

LEARNING OBJECTIVES

• •

After studying this unit, you should be able to:

- List the causes of health problems in the early adult years.
- Describe the adjustments that often must be dealt with in the middle adult years.
- State why preventive health measures are important.
- Describe the changes that occur during the early and middle adult years in terms of family relationships.
- List two reasons a home health aide should encourage the client to exercise.
- List two activities a disabled client can become involved in outside of the home.

Early Adulthood

Adolescence is followed by early adulthood. This is the time of life when formal education is usually completed. Most young adults enter the labor force and begin to assume the responsibilities of daily life.

During early adulthood, most individuals are concerned with bettering themselves. They may change jobs often. Many look forward to better jobs, higher wages, and greater opportunities. As young people make these changes, they must constantly make personal adjustments.

Also, during early adulthood, close personal relationships take on greater significance. Some young adults choose to marry; some also choose to start a family. If both partners are working, they need to arrange their personal lives around their jobs. This effort helps produce harmonious relations with each other. They must learn to share duties and work together as a team.

Today, many young couples choose to delay the start of a family. When they do decide to have children, the mother may find it difficult to leave the work environment. As a result, the child is often left in the care of others. As the family grows, each stage of infancy and childhood brings its own challenges and problems.

Early Adulthood Adjustments

During early adulthood (25–45 years of age), the body normally works efficiently. It remains at a high level of health for about 30 or 40 years, Figure 8-1. The body heals quickly through childhood, adolescence, and early and middle adulthood.

Health problems in early adulthood often accompany parenthood. For example, an infant may be born with a birth defect. The physical problems of the child can create severe psychological stress and financial burdens for the parents. For a woman, the pregnancy itself can endanger her health. Normal pregnancy, pregnancy with complications, and reproductive system disorders can occur in the adult female. Such problems should be cared for by a physician. Other health problems can result

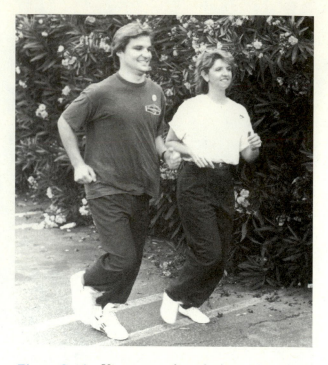

Figure 8-1A Young couple enjoying an outdoor activity—jogging

from conditions related to auto accidents and job-related injuries.

As a **preventive health measure,** all persons should have a physical examination at least every 3 years. The early detection of diseases such as cancer, heart disease, diabetes, and

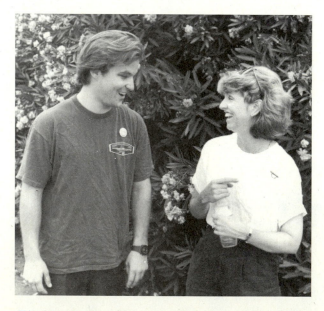

Figure 8-1B Young couple enjoying the company of one another

emotional stress often leads to a better **progno-sis** (outcome). Also, women should do a breast self-examination every month, see Figure 19-3. They should have a vaginal examination that includes a Pap smear every year. The American Cancer Society recommends that a woman undergo a **mammogram** (x-ray of breasts) between the ages of 35 and 39, then every 1 or 2 years from age 40 to age 49, and yearly for women over age 50. It is also recommended that both men and women have a **sigmoidoscopy** (rectal examination with a special tube) every 3 to 5 years after the age of 50.

Middle Adulthood

Society places great demands on a person in the middle adult years (45–65 years of age). It is during this period that people are expected to be highly successful and productive as well as financially secure, Figure 8-2. If a woman has chosen to remain at home with her children, this may be the time when she decides to re-enter the work force.

During the middle adult years, people often assess their accomplishments. Some may question how worthwhile their work or other achievements have been and seek a change. This change may take the form of a different life-style—a separation from their marriage partner, a change in career or place of residence, or loss of a job. Often during this stage of life, individuals are asked to take responsibility for care of their aging parents. The role between parent and children often reverses once one of the parents is unable to manage all of his/her cares. This can be at times a difficult and stressful period in both parent's and children's lives.

Physically, those in their middle adult years will notice some changes. Their hair may turn gray or recede and their eyesight may diminish. Weight gain may occur as a result of a general slowing of metabolism. Hormonal changes that occur during **menopause** may result in mood swings, changes in sleeping patterns, increased anxiety, or other physical symptoms.

Adjustments During the Middle Adult Years

There are several major adjustments that the person in the middle adult years may have to make. These adjustments are in response to a change in some area of their lives.

Family Relationships

The middle years are generally the time when grown children leave the home. Parents who have been very involved in their children's lives may feel at a loss when this occurs (**empty nest syndrome**). As the children mature and gain independence, their own roles and responsibilities may become first priorities, and their ties with their family may become more remote. This can be a time when parents and children form close, adult relationships with each other. This can also be a time of freedom and creativity for the parents as they find they have more time to spend with each other and more time to develop their own mutual interests.

Effects of Exercise

It is very important during the early and middle years of adulthood to become involved in a regular exercise program. At any age, the unexercised body—though free of symptoms of illness—will rust out long before it ever will wear

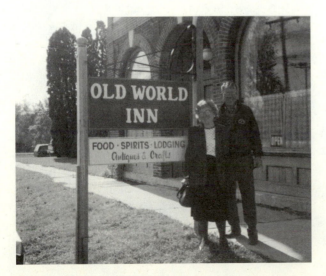

Figure 8-2 Middle-aged couple enjoying a leisure day together

out. Inactivity can make anyone old before their time. Just as inactivity accelerates aging, activity slows it down. Some specialists on aging state that the closest thing to an "antiaging pill" is exercise. One of the best exercises is walking. Some other alternatives to walking are swimming, riding a stationary or moving bicycle, and dancing. If you are working in a home with a young or middle-aged adult, you should try to encourage the client to do some type of exercise within his or her limits. It might be that you are assigned to care for a blind diabetic. There would be no reason you could not walk outside with the client.

Multiple sclerosis, a nervous system disorder, is the major crippler of young and middle-aged adults. The range of activity that these clients can do varies greatly. As a home health aide, you will need to use your creativity and ingenuity to encourage this client to do as much exercise as possible.

Rheumatoid arthritis is also a disease that can afflict individuals in this age group. When working with these individuals, it is better to do exercises with them later in the day. In the morning the client has more pain on movement, but as the day progresses, the pain will diminish. This client benefits greatly from swimming in warm water pools. In certain situations, arthritic clients will benefit from taking a pain pill before starting an exercise routine.

Acceptance of Illness or Disability

It is very difficult for individuals between the ages of 25 and 65 years of age to accept the fact that they need assistance from others to do their activities of daily living (ADLs). At times, the client might express anger at the home health aide because of the disability. The client is usually very frustrated and does not know how to cope with these frustrations. How would you feel if you were 25 years of age and because of a car accident became paralyzed from the waist down? Every case differs. With the assistance of your case manager or supervisor, you will be given special instructions to follow on how to handle these clients.

Emotional Needs

Two of the most important aspects of care of clients with disabilities or disabling conditions are to keep their minds mentally active and to try to meet some of their emotional needs. These individuals have the same basic needs as a healthy individual of the same age, Figures 8-3 and 8-4. It is a little easier to do this task than it was years ago. With modern technology, a client can be transported even if confined to a wheelchair. Special vans are available to help transport these clients. Many restaurant and public places have wheelchair access and also special accommodations for toileting.

Shopping malls and grocery stores sometimes have designated times for these individuals to shop and designated parking. Occasionally these stores will have extra help available to assist these clients in their shopping needs. Many churches have special activities for such individuals to attend, depending on their interest. In some areas of the country, there are activities for the developmentally disabled such as the Special Olympics in which your client may want to become involved. Your role is to encourage your client to participate and attend such functions. In most scenarios, the case

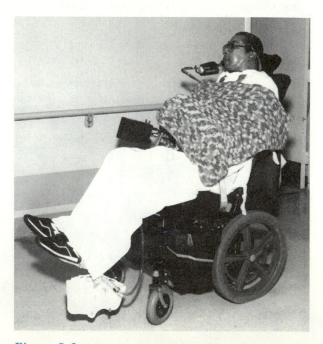

Figure 8-3   Adults confined to wheelchairs have the same basic needs as other adults the same age.

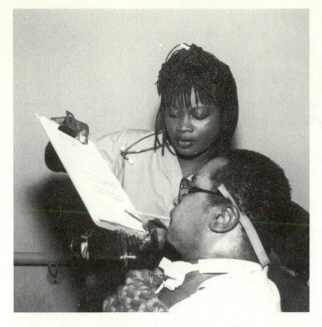

Figure 8-4 A client who is a quadriplegic signs his name holding the pencil in his mouth.

manager initially will arrange for transportation and coordination of these activities. Your role will be to assist the client in getting ready to attend, including having the client dressed properly and having all the supplies needed with the client such as medications, money, and toileting supplies. If the client plans to attend a special family event, you will need to see that the client's hair is clean and stylish and that the client is dressed appropriately for the event.

Usually a member of the family will transport the client to the event. Always check to see if the client has all supplies necessary for the time he or she will be gone. Your goal is to make it as pleasant as possible for the client and also the family members. Be sure the family members know how to operate any special equipment and are instructed on any special care that the client may require.

Retirement

Retirement is a major adjustment for most individuals. Often, an individual's identity and sense of **self-esteem** are closely linked with one's job. Retirement from gainful employment may erode one's self-esteem. It may also remove a person from close relationships formed in the workplace. Retirement for some people is very enjoyable; they have more time for hobbies and travel. Individuals who have not planned for retirement can find it very difficult, especially if they have not planned financially for it or have no hobbies. One must remain mentally and physically active to keep the body at its peak. You have to exercise your brain regularly to prevent deterioration. You also need to exercise the body physically to prevent it from deteriorating. Remember the old saying, "If you don't use it, you'll lose it."

SUMMARY

- Changes that may occur in early and middle adulthood require major adjustment.
- The home health aide should always try to be sensitive to those who are affected by these changes.
- A supportive, caring attitude may help the individual to successfully adapt to shifting life patterns.

- The home health aide needs to encourage the client to attend activities outside of the client's home.
- Retirement can be a positive or negative experience.
- To be mentally and physically healthy, one must exercise the mind and body continuously throughout life.

REVIEW

1. Name three causes of health problems in the early adult years.

2. List three adjustments that may need to be made during the middle adult years.

3. During what period of life does society expect the most from an individual?

4. Why are preventive health measures important?

5. List two activities a home health aide can involve a client in outside of the client's home.

6. List two benefits of regular exercise.

7. The developmental steps of early adulthood is/are:
    a. time the individuals are concerned about bettering themselves
    b. close personal relationships take on greater significance
    c. career choices are made
    d. all of the above

8. Middle adult years are a time when adjustments are made due to:
    a. grown children leaving home
    b. aging parent may be brought into the home
    c. chronic illness may begin
    d. all of the above

9. Multiple sclerosis, a nervous system disorder, is a major crippler of young adults.
    a. true
    b. false

10. Women over 50 years of age should have a Pap smear and mammogram every year as a preventive health measure.
    a. true
    b. false

11. Alcoholism is a problem among adults, as well as among adolescents.
    a. true
    b. false

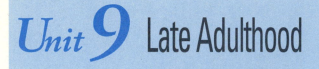

Unit 9 Late Adulthood

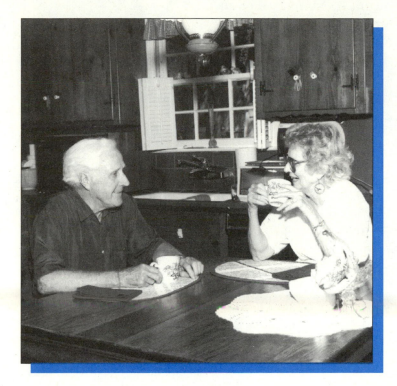

KEY TERMS

Alzheimer's disease   reality orientation   validation therapy
chronological

LEARNING OBJECTIVES

After studying this unit, you should be able to:

- Name some of the physical and emotional effects of the aging process.
- Identify the reasons for establishing regular schedules for elderly clients.
- Identify the effects of Alzheimer's disease.
- Describe the problems of persons confined to bed.
- Describe validation therapy.
- Describe the problems of clients who are nonambulatory.
- List five common chronic diseases of the elderly.

It cannot be definitely stated at what time in life people become old, for age is more a matter of physical and mental aging than it is of **chronological** processes. Tremendous variations exist. Some people are physically and mentally old at age 35, others are still young at the age of 65.

The terms *aging* and *aged* must also be clarified. Aging is a process that begins with conception and ends with death. The term aged means old or mature. Because of today's increased life expectancy, our perceptions of the age at which an individual is old may not be entirely accurate. Today, if a person lives to be 65 and is in reasonably good health, that individual can expect to live 14 to 20 more years. Moreover, women often outlive men by several years. The most recent statistics show that there are at least 31 million Americans over the age of 65. By the year 2000, that number is expected to rise to more than 35 million. These figures have special meaning for anyone entering the field of home health care. Many of these older citizens will probably have need of the services of a home health aide.

In the past, most of the statistics concerning the aged were based on the chronically ill and elderly persons in hospitals, nursing homes, and other institutions. The largest proportion of the aged population, though, are healthy, alert,

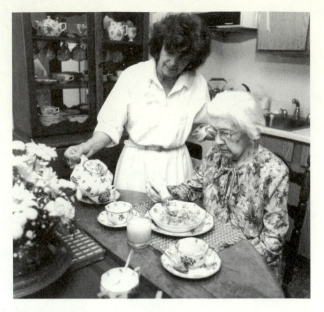

Figure 9-2   Home health aide assisting a client with a meal in client's apartment

able, working, and contributing members of society, Figure 9-1. They have made adequate adjustments to the physical, mental, and emotional changes associated with the aging process. For some of them, home care extends the time in which they can enjoy living at home, Figure 9-2.

What is it like to become old? One person described it in this way: "Smear dirt on your glasses, stuff cotton in your ears, put on heavy shoes that are too big, and wear gloves; then try to spend the day in a normal way." Older people admit that they find it harder to do many of the things they like to do and become impatient with themselves and others just because they find it difficult to accept the loss of their independence. Imagine how an older individual who is in ill health must resent these added problems. A home health aide must become "tuned in" to the special needs of such a person.

Effects of Aging on the Body Systems

As the body grows older, the machinery begins to slow down. The body loses its ability to bounce back after illness. Healing takes longer after surgery, illness, or injury. The body becomes less able to fight off infections.

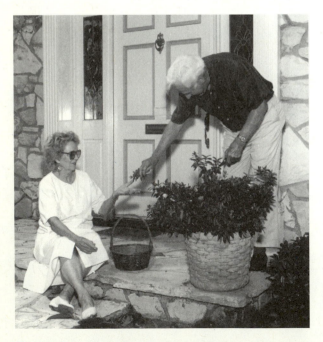

Figure 9-1   An older couple enjoying gardening together

Each body system shows some signs of age, Figure 9-3. The nervous system reacts slower to stimuli. Hearing and sight may fail. Slowed circulation to the brain may cause damage. The nerves of the feet and fingers may be less sensitive. As a result, the body may not sense that the bath water is scalding hot, or that the toes are cold and frostbitten. There may be a buildup of fat in the circulatory system causing the blood vessels to clog up. Slowed circulation weakens the functioning of many other systems. Aging causes the tiny air sacs in the lungs to stretch. This reduces the oxygen exchange and causes the person to feel breathless.

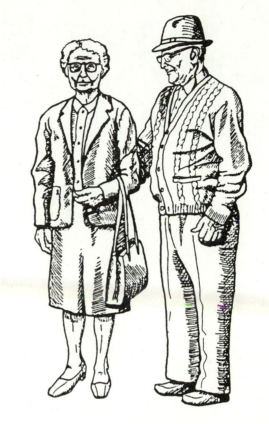

Observable

Hair: Thins and whitens

Vision: Declines; three out of five persons 75+ are affected to some degree, and more often in females than males.

Kidneys: Eventually lose up to 50 percent of their capacity to filter body wastes. This major system shows the greatest decline with age.

Heart: 1st—Between ages 20-90 the amount of blood pumped by the heart decreases 50 percent. 2nd—Muscle fibers contract more slowly. 3rd—Heart and blood vessels are more vulnerable to disease.

Bones: At 40+, the body no longer absorbs calcium efficiently, which contributes to fractures in more than 25 percent of all elderly women.

Joints: 1st—Begin to stiffen, particularly the hips and knees. 2nd—Compressed spinal discs shorten the body and cause a bent posture. Height loss of 1-3 inches is common.

Nervous System: 1st—Hardening of blood vessels create circulatory problems in the brain. 2nd—Aging reduces the speed with which the nervous system can process information or send signals for action.

Circulatory System: Failure in this system is the most common cause of death. Death from cardiovascular disease at age 75 is 150 times higher than at 35.

Nonobservable

Hearing: 1st—Ability to hear high pitches is more difficult. 2nd—Normal sound levels are more difficult to understand.

Skin: 1st—Fine lines around eyes and mouth. 2nd—Lines deepen into wrinkles. 3rd—Skin loses elasticity and smoothness. 4th—Spots of dark pigment.

Lungs: 1st—Between ages 30-75, the amount of air inhaled and exhaled drop by 45 percent. 2nd—Between ages 30-75, the amount of oxygen passing into the blood decreases about 50 percent.

Hormones: 1st—Decline in hormonal flow from the adrenal gland, located atop the kidney, lowers the ability of the elderly to respond to stress. 2nd—For women, menstruation ceases.

Immune System: This system becomes less efficient and therefore lowers the body's resistance to disease.

Muscles: 1st—There is a loss of muscle strength, which reduces coordination. 2nd—Lack of muscle tone causes a sagging of muscles.

Figure 9-3   Changes in the body over time (Reprinted by permission from *Aging in America* by Sandra Zins, copyright 1987 by Delmar Publishers Inc.)

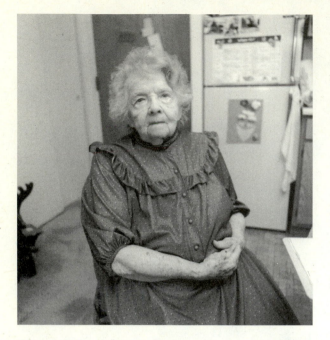

Figure 9-4   Advanced age can cause wrinkling and age spots in the skin.

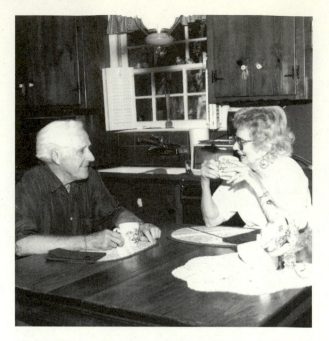

Figure 9-5   An older couple enjoying a cup of coffee together at the start of their day

Another system affected by age is the integumentary system, Figure 9-4. The skin becomes dry and flaky because the oil glands secrete less oil. The body hair becomes thin and starts to fall out. Hair will grow in places on the body, such as the face on women and in the ears on men. In addition, the urinary system filters wastes less effectively. Falls are the most common causes of injuries in the elderly. This is because the bones are more brittle and the muscles less elastic. Many factors of aging cause the healing time to increase. The digestive system is less active. Some foods cannot be digested at all. As a person eats less, there is less available energy. The other body systems suffer from poor nutrition.

The woman produces less vaginal lubrication; it may take an older man longer to achieve an erection. However, none of these changes reduces the sexual pleasure. Generally, sexual activity does slow down as people grow older. Many of the changes that aging brings have more to do with how one looks than how one feels, Figure 9-5.

A home health aide must recognize that older clients have sexuality, including sexual desires. This may cause minor problems, particularly if the client is of the opposite sex. If the client should make a pass or try to take advantage of the home health aide, he or she should firmly say "no." The aide should not shout at clients or angrily scold them. Telling them "no" and walking away is the best action to take. Because the sex drive does continue in later life, it is important for older people to have social contact with members of the opposite sex. Just being with the peer group provides an outlet for sexual needs.

Chronic Illness, Physical Health Problems, and Aging

Although the problems associated with chronic illness and those associated with aging and the aged are not identical, the two areas overlap extensively. Aging in itself is not necessarily accompanied by chronic illness; most of the disabilities and limitations experienced by elderly persons are a result of chronic, progressive disease and not a result of aging alone. Figure 9-6 identifies some of the health problems common among the aged. Many conditions result from a natural aging process; others arise from chronic health problems developed earlier in life.

CONDITION	SYMPTOMS AND TREATMENT	HOME CARE REQUIRED
Glaucoma	**Symptoms:** Accompanied by loss of peripheral vision, headache, dull pain. May be acute or chronic and usually affects both eyes. It is caused by an increased amount of pressure within the eye. **Treatment:** The condition is treated with medication and surgery.	The home health aide should assist the client in the activities of daily living. Adjust the home environment to accommodate the client's "tunnel vision." Encourage client to take medication as prescribed.
Cataracts	**Symptoms:** Accompanied by gradual loss of vision. The client's vision becomes blurred, distorted, and at times he or she sees double. A gray opaque or milky substance appears on the lens of the eye. **Treatment:** Laser—outpatient clinics Surgery may restore partial or total vision. Surgery cannot be performed until the cataract is "ripe." Contact lenses may be implanted into the eye itself.	The client may be fitted with contact lenses, glasses, or implants into the eye itself. The home health aide may assist in the care of the lenses or assist the client with the eyeglasses prescribed. If client has only partial vision, the aide assists in the activities of daily living as recommended by the doctor or supervisor.
Deafness	**Symptoms:** A person may gradually suffer mild to total loss of hearing. Deafness may be the result of an ear injury, a congenital defect, or simply be a process of aging. **Treatment:** A hearing aide may be prescribed. In some cases surgery may restore partial or total hearing.	The home health aide should follow the care plan. It is important to speak clearly, slowly and distinctly when communicating with a deaf person. The aide may assist the client with care of the hearing aide. Make sure that the batteries are working and that the volume control is operating.
Parkinson's disease	**Symptoms:** Accompanied by tremors of the hands, stiffness and rigidity of muscles, masklike expression on face, shuffling bent forward gait, cog-wheel rigidity, problems with speech due to inability to move muscles of face to pronounce words. There is no decrease in awareness or IQ. **Treatment:** Medications may be prescribed to control the condition. In some cases surgery is performed to reduce tremors.	The home health aide should assist the client in the activities of daily living. Encourage the client to do as much as possible. Allow adequate time to eat and dress, as all simple tasks will need longer time to be accomplished. Do not rush this client; allow the client to work at own speed. Give emotional support as needed, as these clients become frustrated and depressed frequently over their disease. Medications need to be taken as prescribed and side effects of the medications must be noted. Remember, however, they are not mentally ill. Their minds are just as sharp as they were before the onset of disease.

Figure 9-6 Medical conditions common among older adults

Continued on the following page.

CONDITION	SYMPTOMS AND TREATMENT	HOME CARE REQUIRED
Fractures	**Symptoms:** A fracture is a break in a bone. After an accidental fall, a person may complain of pain. Swelling may occur around the injured part. Fractures among the aging are the result of loss of muscle tone and brittle bones. The most frequent sites for breaks are the shoulder, arm, wrist, collarbone, and hip. **Treatment:** Treatment is determined by the location and severity of the break. Some breaks are put in a light plastic cast, others are set surgically using metal pins; in some cases a joint may be replaced.	The dietitian may order a high-calcium diet. The aide can provide this and make the environment safe so that other falls can be prevented. The aide follows any other instructions given by the case manager. The aide should observe the color and temperature of the affected extremity. Look for signs of blood on the cast. The client may complain of pain inside the cast. These signs should be reported at once. Use care in transfer techniques.
Arthritis	**Symptoms:** There are many types of arthritis. The person complains of pain, especially on movement, and also will have some stiffness and muscle spasms. Arthritis is an inflammation of the joints; in some cases there is a change in the structure. The fingers become bent and gnarled. There is often heat and swelling of the joints. **Treatment:** Bed rest in acute stages. There is no cure, but it may be controlled by medication. Heat treatment may be prescribed. Splints may be applied to prevent permanent deformities.	The client should be encouraged to be as active as possible. Active or passive range of motion exercises should be done as prescribed. Application of splints or other devices to prevent deformities as ordered. Weight needs to be controlled. Arthritic clients should have a well-balanced, nutritious diet.
Cerebral vascular accident (Stroke or CVA)	**Symptoms:** Effects may be slight to severe, temporary, or permanent. The client may suffer from numbness of face, arms, or legs; loss of speech or difficulty in speaking or understanding speech; dimness or loss of vision, particularly in one eye; double vision, dizziness, change in personality, inappropriate behavior; paralysis of one half of body. **Treatment:** CVA clients are started on physical therapy as soon as possible. Surgery may help in a few selected cases. Good rehabilitation program. Medication may be of some help.	The home health aide must show patience and kindness while following case manager's instructions. It is important to assist the client in self-help. Clients with arterial problems are usually placed on a low-sodium diet. Skin care is extremely important for the client. Special mouth care is also vital. For clients suffering emotional disturbances or confusion, the aide is expected to watch them carefully so they will not harm themselves. These clients are often impatient.

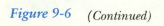

Figure 9-6   *(Continued)*

CONDITION	SYMPTOMS AND TREATMENT	HOME CARE REQUIRED
Colds, viruses, pneumonia	**Symptoms:** A person suffers upper respiratory discomfort, often accompanied by high temperature, chest pains, and labored respirations. Pneumonia may be a complication of colds or flu. It may be viral or bacterial. **Treatment:** Medication may be prescribed. Oxygen is sometimes needed. A vaporizer may be set up in the person's room. Bed rest and diet modifications.	An aide may be asked to take vital signs regularly and report changes to the case manager. Fluid intake is usually increased; a high-caloric diet may be recommended. The client should be kept comfortable. Aseptic techniques should be used in handling linens, tissues, and body wastes.
Heart disease (coronary occlusion, heart block fibrillation, emboli, congestive heart failure)	**Symptoms:** A client may have shortness of breath, pain in chest radiating down the left arm (mild to severe), edema of the ankles and in the lungs, severe indigestion, chronic fatigue, heart palpitations, and blueness of lips and extremities. **Treatment:** Medications as prescribed, bed rest, oxygen, rehabilitation within limits ordered by doctor, psychological support.	When caring for a client with a heart condition, the aide should observe the client for changes in color, pain, or sudden changes in vital signs. Medical instructions should be carefully followed. Clients are usually on a low-salt and low-cholesterol diet. These clients should be encouraged to follow their exercise program as stated on their care plan. It is important to help the client maintain a positive outlook.
Chronic obstructive pulmonary disease (COPD)	**Symptoms:** Symptoms tend to develop slowly over the years. The client may tire easily at first. A nagging productive cough and shortness of breath on minimal exercise may follow. The client's color may appear gray with bluish (cyanotic) lips. Once emphysema has developed, it is irreversible. Efforts must be made to slow its progress. **Treatment:** Oxygen (O_2) therapy, no smoking, avoid exposure to respiratory infections. Flu shots are recommended. IPPB (intermittent positive pressure breathing) using a breathing machine which combines oxygen with medication. Special nasal sprays to open or dilate bronchi and increase oxygen supply to body.	The COPD client must limit physical activities. The home health aide should observe the client for signs of distress and follow medical instructions as given. Keep visitors from smoking so that the air is not contaminated. The fluid intake may be increased to liquify sputum and help client to cough up the sputum. Portable O_2 tanks allow the client more mobility.

Figure 9-6   (Continued)

Continued on the following page.

CONDITION	SYMPTOMS AND TREATMENT	HOME CARE REQUIRED
Osteoporosis	**Symptoms:** The bones break under the slightest trauma or injury. Low back pain and backaches may be the first symptoms. In later stages, a "dowager's hump" may appear (this is a rounded hump between the shoulder blades often seen in older women). **Treatment:** Adequate intake of calcium throughout life span. Exercise regularly. Drink moderately. Don't smoke. If at high risk (white or Asian, small boned, family history of osteoporosis), take estrogen supplements during and after menopause as prescribed by a physician.	The aide must help the client to avoid accidental falls. Extreme caution and attention to the client's safety is crucial. Balanced diet with increased calcium intake. Have client follow medication and exercise regimens prescribed by the doctor.

Figure 9-6   *(Continued)*

Care of the Nonambulatory Client

A client who is confined to bed needs special care no matter what the reason for the bed rest may be. Inactivity, especially in the elderly, leads to conditions such as constipation, pneumonia, and pressure areas. Constant pressure on certain skin areas can easily lead to the formation of bedsores. Lying in the same position for a long time, poor posture, or sitting in a wheelchair can cause the muscles to become weak and deformed. The deformed condition (a muscle contracture) becomes permanent if not corrected early. The following care techniques help prevent complications of long periods of bed rest:

- Change the client's body position and reposition at least every 2 hours.
- Massage the skin around the bony prominences to prevent pressure sores.
- Keep the client's skin clean and dry.
- Place a bed cradle over the client's feet to take the weight of the bedcovers off the feet.
- Use proper positioning and pillows to align the body.
- Assist the client to do range of motion exercises.
- Record the frequency of the client's bowel movements to check for constipation. The doctor may order an enema if the client is constipated. Diet changes may include an increase in high fiber foods and increased fluid intake, as well as increased mobility.
- Provide the client with a radio, television, or some form of entertainment. Diversion reduces boredom and takes the client's mind off the pain and discomfort.
- If limited use of a wheelchair, walker, or cane is permitted, encourage the client to use it.

Emotional and Psychological Effects of Aging

Individuals over 65 years of age are healthier than ever before in our society. The majority of individuals, once they reach the age of 65, have at least 10 to 20 more years to live. The age group of 85 years and older is one of the fastest growing segments of our population. The losses that have been associated with aging years ago are now generally attributed to disuse. The individuals who have good health at the age of 85 generally have practiced good health habits throughout life. Between the ages of 65 and death, a person usually has to deal with many changes in living styles. One of the major losses might be death of a spouse. Loneliness then becomes a reality for the survivor. After being a partner with another person for at least 50 years, this becomes quite an adjustment. The remaining spouse would like to do some work outside of the home or even in the home, but in many cases is physically unable to do so. The only visitors who might come to see the client will be you, *the home health aide and your smiling face.*

Another major concern is finances; many clients are on fixed incomes and have to watch their money very closely to pay their routine bills. Many of them do not have sufficient funds to pay their rent and buy adequate clothing and nutritious foods. They may not have any relatives living close to assist them. One other major concern is what will happen to them if they get sick. Who will care for them? This is where the home health aide comes in. You are the person to assist them to stay in their home as long as possible. The majority of clients you will care for will be living alone and depending on you for many services. Understanding a client's home situation helps in evaluating related health problems.

General Effects

Aging should be expected as a normal part of the life process. However, depression and sadness often accompany aging. The depression felt by many older people comes from the discouragement of having nothing to do that gives them a feeling of success and achievement. Older persons must be encouraged to find new outlets, Figure 9-7. If they can no longer drive, then when riding in the car they should be reminded to look around and see the changing of the seasons, watch people walking, enjoy the children playing along the way. If older persons spend all of their time regretting what they cannot do, there will be no time to expand their horizons and they will surely become depressed. It is good for all mature adults to become involved with their local senior citizen's group and their noon meal program. If needed, the case manager could arrange transportation to take the client to the activities and meals. Some communities have special days that they make special accommodations for the senior citizen or the disabled to shop at their stores and give them extra discounts on merchandise purchased that day.

A person who was once active in the garden but can no longer perform the heavy work in-

volved should be encouraged to have a windowsill garden. A person who enjoyed reading but whose eyesight is failing can get tapes and records of "listening books" from the library and keep up on new literature through the sound medium.

Setting up a daily schedule is important in old age. A regular pattern of rising, dressing, eating, doing chores, working on hobbies, and visiting with friends and family should be arranged. This kind of planning allows for variety and keeps the person from sinking into a depression where sleep becomes a way of escaping from boredom. When an older person sleeps away the day, it is hard to get a restful night's sleep. This causes anxiety and sets up a cycle of fear, anger, and resentment. The elderly must find a rhythm of daily activity that lets them feel alive, useful, and content, based on their physical capacities.

Some elderly persons become mentally confused. This confusion may be the result of pneumonia, cardiac failure, too much medication, abuse or misuse of alcohol, strokes, dehydration, anemia, malignancy, or some other physical process or disease. Even a minor change in the individual's environment may bring about a state of confusion. The home health aide

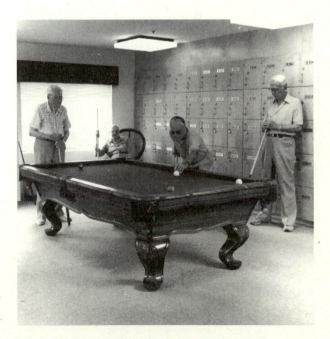

Figure 9-7   These senior citizens are very involved in a game of pool.

should make every attempt to provide a secure, supportive environment for confused clients.

More about Growing Old

Geriatrics, according to the dictionary, is that branch of medicine that deals with the structural changes, physiology, diseases, and hygiene of old age. That covers a wide area. What does the term *geriatric* mean to the home health aide? When does an individual qualify as a geriatric patient—at age 50, 60, 70, or older? What are the structural changes that can and do occur? What are the vital processes, or physiology, of aging? Which are the diseases most often associated with the geriatric patient? What is meant by the hygiene of old age?

These are not easy questions and there are no answers that apply to every older individual. As has been noted before, it is not possible to generalize. Each and every person goes through the aging process in his or her own way. Environmental, financial, and hereditary factors play a large part in what happens to any one person.

Let us start with the home health aide's role, responsibilities, and reactions to the aging disabled client.

The majority of clients for whom you will provide care will be geriatric clients. The combinations of physical ailments, personality types, and environmental conditions are impossible to predict. This places a great deal of responsibility on the home health aide. Remember, one of the major traits a home health aide must develop is flexibility. (It might be mentioned here that physical and emotional flexibility is not a trait you can expect of your clients. You must keep in mind that as individuals grow older, they lose the ability to "go with the flow" or to adjust rapidly to new and changing conditions. They also lose physical flexibility, their bones are brittle, muscles may be weak, and diseases such as arthritis and osteoporosis limit movement. Thus, they can't bend, move, or function as well as younger persons.)

Devise a care plan for the client described in Case Study 1. The client lives in a two-story house; the bedrooms and bath are upstairs. The doctor advises no more than one trip upstairs per day. There is a toilet on the main floor. The client must be assisted in bathing. Laundry must be done. Beds need to be changed and meals prepared. A medications chart has been set up by the visiting nurse. (The aide is to work 4 hours per day, 5 days a week.)

Write a story about a typical day's activities in this home. Some of the areas you might want to include are: how the couple relate to each other and to you; successes or failures in getting them to eat properly; whether the medications were taken properly; how the wife responded to personal care; the energy level of the wife; the mental status of the husband; what you said or did to build their self-confidence; any progress in getting them to agree to removing some of the accumulated "stuff." (You would always want to be sure the client understood and agreed to having any of the accumulated items thrown away. Remember "one man's trash is another man's treasure." Often what may look like junk to an outsider is an object with great sentimental value to the owner.)

One of the hardest adjustments that an elderly person must make is that his body just isn't functioning as well as it did only a few months earlier. It takes longer to get up from a chair; it is harder to take care of hair grooming; and it becomes a chore to plan meals and prepare and clean up after them. As body functions become less efficient, an individual becomes fearful. "What if I should fall?" "Did I take my medicine?" "Did I turn off the iron?" Fear is a negative emotion, and it feeds on itself. Suddenly, aging individuals can become afraid of anything and everything. They become uncertain about writing checks to pay bills and worry whether they did actually pay the bills. They wonder if they have enough money to last the rest of their lives. Then, when an illness strikes, they become even more fearful. One elderly client said she felt like the song "Ole Man River"—"Tired of livin' and feared of dyin'." One job of a home health aide is to help the client regain self-confidence, reminding the client of how much progress they have made.

Often elderly individuals become depressed. They remember how active they were just a short time ago and compare their active days to the restricted lives they now lead. This is

Case Study 1:   Spouse Dependency

Here is an example of an actual situation faced by a home health aide. CLIENT: Woman, 83 years of age, mildly diabetic with high blood pressure, angina, and arthritis, develops a gastric ulcer due to medication to ease the arthritic pain, is anemic, is diagnosed as having hardening of the arteries, and her spine is disintegrating, causing great pain.

Until recently, this woman has been functioning at a reasonable level, caring for her 84-year-old husband and herself in their own home. Suddenly she becomes aware that her husband is short of breath, his sleep pattern has changed, his walk is slow and appears to be painful. He says he just doesn't feel well. This change in her husband causes her to become fearful. What will she do if he dies? In her own words, she can't sleep at night because she is afraid that her husband will die at night. He isn't sleeping; she isn't sleeping.

They depend on each other. She feels inadequate and is fearful that she is losing her mind. It becomes a chore to decide what to eat so she stops planning and cooking regular meals. As a result, neither of them eat nutritionally proper food. They both become weak. He sits in a chair all day watching television and nodding off to sleep. She finds herself becoming dizzy and falling down. She is restless and unable to find a comfortable spot for herself. It is hard for her to get dressed in the morning. Over a 4-month period, she has been out of the house only to go to the doctor or the grocery store, perhaps only two times a month in all. They start bickering with each other, each blaming the other for anything and everything. Both are getting weaker each day. As one sees the other not functioning, fear grows. Are they dying? If so, what will happen to the other one?

What else is going on in that situation? The housework is not being done. Dust and clutter are everywhere. Neither has the energy to vacuum. The kitchen is a mess. Dishes are not washed because she is too tired and possibly because she can't see too well. Although there is a clothes washer and dryer in the basement, she is unable to go up and down the stairs to do the laundry. He wears his clothes until they are stiff with dirt. Finally, he takes the dirty clothing to the basement and does the washing. The clothing is stained with bits of food that have dropped. The stains don't come out because he either can't see the stains or he hasn't the strength to take the extra effort required to remove them.

Neither of them is willing to throw out anything. So the house is piled high with "things"—old, stained, and torn clothing, bedding, and pillows; unopened gifts; and furniture that should have been discarded. They have every television set ever brought into the house, as well as coats, shoes, and clothing from the past 20 years. They do not have the strength to get such junk out of the house.

She is taking five kinds of medicine, including nitroglycerine, ulcer pills costing $1.45 each, two separate medications for blood pressure, and pain pills (cortisone and muscle relaxants) to ease the arthritic and spinal discomfort. She can't remember which pills she has taken and when she is due for another.

Neither of them eats very much. She says she has no appetite and everything tastes like sawdust. She is controlling the diabetes by watching her intake of sugar. So far she has kept her blood sugar within the normal range and her blood tests are within normal limits. However, her hemoglobin count is down, the cholesterol count is up, and her blood pressure is too high. She also is chronically constipated and has hemorrhoids.

She has just returned from the hospital where the ulcer was diagnosed when the home health aide is assigned to the case.

Continued on the following page.

Case Study 1 *(Continued)*

The home health aide's primary responsibility is the 83-year-old woman. Where does she start? What are the limits of her responsibilities?

Ideally, the supervising nurse or nutrition therapist will determine what foods should be consumed. This is particularly true in a case in which there are so many special requirements. Many factors must be considered. Since the client is a diabetic, she will need a diet that is balanced and low in sugar. Since she has an ulcer, the diet must be bland and must not include acidic foods. In addition, she must be encouraged to eat many small, frequent meals instead of several large ones. Because she has high blood pressure, she needs a sodium-free diet. Although her cholesterol level indicates that her diet should not include red meat, liver, cream, whole milk, and butter, her low hemoglobin indicates that she eat red meat and liver, as well as apricots and other foods high in iron. Although her ulcer indicates that she should eat bland foods, her chronic constipation requires a diet high in bulk and fiber. Finally, her poor appetite needs to be counteracted with small, good-tasting, attractively served meals.

As you can see, filling all of these needs will not be easy. The client has lost her appetite. A skilled dietitian or nutritional therapist should be consulted to set up appropriate menus for this client.

It should also be noted that certain of the prescriptions are to be taken at different times: either before, after, or at the same time meals are given. Check with the supervising nurse for the correct time each drug should be taken.

(Using the diets listed in the unit on nutrition, plan a suitable menu for 2 days under the above-listed circumstances.)

This client lives on a fixed income which averages approximately $15,000 a year. Basic medical expenses are covered by Blue Cross/Blue Shield and Medicare. Let us look at the way this money is spent:

Total Income (Social Security and investments)		$15,000.00
Property taxes	$2,000.00	
Food ($60.00 per week)	3,120.00	
Insurance (car and house)	1,350.00	
Monthly car payments (gas/oil)	2,000.00	
Medical insurance (Blue Cross/Blue Shield/Medicare $200.00 deductible)	2,400.00	
Clothing/shoes	600.00	
Oil heat	1,300.00	
Electricity	300.00	
Water	140.00	
Telephone	280.00	
Newspaper/magazine subscriptions	275.00	
Total budgeted expenses		$13,765.00
$200.00 prescriptions not covered by major medical, emergencies—new tires for car, replacements of furniture or other unbudgeted items	$1,235.00	

Home health care is *not* covered by the insurance plan so that means that if the total costs through the health care agency amount to $120.00 per week, this client will be left with no emergency money cushion after only 10 weeks of home health care. Just imagine if the client had to have three shifts of home health aides 7 days a week. That alone can run as much as $1,500 in just a week.

particularly true when illness or a physical condition is also present. Depression feeds on itself and as they become more depressed, they feel worse physically. Their appetites become poorer, they give in to the fear of dying. These feelings of hopelessness lead to helplessness.

It has been proven that laughter can be good medicine in cases such as this. Norman Cousins, who was diagnosed as having a terminal illness, had a very positive attitude about himself and about life in general. He refused to become depressed and give in to his illness. He deliberately set out to find things that would make him laugh because he discovered when he laughed he felt better.

Recent experiments in nursing homes have reinforced the idea of laughter being good medicine. Patients were shown movies and videotapes of Charlie Chaplin films, Buster Keaton, the Keystone Kops, Laurel and Hardy and the Marx Brothers—all of whom, it should be noted, produce the "slapstick" variety of comedy.

Recent research has shown that depressed people respond positively to sunlight. Experiments have proven that clinically depressed individuals who spend several hours a day in a specially lighted room have shown remarkable improvement and have expressed how much better they feel. If such treatment works for those who are psychologically impaired, just imagine how helpful "sunlight" treatment might be for a homebound client. Pet therapy and music therapy are also effective with the older client.

Write a brief description of an imaginary encounter with the client described in Case Study 2, in which she accuses you, the aide, of stealing her watch. (You find the watch later in the kitchen cabinet.)

Write a second brief description of a situation where the same client told you what a miserably rude and uncaring person the previous aide had been. What else would you do besides document this?

The New York Bell Telephone Company provides some special services for handicapped individuals. For example, for this client, the agency requested specially magnified dials for the phone so that, even with limited vision, the client can dial her phone. In addition she has been given "operator assistance" at no extra charge. If she needs to make a call and does not know the number, all she has to do is dial "0" and the operator will look up the number and complete the call.

There is also available a "medic alert" which is a button the client wears at all times. In case she should fall while alone, she can press the button and an emergency number will be dialed automatically. The phone will continue ringing the emergency number until someone answers and receives the message that there is an emergency at the client's address.

Another service available through the telephone company is a remote phone which the client can place in a bag on her walker. No matter where she is, she will have a phone within reach. For the individual who is alone in a home or apartment for any period of time during the day, these services are quite important.

Another service available in some areas is "medi-cab." For a very small sum (perhaps only a dollar each way), a client will be picked up and taken, for example, to medical appointments or to senior citizen functions. When the appointment is over, the medi-cab will return the client to her home. The home health aide or companion rides without charge.

Alzheimer's Disease

An illness that has received much publicity in the past few years is **Alzheimer's disease,** a progressive, degenerative disease that attacks the brain and results in impaired thinking, memory, and behavior. It affects an estimated 2.5 million American adults. There is no known cause for this debilitating illness, characterized by loss of memory and diminished mental capacity. The disease eventually leads to a state in which the person has no control of mental or physical functions. Changes occur in nerve cells in the outer layer of the brain, producing almost unnoticeable symptoms at first. As the disease progresses, simple forgetfulness increases to greater memory loss. There are changes in thought patterns and personality. Those affected can no longer care for themselves or communicate their needs to others, Figure 9-8. When it was

Case Study 2:   Client Alone

This client is a 76-year-old woman living alone in a co-op apartment. She has an inoperable brain tumor and suffered a CVA. After hospitalization and 3 months of rehabilitation at a nursing home, she is released to her home. The only relatives live out of state or out of the country. The medical recommendation is that 24-hour home health aide coverage be initiated. This requires the rotation of three aides daily, 7 days per week; visits from case manager; visiting nurses; a physical therapist 3 times a week; a speech therapist 3 times a week; and an occupational therapist 3 times a week.

The environment is a one-bedroom apartment in a pleasant suburban area. Prior to the CVA, the client's husband died. Following his death, the client first showed signs of mental disorientation when she collected every container, carton, wrapper, can, or bag that was brought into the house. She could not bring herself to throw out anything. As a result, the apartment was stacked high with boxes, cartons, piles of newspapers, magazines, and mail, leaving only an aisle in which to move from room to room.

Before the client was brought home, her attorney had arranged to have the apartment cleared out so that there would be room for a wheelchair, chair commode, and walker, as well as room for an aide to walk beside the client as she became more mobile.

During the first 2 months, three aides a day were provided by the agency. For the first few weeks, the client was so happy to be at home that she made no complaints about anything. The agency supervisor spoke daily with each aide. She discovered that the client was gossiping about each of the aides to the other two—making critical remarks and comparing them unfavorably. The client was also showing favoritism by offering extra money to one aide. (The aide immediately reported this to her supervisor, who called the client

and explained that such behavior on her part was improper.)

At about this time, the client became very critical of the aides and called the supervisor to complain on a daily basis. The supervisor spoke with the aides individually and heard their side and recognized that it would be best to change their assignments. At first, when a new aide was assigned, the client would be very enthusiastic and tell the supervisor how wonderful the aide was. However, after 2 or 3 weeks, she would claim that money was missing or that the aide came in late or was lazy or just wasn't a nice person. The night time aide reported to the supervisor that the client told the aide to go to sleep as she wouldn't need her. Then she became aware that the client was trying to go to the bathroom by herself. Finally it was decided that the night time aide really wasn't needed and the client agreed to try coping alone for one, then two, then three nights, and finally a full week without an aide at night. At this point the client was progressing very well and again it was determined by the doctor and the agency supervisor that the aides' hours be cut back.

It has now been a year since the client was released from the nursing home. She no longer needs the wheelchair or commode and can use the walker very well. She prepares her own breakfast and dresses and undresses herself. Arrangements have been made for a neighbor to prepare her evening meal and do the grocery shopping. An aide comes in between 9 AM and 1 PM Monday through Friday to go to the laundry room and do the laundry, change the bed, and assist with activities of daily living. This aide also prepares lunch, goes with the client to her appointments with the doctor and dentist, and takes the client out of doors when the weather permits.

The client has reported to the supervisor that she truly enjoys this aide because she re-

Case Study 2 (Continued)

ally listens when the client talks. The aide explained to the supervisor that she asks the client questions about where she and her husband used to go on vacation, what movies or plays she saw—she gets the client involved in reminiscing about pleasant, past experiences. At the same time she will take out a dresser drawer and have the client "help" her rearrange, throw away, and clean the drawer. This aide has unlocked the secret of pleasing the client, who loves to talk. She has proved to be a creative and thoroughly professional aide.

What would happen if this client noticed that her eyesight was failing? After a visit to the ophthalmologist, she learns that not only are cataracts developing, but, following the stroke, there was damage to the blood vessels of the eyes which is now getting worse. The doctor tells her that there is no corrective surgery and her eyesight will gradually fade completely.

1. She will require full-time aides.
2. She should start taking lessons in Braille so that she can read for pleasure.
3. While she is still able to get around easily, she could enroll in programs for the blind offered through the Lighthouse so that she would be better prepared to function and become as independent as possible when her eyesight is gone.

This client's annual income from investments and social security comes to just over $50,000 per year. During her first year of illness her medical expenses alone were over $100,000. Fortunately much of that was covered by insurance.

Health care not covered by insurance during past year	$35,955.00
Maintenance fees (co-op apartment)	7,200.00
Electricity	580.00
Telephone	425.00
Food	2,800.00
Pharmacy (prescriptions and medications)	818.00
Insurance (health and property)	2,700.00
Charities (church, etc.)	2,000.00
Clothing	400.00
Dental care (not covered by insurance)	2,600.00
Transportation (cabs to doctor appointments)	345.00
Attorney's fees	2,000.00
(No taxes were due this year because of excessive medical expenses.)	
Television repair contract	230.00
	$58,478.00

This meant that she had to use nearly $8,000 of her capital to pay the bills for the past year. As a result, her income next year will be lower.

During the period when three, and later two, aides were assigned to work with this client, the need for accurate observing, reporting, and documenting was of more than normal importance. This client was a manipulative person, and each aide needed to be sure that the record of her own activities was complete so that if the client complained about tasks not being done, the record would stand to refute that accusation. It was also important that activities and tasks were clearly recorded so that each aide could quickly learn what the aides on the preceding shifts had done, and what the client's actions had been. In this way, tasks would not be duplicated or omitted, and tips on successful interventions and methods could be passed on from aide to aide.

STAGE	SYMPTOMS	CARE PLAN
I.	Forgetfulness. Lack of spontaneity. Poor judgment. Poor time orientation. Cannot organize work. Unable to subtract or add.	Be supportive, provide reminders, make lists. Client is still competent in the activities of daily living. Client can work, drive, and socialize.
II.	Confusional stage. Increase in memory lapses: forgets appointments, fails to pay bills. An increase in anxiety and tension—fear of new situations.	Sew labels in clothes; provide ID bracelet or prepare ID card to be kept in the wallet or purse. Supervise and structure travel. Avoid crowds, remove the client from stressful situations.
III.	Inability to function independently. Progressive loss of motor skills. Increasingly uncomfortable in complex situations where much activity is taking place. No longer able to hold job. Has tantrums, and very little emotional control—may run away.	Help client with money matters: shopping, choosing clothes, etc. Client may have difficulty using eating utensils, so finger foods should be given. Accept clients as they are, not how they "should be." Clients must be treated with dignity.
IV.	Personal carelessness. Refuses to bathe. May refuse to eat, is restless, and may have sleep disturbances. May try to get dressed in the middle of night to go to work. Unable to button clothing, tie shoes, and dress appropriately. Unable to make decisions. Is very absorbed into oneself.	Do not allow the client to drive. Provide slip-on shoes and simple clothing. Assist with eating and dressing. Protect client from self-harm.
V.	Crying episodes common. Hyperactivity increases. Days and nights completely confused. Decreased attention span, unable to follow instructions. Starts to become incontinent of both bowels and bladder. Unable to feed self and shows no interest in food. Likes to follow others—shadowing. Has changes in walking ability. Has frequent movements of mouth. Wants to feel and touch objects constantly. Repeats words and sounds over and over again. Starting not to recognize familiar people.	Keep client as comfortable and calm as possible. Client requires full-time custodial care. Speak slowly and clearly, giving only one suggestion at a time. ("It's time to take a bath," "Take off your shirt," "Take off your shoes," etc.) Handle one item at a time to avoid making the client feel threatened. If a caretaker demands instant responses, the client will become terribly distressed and stubborn. The aide must *always* remember the client is not in control of his emotions, therefore, the aide must retain *self-control.* Keep client clean and dry. Feed client small amounts as often as possible or provide liquids and liquified or pureed foods.
VI.	Incontinence of bladder and bowel. Inability to speak or feed self. Increased agitation, complete helplessness.	Client will require 24-hour supervision and care. Dependent on others to do all activities of daily living. Client will need to be fed pureed food and observed closely for choking. The client will need to be turned and repositioned every two hours to prevent pressure sores. The client needs to be bathed frequently and linens on bed need to be kept clean and dry. The client will lose consciousness and slowly go into a coma and die.

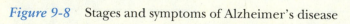

Figure 9-8   Stages and symptoms of Alzheimer's disease

first described by Dr. Alois Alzheimer in 1907, it was considered a rare disease. Today, it is the most common form of dementia. It is usually diagnosed by behaviors that the client displays. On autopsy, the Alzheimer's brain shows the presence of abnormal nerve tangles and clusters in the part of the brain that has to do with memory and intellectual functions. Alzheimer's disease is more likely to occur as a person gets older. Although less than 1% of people over 65 are affected by the disease, it is present in an estimated 25% of those 85 or older. There are also other forms of dementias, but the care of the dementia client, no matter what the type, is the same.

Since Alzheimer's disease is the most common form of irreversible dementia, let's take a closer look at what it does to a client and family members. There is no known effective treatment when the disease reaches its advanced stages. Sedatives are prescribed to lessen agitation and perhaps allow the client to rest. Remember always that clients deserve to be treated with dignity and every effort should be made to keep the client functioning at the highest level possible.

On the average, once Alzheimer's disease has been diagnosed, it may be 12 years until total degeneration occurs. It starts with simple memory lapses similar to that experienced by most individuals, Figure 9-9. All of us have put an item down and forgotten where we put it. At one time or another, we've started into another room to perform a task and suddenly been unable to remember why we went there. We have all parked in a large parking lot and forgotten where the car was. Everyone has had such episodes, and they are momentarily frightening. These memory lapses occur more and more often to those with Alzheimer's disease. As the disease progresses, they forget to pay bills, don't realize they have invited guests for dinner, arrive somewhere and don't know where they are or what they are doing there.

At this stage, Alzheimer clients become anxious, tense, nervous, and very uncomfortable. They can still perform all the basic activities of daily living, but should be supervised by family members in more complex social and daily situations. Financial supervision should be given and structured and supervised travel should be arranged. At this point it will probably be necessary to sew address labels in the client's clothing or provide identification bracelets in the event that the individual wanders off or becomes disoriented.

In the next stage, the client can no longer function independently. The family must take over financial affairs, shopping, and even choosing proper clothing. The client may forget to bathe and become careless about personal appearance. It may be that some clients are extremely fearful of being in water. Driving a car at this stage can be very dangerous. If a client continues to want to drive, it is up to the caregiver to prevent the client from driving. Crying episodes, hyperactivity, and sleep disturbances may arise at this time and around-the-clock care becomes necessary.

As the disease progresses, the client loses the ability to dress, feed himself or herself, bathe, and go to the toilet. This may first be noticed when the client puts on daytime clothing over pajamas or is unable to tie his shoes. The brain and body no longer function as a unit.

The caregiver can become extremely frustrated with the Alzheimer's disease client, Figure 9-10. The caregiver should try to imagine the frustration of the client, Figure 9-11. During the course of the illness the client sometimes seems fully aware, recognizes family and friends, and makes "sense." These "windows of reality" become smaller and smaller as the condition progresses. It finally reaches a point where the client becomes nonfunctioning and requires around-the-clock custodial care.

- Memory loss
- Difficulty in finding the right word to use in conversation
- Difficulty in speaking or understanding what is said
- Poor judgment and loss of logical reasoning ability
- Loss of mathematical ability
- Change in visual perceptions
- Inability to recognize faces or objects

Figure 9-9   Early signs of Alzheimer's disease

- Problem-solving ability
- Patience
- Caring attitude
- Empathy
- Ability to relate to clients and to family members

Figure 9-10 To care for the Alzheimer's disease client, the home health aide must possess these essential characteristics.

There is no point in trying to force the client to "make sense" or to become angry because the client is forgetful, personally sloppy, or appears to be "stubborn." What the home health aide and the family must understand is that the victim of Alzheimer's disease has no control over what is happening. They cannot force the client to admit to confusion. They must accept the person just as he or she is. The client must have the freedom to be old and confused. Don't make a tug-of-war over meals and sleeping time. All an aide can do is make sure the client is clean, fed, warm, and safe. Trying to reason with a client with Alzheimer's disease is similar to asking a client who has no legs to walk.

Alzheimer's clients must be weighed on a regular basis and any significant changes in weight—more than 5 lb either way in 6 weeks—must be reported. If a decrease in weight occurs, changes in eating patterns may be required, such as smaller, more frequent meals, or the use of finger food so that the client can self-feed. As the disease progresses, regular eating patterns may be refused by the client. They become confused with the knife, fork, or spoon and will have to be fed by the aide. If the client refuses to eat, it may be necessary to turn to finger foods, liquid nutritional supplements, or puréed foods.

Alzheimer clients may become incontinent. Regular toileting schedules can be set up when incontinence first occurs; this gives the client more dignity. Be sure the bathroom is clearly marked and the client knows where to go. Don't try to limit fluids because dehydration might occur. When incontinence cannot be controlled by medical treatment or regular toileting, products can be recommended by the nurse. Protective panties or briefs can protect the furniture and avoid embarrassment to the client. Adult disposable briefs can be used at night or for the bedbound client. There may come a time when an in-dwelling catheter will be required.

When working with the Alzheimer's client, a home health aide must remember to keep everything as simple and as unchanging as possible. It is difficult for the clients to adjust to change. They like doing the same things, at the same time, with the same individuals every day. They like to wear the same clothing every day and do the same activity every day. They also like an environment that is simple with few decorations. When serving meals, it is better to serve them one food at a time and not to give them choices. As the disease progresses, you will need to give simple instructions to them on simple tasks such as eating. Tell them to pick up the spoon, then place the spoon with the food in the mouth, chew the food, and then tell them to swallow the food. Then repeat the instructions over again.

Validation Therapy

Validation therapy or communication technique is used for moderately to severely disoriented clients with diagnosed dementia. The goal of the program is to increase self-esteem and validate feelings. The basic premise is that if the client wishes to remain in the past that should be allowed and no attempt be made to reorient the client. An example of this type of communication technique is: Molly, age 80, is telling the aide after her bath and shampoo, not to set her hair, as her mother will be coming to do it. You know her mother died 20 years ago. Instead of telling her that her mother is dead, which would make her feel bad, the aide asks her something about her mother such as her mother's name or her mother's hobbies. This will help relay a message to Molly that you are concerned with her wishes and will make her feel good about herself. Once clients have Alzheimer's or another type of dementia, the ability to reason with them has diminished. If you try to reason with them, you will cause them to become more agitated and more combative.

THE ALZHEIMER'S DISEASE	
CLIENT	**HHHA ACTIONS/RESPONSIBILITIES**
Has difficulty communicating . . .	• Approach the client with a friendly facial expression • Be calm • Stand in front of the client • Try to maintain eye contact; touch the client to attract attention or regain it • Speak in a low, calm, reassuring tone of voice (if the client has a hearing problem, follow the instructions in the care plan) • Speak slowly and give the client time to answer • If necessary, repeat the statement or question—do not change the wording • Keep the language simple and express only one idea at a time • Lead the client in answering if he can't find the right words—point to objects to provide cues • Do not become impatient

Has difficulty walking . .	• Provide a safe environment
	   —Remove scatter rugs
	   —Do not wax floors
	   —Pick up and put away objects the client may not see and thus trip over such as small footstools, doorstops, plants, pet toys, and dishes
	   —The client is to use only chairs with arms for support
	• Show the client what you want him/her to do and provide support
	• Do not hurry the client
	• If the client is unsteady and is using an aid (cane, walker) do not let the client out of your sight
	• Be sure the client's shoes fit properly
	• Always use proper body mechanics when helping the client
	• Keep the client walking as long as possible (as the disease progresses)

Experiences changes in eating patterns . . .	• Meals must be served at the same time each day • Meals should look appetizing and be served at the proper temperature • Give the client one course and one utensil at a time; do not give the client a choice of foods • If the client must be fed, do so slowly and cut the food into small pieces • Nutritious snacks should be kept on hand • Always encourage fluids • As the client loses the ability to chew, soft foods are introduced; a blender can be used to liquify foods • As the client loses the ability to use utensils, finger foods can be used • Maintain the diet plan included in the overall care plan

Figure 9-11   Guidelines for working with the Alzheimer's disease client (up to terminal stage) (Adapted from "How to Care for the Alzheimer's Disease Patient: A Comprehensive Training Manual for Homemaker-Home Health Aides" copyright 1986 by the Foundation for Hospice and Homecare)

Continued on the following page.

CLIENT	HHHA ACTIONS/RESPONSIBILITIES
Tends to wander . . .	• Weigh the client regularly (at least once weekly) and record the weight • Be sure the client wears an ID bracelet or necklace • Sew labels to each piece of clothing—labels should have the name of the client, address, and telephone number • Keep doors locked; make sure the bell or chimes are in working order • Place large print signs on doors—"DO NOT GO OUT," "TURN AROUND" • If the client insists on going out, do not argue—go with him (lock the door and take keys) • After a few minutes, suggest returning to the house to rest • Try to distract the client from leaving—try another activity you know the client enjoys (Alzheimer's Disease clients often respond to music) • Keep a recent photograph of the client at hand in the event the client does wander off and is not in the immediate neighborhood • If the client does leave unnoticed and you can't find him—call family members, police, and your agency
Experiences incontinence . . .	• Remember that the client cannot control this behavior • Do not scold or punish the client • Treat the client with respect • Set up a regular schedule for toileting and follow it • Encourage fluids as usual to prevent dehydration • Mark the bathroom clearly with a large print sign and a picture • Keep the client clean and dry; use simple washable clothing • Recognize the client's verbal and nonverbal language • Check the skin regularly for signs of irritation
Exhibits restlessness and agitation in late afternoon (sundown syndrome) . . .	• Decrease the level of activity in late afternoon to reduce potential stress • Play soft, soothing music • Do not try to reason the client out of this behavior—the client has no control over his/her actions • Do not institute sudden changes into the routine which will confuse and upset the client • Appointments and trips should be scheduled for morning and early afternoon • Do not restrain or argue with the client • Try to distract the client with quiet, simple activities • Make sure the client has adequate exercise during the day
Experiences sleeping disturbances . . .	• The client may exhibit less need for sleep • Try to keep the client active during the day so he/she will feel the need for sleep • The client should drink caffeine-free beverages • Establish a bedtime routine and follow it • Make sure the client is toileted before going to bed

Figure 9-11   (Continued)

CLIENT	HHHA ACTIONS/RESPONSIBILITIES
	• Make sure there are no loud noises; soft music may help • The client may feel more secure with a night-light • Keep a night-light on in the bathroom and keep the door open
Needs help with bathing and oral hygiene . . .	• Permit the client to do as much as he/she can—suggest steps if necessary • Ensure the client's safety when bathing—use hand holds, nonslip mats, tub seats, etc. • Organize all the necessary equipment before you bring the client to the bathroom • Stay calm and pleasant; try to make this a pleasurable experience for the client • Do not leave the client alone when bathing • Schedule bathing when the client is least agitated • Do not force the client into bathing; wait until the client is calm and try again • Give the client a sponge bath if all attempts to tub bathe or shower fail • Cleanliness must be maintained—consult with your supervisor if the client continues to exhibit resistance to bathing • If the client cannot provide oral care, even with coaxing, brush his/her teeth yourself or clean the dentures
Experiences delusions, hallucinations and inappropriate (catastrophic) reactions to normal events . . .	• What the client sees or hears is real to him • Do not argue or reason with the client • Maintain a calm, ordered environment • Reassure the client that you are there to protect him • If the client becomes violent, stay out of his/her way • If the client becomes agitated, try to distract him/her with an activity you know he/she likes; a small snack of a favorite food may distract him/her sufficiently to restore calm • If the client attacks you verbally, do not take it personally • The client may accuse you of stealing; again, do not take it personally
Exhibits improper sexual behavior . . .	• Remember, the client is confused and disoriented • Do not overreact—remain calm • Do not scold or argue with the client • Do not try to reason with the client • If the client undresses, provide a robe or redress him/her • If the client is in public when inappropriate behavior takes place, distract the client and remove him/her from the scene • Plan ahead ways you can distract the client • Provide appropriate touching to show that you care for and value the client

Figure 9-11 (Continued)

The majority of clients with dementia you will be caring for in the home will be in the middle stage of the disease. The following list will give you hints on how to care for them. Please remember that every client is unique and the following are only general suggestions on how to manage their care.

1. Don't argue or confront a client.
2. Promote frequent periods of rest.
3. Do not restrain unless absolutely necessary.
4. Limit intake of liquids that contain caffeine.
5. Play music for the client rather than have client watch television.
6. Keep decorations simple.
7. Serve meals at the same time every day.
8. Don't try to reason with the client.
9. If client becomes upset over something try to distract with something else.
10. Let client wander in a safe area.
11. Maintain eye contact with client.
12. Demonstrate how to do a task before letting the client do it.
13. Give very short simple instructions to client.
14. Limit outings to small groups of people. Avoid large crowds.
15. Involve client in activities that are simple— looking through a scrapbook or a magazine.
16. Keep the environment as unchanging as possible.
17. Have finger foods available during the day.
18. Take to bathroom at frequent intervals.

There are support groups in many communities. Family members can meet to share common problems and learn more about how to cope with their parent or relative as well as face up to their own feelings and fears.

In some areas there are special "day-care" centers where Alzheimer's disease clients can be taken for a few hours a day. These centers are well supervised and clients will often entertain each other by talking, playing cards, playing the piano, or singing. Since the progress of the disease is uneven, clients may have "good" days or weeks when they function reasonably well at such centers. On the other hand, if the group activities have a bad effect on the client and make him or her more agitated or fearful, the activity should be stopped immediately.

The home health aide helps the family members by providing respite care. That is, while the home health aide provides care, the family may take advantage of these few hours to take care of errands or just experience the freedom from caregiving responsibilities.

Reality Orientation

Activities for clients with mental impairments should be maintained at as normal a level as possible. It may be helpful to provide simple memory aids to assist the client in day-to-day living: a prominent calendar, lists of daily tasks, written reminders about routine safety measures, and other "memory joggers." This process if know as **reality orientation.**

A legend attributed to the Native Americans states that, to understand how another person feels, you should walk a mile in that person's "moccasins." Too often, people do not stop to think about how other people feel and often expect others to react as they would. As people grow older, their normal response time slows down. This does not make them less worthwhile as individuals. They know they do not respond as quickly, think as fast, or move as fast as they once did. This is frightening to the elderly and they also resent it.

The elderly may often seem to dwell in the past. They are sometimes confused and may

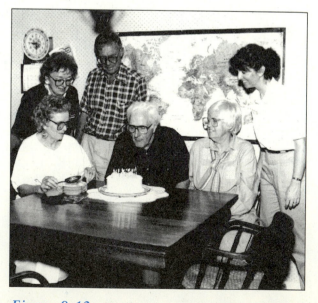

Figure 9-12   Birthday celebrations are very important family gatherings at any age.

think a grandchild is their son or daughter. They may forget what day it is or what task they are doing. Forgetting what they are doing can be dangerous. Suppose an older person puts the teakettle filled with water on the stove to heat and then goes to another room and forgets about it. The teakettle could boil dry and explode, or the gas stove pilot light could be extinguished causing gas fumes to fill the home.

Someone once said, "We can foresee the needs and the problems of aging, but we cannot forefeel them." Therefore, we need imagination, much patience, kindness, and understanding in order to give the elderly the service and care which really meets their needs, Figure 9-12.

SUMMARY

....

- Each stage of life offers its own rewards and has its own special problems.
- As the body ages, it is slower to return to wellness after injury or illness.
- Depression, loss of self-esteem, loneliness, anxiety, and boredom can become more common as elderly persons face the process of aging and illness.
- The deaths of relatives and friends, as well as other crises, add to the problems of old age.

- The home health aide must draw on many areas of learning in order to provide the care needed for each client.
- The home health aide must keep in mind that clients with dementing conditions cannot be cured, but special techniques can help minimize symptoms and make their care more manageable.

REVIEW

1. Name two emotional problems that the elderly may have to deal with.
2. What are the characteristics of Alzheimer's disease?
3. Name three memory aids used to help orient elderly clients.
4. Lists four common ailments of older clients.
5. Explain validation therapy.
6. List three common problems of clients who are nonambulatory.
7. Which of the following is not associated with the aging process?
   a. increased size of muscles
   b. brittle bones
   c. stiff and swollen joints
   d. decreased strength
8. The rate of aging in an individual is influenced by:
   a. nutrition and diet
   b. environment
   c. genetic factors
   d. all of the above
9. Which of the following changes would you not expect to occur in the elderly?
   a. facial hair on female's face
   b. decreased sense of taste
   c. decreased sense of pain
   d. all of the above are to be expected in the elderly

10. Which of the following are possible signs of a stroke in a client?
    a. numbness of face and arm
    b. difficulty in speaking
    c. dizziness
    d. paralysis of one half of the body
    e. all are correct

11. Signs of emphysema are:
    a. productive nagging cough
    b. red color to face
    c. pain in all extremities
    d. heartburn
    e. all are correct

12. In the last stage of Alzheimer's disease the client:
    a. may need to be fed
    b. may not recognize family members
    c. may have no control of bowels and bladder
    d. all of the above

Section 4

Promoting Health and Understanding Illness

Units

10   Mental Health

11   Nutritional Guidelines

12   Principles of Safety and Body Mechanics

13   Understanding Illness

14   Preventing the Spread of Disease

15   Caring for the Client with an Infectious Disease

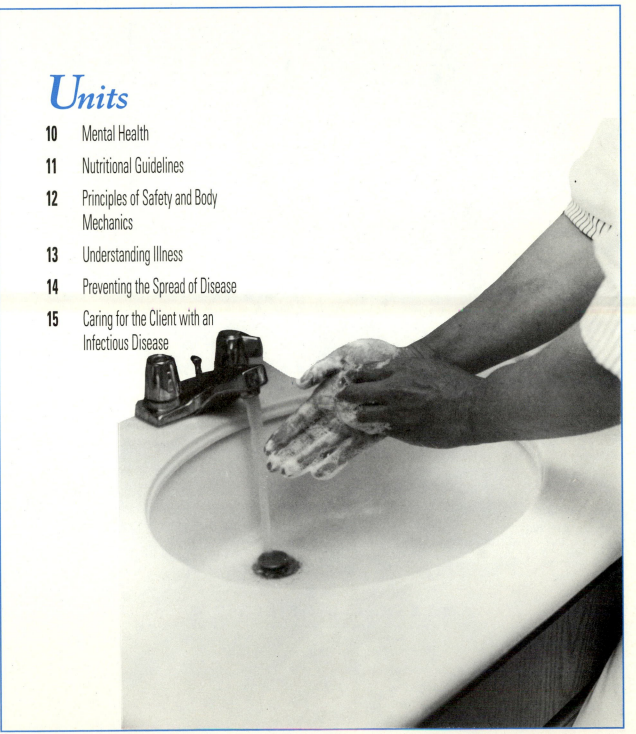

Unit **10** Mental Health

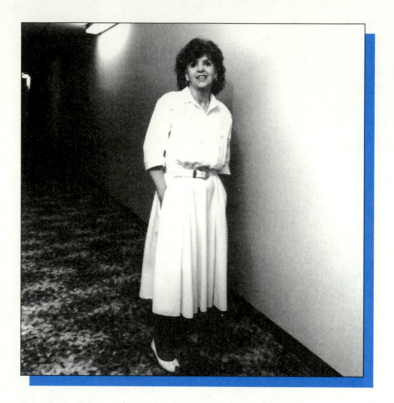

KEY TERMS

adjustment
anxiety
compensation
defense mechanism
denial
displacement

emotion
external stimulus
fantasizing
internal stimulus
mental illness
phobia

projection
psychology
rationalization
wellness
withdrawal

LEARNING OBJECTIVES

After studying this unit, you should be able to:

- Identify an example of a defense mechanism.
- Identify several common emotions.
- Identify how a physical response can result from an emotional reaction.

- Define psychology, mental health, and adjustments.
- Differentiate between external and internal stimuli.

Psychology is the science of human behavior. It is the study of the way the mind works and how emotions and feelings affect human behavior. Just as no two bodies are exactly alike, no two minds react in the same way. **Adjustment** is the change a person makes in behavior in order to deal with a situation. A person is mentally healthy if he or she can see reality as it is, respond to its challenges, and develop a reasonable strategy for living. A mentally healthy person has compassion or feelings for other people. A mentally healthy person can accept limitations and possibilities of reality. For example, an 80-year-old, mentally healthy person, knows he cannot run as fast as he could at the age of 25 and accepts the change in his capabilities. When chronic illness occurs, a well-adjusted person may feel stressed, even overwhelmed at times. A well-adjusted person is able to handle the daily problems of living, taking bad times in stride and coping with crises. The well-adjusted person has a good self-image and can be flexible when meeting new or difficult obstacles. It takes less time for a well-adjusted person to recover from a difficult situation. People can adjust easily to some situations and not to others. A person does not have to be strong all the time. The mentally healthy person is able to make life work in a way that is both personally and socially acceptable.

To understand basic psychology it is necessary to review the nervous system. The brain acts as the body's communication center. All messages (called stimuli) from the five senses are carried to the brain where they are received and acted on. There are both internal and external stimuli. Example: The stomach is empty so the nerve endings in the stomach send a message to the brain. The brain translates the impulses, and the individual thinks, "I'm hungry," and looks for food. This is an **internal stimulus.** On the other hand, on entering a room where food is being cooked, a person might smell a pleasant aroma or see an attractive piece of fruit. The sight and smell of the food can stimulate the nerve endings and the person might think, "I'm hungry," and eat the food even though it was not mealtime. This is an **external stimulus.**

Internal stimuli cause automatic or unconscious reactions within the body. External stimuli come from outside the body and bring about a conscious reaction. Psychology relates to both internal and external stimuli. In some conditions, chemical imbalances within the body or brain and nerve cell damage can cause changes in behavior. In other cases, environmental conditions may have a direct effect on emotional health.

Understanding Emotions

Emotions are common to all people and are neither good nor bad. An **emotion** is a strong generalized feeling. The way a person shows emotion may be healthy or unhealthy. There is a wide range of acceptable levels of emotional behavior. Well-adjusted people most often use emotions in a healthy way to serve their purposes; they can control emotions so as not to harm themselves or others. Fear, anger, and grief are necessary to all people. Those who claim that they "never lose their temper" or have "never been afraid" or "do not feel grief" are fooling themselves. Whether emotional behavior is healthy depends on where and how the person expresses these emotions. Anger and happiness can be healthy reactions in some situations while not in others.

Emotions may cause physical reactions. Anger and fear sometimes cause the heart to beat faster, respirations to increase, and chemical changes to take place within the body. The mouth may become dry, the person may become pale and start to shake. Such physical changes are common and usually of short duration. Emotions can trigger the release of hormones and produce unusual results. For example, a 34-year-old man was traveling in an airplane that crashed. The plane burst into flames and hundreds of people were trapped inside. This man, who was injured himself, pulled ten individuals from the plane before he collapsed. Despite his upset mental and physical state, his body was able to function at an unusually high level.

Individuals develop a pattern of emotional response. This may be a hereditary characteris-

PHYSICAL STAGE	YEAR OF OCCURRENCE	TASKS TO BE MASTERED
Oral-sensory	Birth–1 year (Infant)	To learn to trust (Trust)
Muscular-anal	1–3 years (Toddler)	To recognize self as an independent being from mother (Autonomy)
Locomotor	3–5 years (Preschool years)	To recognize self as a family member (Initiative)
Latency	6–11 years (School-age years)	To demonstrate physical and mental skills abilities (Industry)
Adolescence	12–18 years	To develop a sense of individuality as a sexual human being (Identity)
Young Adulthood	19–35 years	To establish intimate personal relationships with a mate (Intimacy)
Adulthood	35–50 years	To live a satisfying and productive life (Generativity)
Maturity	50+ years	To review life's events and examine how they have influenced the development of a unique individual (Ego integrity)

Figure 10-1   Tasks of personality development according to the stages defined by Erikson (From Hegner and Caldwell, *Nursing Assistant, A Nursing Process Approach,* 6E, copyright 1992 by Delmar Publishers Inc.)

tic. Some babies, for instance, seem calmer and happier than others. The social environment of a family determines whether a baby's early experiences are pleasant or unpleasant. As years pass, the child's successes and failures in daily life influence the child's emotional patterns. The child who is healthy and who is given tender, loving attention from birth has a good chance of growing up to be well adjusted. The stages of personality development are listed in Figure 10-1.

The type of emotion (pleasant or unpleasant) that a person feels most of the time often determines disposition. A disposition is the usual mood of an individual. An optimistic person probably feels more pleasant emotions and, therefore, has a brighter outlook than a pessimist. The aide who has a cheerful outlook may transfer this pleasant mood to the client. Words, tone of voice, actions and facial expression show how a person looks at life. This often exposes the person's inner feelings. Pessimists may be just as well adjusted as optimists but their viewpoints differ.

People have mood changes or emotional cycles. It is normal to feel high or low from time to time. In some people, this mood swing is more noticeable than in others. The well-adjusted person is able to function in both highs and lows. A less stable person has extremes of highs and lows. Emotional cycles can be affected by the time of day or season of the year or the weather. For example, some people are happiest and function best early in the day. Others, who are sometimes called "night people," are more alert in the evening hours. Many people also allow the seasons to affect their feelings. Some dislike the winter and feel depressed; others dislike the summer months.

Mentally healthy people learn to make their emotions work for them. One can deal with unhealthy emotions in a positive way. When a home health aide gets angry with a client, the aide cannot have a tantrum. Strong outbursts of emotion are not acceptable while on duty. Sometimes anger must be expressed, but it should be done in a way which is constructive. A home health aide must not only deal with her own emotional needs, but must also be aware of the emotional needs and reactions of the client. This requires a great deal of self-control and self-discipline. The home health aide must be sensitive to the emotions of the client. Clients are often frightened and worried about their health. The home health aide must be kind and understanding and think of the client's needs first. Illness can cause temporary changes in the client's personality. This often requires the client to make adjustments. It takes time to accept the physical changes caused by a disease. The home health aide must be willing to allow clients to express their emotions. The well-adjusted aide will be able to endure the client's emotional storms without becoming a part of them, Figure 10-2.

Defense Mechanisms

Defense mechanisms are specific techniques used to protect oneself from unpleasantness, shame, anxiety or loss of self-esteem. Some are common and are unknowingly used when a person feels uncomfortable.

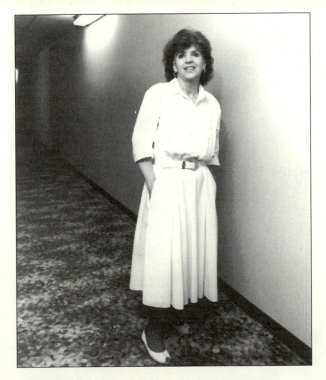

Figure 10-2   A well-adjusted aide will listen to the client's family problems but will not get involved in family disagreements.

Rationalization is the use of excuses to substitute for the real reasons behind an action. An example of this would be a girl trying out for a lead in the school play and not being accepted. She might say, "I had a headache and just couldn't do my best at the tryouts."

Projection is blaming someone else to cover up personal failure. The child who fails a math test might say, "The teacher hates me. That's why I failed."

Displacement is taking anger or frustration out on someone else. A woman might be very angry at her husband but too afraid to let it show. Instead, she exhibits her anger with one of her children by overreacting to a minor incident or by scolding the child.

Fantasizing or daydreaming is a way of avoiding reality. A woman who is 30 pounds overweight and on a weight-reducing diet might fantasize that she won a beauty contest. If the fantasy helped her stay on the diet, it could have positive effects. However, fantasies often just delay action needed to make a change.

Withdrawal or isolation is removing oneself physically from an uncomfortable or frightening situation. Children who hear and see their parents fight might go to their room and close the door.

Denial is the defense mechanism used to avoid facing the truth. Glen Cunningham, the first man in history to run the mile in four minutes, was severely burned and was told by doctors that he would never walk again. He refused to believe the doctors—he denied being severely injured. In this case, denial was a positive reaction and the man overcame hardships to reach success. However, if a child lost a parent in an accident and denied the truth, it could cause deep psychological problems.

Compensation is making up for a weakness by becoming very good in some other area. The physically weak person may become a good student to compensate for not being good in sports.

Most people are anxious and concerned from time to time. **Anxiety** is an unpleasant emotional or psychological state of constant fear or apprehension. Anxiety can be severe and cause a person to stop functioning. There are people who are afraid to board an air-

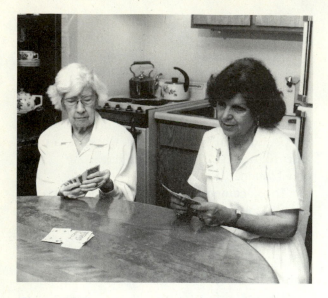

Figure 10-3 A home health aide playing cards with her client. Emotional and social needs of the client are very important.

plane. They have such a **phobia** (fear) that they refuse to go near a plane. Others may be uncomfortable about flying but decide to fly despite their fear.

Another way of coping with anxieties is to use humor. It is a positive way of dealing with negative feelings without causing distress. At times it is better to laugh at a mistake than to take it too seriously.

The home health aide does have to make many adjustments throughout the day. There are always new problems that arise and choices to be made. Well-adjusted people accept the fact that they will make errors of judgment. Making mistakes is part of life. Adjustments come about easier when people accept that they are not perfect. They learn to do the best they can with what they have, Figure 10-3.

Stress

The "stress response" is a normal response felt by all individuals when demands are made on the body. It is a healthy response and helps the body resist and avoid real physical danger. As a home health aide you will be under different types of stress—some physical and some mental. Ongoing stress affects the aide's ability to respond to new daily stressors. Each person has a breaking point with stress. A series of too-rapid or too many changes can push an aide to a

breaking point. That is why it's important to have some individual plan to reduce stress. Some examples of stress relievers are: regularly exercising, thinking and talking positively, avoiding alcoholic beverages, expressing your inner feelings to another individual, meditating, being nice to yourself and rewarding yourself with a new pair of shoes or favorite tape, balancing work with play, enjoying hobbies such as knitting or sewing, and eating proper foods.

Effects of Emotions on Health

Wellness means different things to different people; people feel better on some days than on others. Temporary discomforts are not necessarily a health hazard or danger. Life can be compared to a roller coaster ride—it has its ups and downs. After a very hard day at work, an argument with a close friend, or the death of a loved one, people may feel unwell. A tension headache caused by an emotional crisis can make a person feel ill for a short time. When the upset is resolved, the person forgets the pain and feels well again. Persons who are acutely or chronically ill also have good and bad days. To a great extent these changes are related to their emotional outlook. When routines have gone smoothly or when a special friend has called or visited, a person may feel very well despite physical problems. On a day when the home health aide comes late and is in a bad mood, the client may complain of feeling much worse than the physical condition warrants.

No two people react the same to external stimuli. The stress situation causing one person to feel unwell may have no effect on another person. People react to personal crisis in their own way. It has been proven that an emotionally depressed person is more likely to catch a cold or develop a physical disorder. Wellness may be described as freedom from discomfort—both physical and mental. Emotional health may strongly influence a person's state of wellness.

Depression is an unusual feeling of sadness and often hopelessness. Signs that a client may be depressed are no interest in activities, withdrawal from others, loss of appetite, poor personal appearance, loss of interest in pleasurable activities, increase or decrease in sleep, inability to make decisions, and conversation centering around one's failures in life. Another sign of depression is when a client may think and also talk about suicide. A home health aide should report to the supervisor if the client does give clues to the aide that he or she is suicidal. One never knows if the client is serious or not. Signs that the client may be thinking of suicide are: giving away favorite items; talking about "killing" oneself; talking about death and that they might not be around very long; obtaining a weapon such as a gun, strong rope, or a collection of pills; and a strong interest in life insurance policies or changing their wills.

Mental illness and developmental disabilities have been handled in many different ways over the years. **Mental illness** refers to those who are unable to cope with life because of severe emotional problems and cannot act normally.

At one time, those who were mentally ill were regarded as being possessed of the devil and were greatly feared. In Medieval England, the mentally ill were thrown into a prison-like hospital. They were literally discarded, ignored, and forced to survive under impossible conditions. They were treated with less care than animals on a farm. The screaming, crying, and yelling of these poor creatures caused the London mental institution's nickname, Bedlam, to mean a place of noisy confusion.

Developmentally disabled children were sometimes hidden away in the family attic or basement because the family was ashamed of them. Gradually, however, society came to realize that the mentally ill and developmentally disabled are human beings with the same physical and emotional needs as the general population. Special institutions were opened where families could take their severely retarded or emotionally disturbed relatives.

Within the past 20 years, many of these institutions have been closed. Some "half-way houses" were started so that the mentally ill could live with others who were being returned to the "real world." In these houses they lived under the supervision of psychiatrists, psychologists, and house supervisors.

Some of these "half-way houses" have proven successful. However, the majority of the mentally ill were simply released in the hope that family members would provide shelter and take care of them. Many have ended up on the street.

Group homes have also been set up for the developmentally disabled so that they can live in a family-like situation and work together to provide for their common needs. However, there are not enough half-way houses or group homes.

A great many emotionally ill and developmentally disabled individuals live with their families. When caring for such persons, an aide must be well briefed by the supervisor and must follow instructions very carefully.

Several in-service courses should be taken before an aide works with the mentally ill or with a developmentally disabled individual.

SUMMARY

....

- The aide should develop an awareness of the ways in which emotions affect behavior.
- Psychology is concerned with making reasonable adjustments. The human body and mind are both able to adapt to new situations.
- A home health aide's job is important in helping a client adapt both physically and mentally by giving proper care.
- Although each individual is different, there are reasonable limits of acceptable behavior for all.
- Each person experiences the same emotions—fear, anger, joy, sorrow, contentment, pleasure. However, people may show their emotions in different ways. As long as emotional responses are within reasonable limits they are acceptable. In other words, a person's emotional responses should not cause personal harm or injury to others. Mood swings are normal to all persons.
- The aide should keep personal emotions in balance when caring for a client. At the same time the aide must recognize the emotional needs of the client.

REVIEW

1. List four common emotional reactions.

2. What is the difference between an internal stimulus and an external stimulus?

3. Explain how a physical response can result from an emotional reaction.

4. Name five defense mechanisms. Give an example of each.

5. Define mental health and adjustment.

6. Match Column I with Column II (mental mechanisms)

    Column I

    ___1. rationalization
    ___2. fantasizing
    ___3. compensation
    ___4. displacement
    ___5. withdrawal

    Column II

    a. removing oneself physically from a situation
    b. using excuses to substitute for the real reasons behind an action
    c. making up for a weakness by becoming very good in some other area
    d. taking anger out on someone else
    e. daydreaming

7. Characteristics of a mentally healthy person are:
    a. sees reality as it is
    b. responds to change
    c. sets reasonable strategies for living
    e. all are correct

8. Group homes have been set up for the developmentally disabled so that they can live in a family-like situation.
    a. true
    b. false

9. No two individuals react the same to a stressful situation.
    a. true
    b. false

10. An anxiety is an unpleasant emotional state of constant fear.
    a. true
    b. false

Unit **11** Nutritional Guidelines

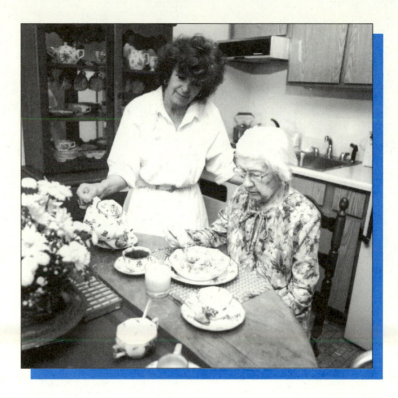

KEY TERMS
....

bland diet

calorie-controlled diet

clear liquid diet

degenerative disease

diabetic diet

diuretic

empty calorie

food pyramid

full-liquid diet

high-bulk diet

low-residue diet

low-sodium diet

malnutrition

Meals on Wheels

nutrition

soft diet

vegetarian

LEARNING OBJECTIVES
....

After studying this unit, you should be able to:

- List the six food groups on the food guide pyramid.
- Identify the special diets used for at least five medical conditions.
- Name six things to keep in mind when planning and preparing meals.

- Name eight special diets that may be prescribed for your client, and describe the types of foods that are usually permitted for each.
- Identify the special diet a client with acquired immunodeficiency syndrome (AIDS) would require.

Nutrition is the sum of a combination of processes by which the body receives and uses food and nutrients. The body needs food for energy, cell growth, and to feel comfortable and satisfied. The single most important use of food is to provide proper nutrition to the body.

Since the field of nutrition is so very complex, it is recommended that home health aides take in-service courses to learn more about this vital health area. One of the most rapidly growing fields in health care is nutrition. Hospitals have nutritionists on staff as do other health care facilities such as nursing homes. It is becoming a common practice for hospitals and nursing homes to provide a nutritionally sound plan to patients as part of their discharge instructions. The nutritionist takes into account the age, weight, sex, and medical condition of the patient when setting up a food plan. It is the responsibility of the home health aide to follow this plan.

Some dietitians recommend that the average diet consist of the following:

30% fat
15% protein
10% simple sugars (such as fruits)
45% complex carbohydrates

They further suggest that the amount of fiber, found in whole grains, leafy vegetables, fruits, beans, and peas, be increased in the daily diet. It is thought that fiber flushes out food wastes and may help to prevent cancer of the colon.

In addition, these nutritionists feel that the average individual should have a regular exercise program. A half-hour walk three times a week would be beneficial to keep the body trim. Nutritional therapists know that individual diets must take into account a person's ethnic background and food likes and dislikes. Also to be considered is any physical condition that prevents a client from eating certain foods and requires certain foods as part of the care plan.

Food Guide Pyramid

The foods recommended in the food pyramid are the fruit group; vegetable group; milk, yogurt, and cheese group; bread, cereal, and rice group; meat, poultry, and fish group; and the fats, oils, and sweets group. Each individual needs the nutrients that can only come from a proper balance of the **food pyramid,** Figure 11-1.

Dietary Guidelines for Americans*

- Eat a variety of foods.
- Maintain healthy weight.
- Choose a diet low in fat, saturated fat, and cholesterol.
- Choose a diet with plenty of vegetables, fruits, and grain products.
- Use sugars only in moderation.
- Use salt and sodium only in moderation.
- If you drink alcoholic beverages, do so in moderation.

These guidelines call for moderation—avoiding extremes in diet. Both eating too much and eating too little can be harmful. Also, be cautious of diets based on the belief that a food or supplement alone can cure or prevent disease.

Your good health may depend on your learning more about yourself. Are you at your healthy weight? Are your blood pressure and your blood cholesterol levels too high? If so, diet or medicine your doctor prescribes may

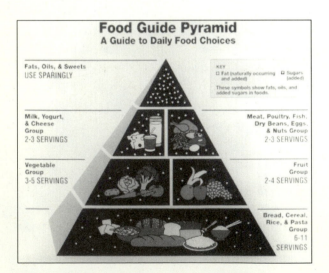

Figure 11-1   Food pyramid—a guide to daily food choices

*Courtesy of U.S. Department of Agriculture

help reduce them. Generally, the sooner a problem is found, the easier it is to treat.

The foods Americans have to choose from are varied, plentiful, and safe to eat. These guidelines can help you choose a diet that is both healthful and enjoyable.

Eat a Variety of Foods*

You need more than 40 different nutrients for good health. Essential nutrients include vitamins, minerals, amino acids from protein, certain fatty acids from fat, and sources of calories (protein, carbohydrates, and fat).

These nutrients should come from a variety of foods, not from a few highly fortified foods or supplements. Any food that supplies calories and nutrients can be part of a nutritious diet. The content of the total diet over a day or more is what counts.

Many foods are good sources of several nutrients. For example, vegetables and fruits are important for vitamins A and C, folic acid, minerals, and fiber. Breads and cereals supply B vitamins, iron, and protein; whole-grain types are also good sources of fiber. Milk provides protein, B vitamins, vitamins A and D, calcium, and phosphorus. Meat, poultry, and fish provide protein, B vitamins, iron, and zinc.

No single food can supply all nutrients in the amounts you need. For example, milk supplies calcium but little iron; meat supplies iron but little calcium. To have a nutritious diet, you must eat a variety of foods.

One way to ensure variety—and with it, an enjoyable and nutritious diet—is to choose foods each day from five major food groups. Individuals who do not eat foods from one or more of the food groups may want to contact a dietitian for help in planning how to meet nutritional needs.

A Daily Food Guide*

Eat a variety of foods daily, choosing different foods from each group. Most people should have at least the lower number of servings suggested from each food group. Some people may need more because of their body size and activity level. Young children should have a variety of foods but may need small servings.

*Courtesy of U.S. Department of Agriculture

Food Group	Suggested Servings
Vegetables	3–5 servings
Fruits	2–4 servings
Breads, cereals, rice, and pasta	6–11 servings
Milk, yogurt, and cheese	2–3 servings
Meats, poultry, fish, dry beans and peas, eggs, and nuts	2–3 servings

People who are inactive or are trying to lose weight may eat little food. They need to take special care to choose lower calorie, nutrient-rich foods from the five major food groups. They also need to eat less of foods high in calories and low in essential nutrients, such as fats and oils, sugars, and alcoholic beverages.

Diets of some groups of people are notably low in some nutrients. Many women and adolescent girls need to eat more calcium-rich foods, such as milk and milk products, to get the calcium they need for healthy bones throughout life. Young children, teenage girls, and women of childbearing age must take care to eat enough iron-rich foods such as lean meats; dry beans; and whole-grain and iron-enriched breads, cereals, and other grain products.

Supplements of some nutrients taken regularly in large amounts can be harmful. Vitamin and mineral supplements at or below the Recommended Dietary Allowances (RDA) are safe, but are rarely needed if you eat a variety of foods. Here are exceptions in which your doctor may recommend a supplement:

- Pregnant women often need an iron supplement. Some other women in their childbearing years may also need an iron supplement to help replace iron lost in menstrual bleeding.
- Certain women who are pregnant or breast-feeding may need a supplement to meet their increased requirements for some nutrients.
- People who are unable to be active and eat little food may need supplements.
- People, especially older people, who take medicines that interact with nutrients may need supplements.

Choose a Diet Low in Fat, Saturated Fat, and Cholesterol*

Most health authorities recommend an American diet with less fat, saturated fat, and cholesterol. Populations like ours with diets high in fat have more obesity and certain types of cancer. The higher levels of saturated fat and cholesterol in our diets are linked to our increased risk for heart disease.

A diet low in fat makes it easier for you to include the variety of foods you need for nutrients without exceeding your calorie needs because fat contains over twice the calories of an equal amount of carbohydrates or protein.

A diet low in saturated fat and cholesterol can help maintain a desirable level of blood cholesterol. For adults this level is below 200 mg/dL. As blood cholesterol increases above this level, greater risk for heart disease occurs. Risk can also be increased by high blood pressure, cigarette smoking, diabetes, a family history of premature heart disease, obesity, and being a male.

The way diet affects blood cholesterol varies among individuals. However, the blood cholesterol level does increase in most people when they eat a diet high in saturated fat and cholesterol and excessive in calories. Of these, dietary saturated fat has the greatest effect; dietary cholesterol has less.

Suggested goals for fats in American diets are as follows:

Total Fat. An amount that provides 30% or less of calories is suggested. Thus, the upper limit on the grams of fat in your diet depends on the calories you need. For example, at 2000 calories per day, your suggested upper limit is 600 calories from fat (2000 × .30). This is equal to 67 grams of fat (600 ÷ 9, the number of calories each gram of fat provides). The grams of fat in some foods are shown in the display.

Saturated Fat. An amount that provides less than 10% of calories (less than 22 grams at 2000 calories per day) is suggested. All fats contain both saturated and unsaturated fat (fatty acids). The fats in animal products are the main sources of saturated fat in most diets, with tropical oils (coconut, palm kernel, and palm oils) and hydrogenated fats providing smaller amounts.

Cholesterol. Animal products are the source of all dietary cholesterol. Eating less fat from animal sources will help lower cholesterol as well as total fat and saturated fat in your diet.

These goals for fats are not for children under 2 years, who have special dietary needs. As children begin to eat with the family, usually at about 2 years of age or older, they should be encouraged to choose diets that are lower in fat and saturated fat and that provide the calories and nutrients they need for normal growth. Older children and adults with established food habits may need to change their diets gradually toward the goals.

These goals for fats apply to the diet over several days, not to a single meal or food. Some foods that contain fat, saturated fat, and cholesterol, such as meats, milk, cheese, and eggs, also contain high-quality protein and are our best sources of certain vitamins and minerals. Low-fat choices of these foods are lean meat and low-fat milk and cheeses.

For a Diet Low in Fat, Saturated Fat, and Cholesterol*

Fats and oils
- Use fats and oils sparingly in cooking.
- Use small amounts of salad dressings and spreads, such as butter, margarine, and mayonnaise. One tablespoon of most of these spreads provides 10 to 11 g fat.
- Choose liquid vegetable oils most often because they are lower in saturated fat.
- Check labels on foods to see how much fat and saturated fat are in a serving.

Meat, poultry, fish, dry beans, and eggs
- Have 2 or 3 servings, with a daily total of about 6 oz. Three oz of cooked lean beef or chicken without skin—the size of a deck of cards—provides about 6 g fat.
- Trim fat from meat; take skin off poultry.
- Have cooked dry beans and peas instead of meat occasionally.
- Moderate the use of egg yolks and organ meats.

*Courtesy of U.S. Department of Agriculture

Milk and milk products
- Have 2 or 3 servings daily. (Count as a serving: 1 cup of milk or yogurt or about $1\frac{1}{2}$ oz of cheese.)
- Choose skim or low-fat milk and fat-free or low-fat yogurt and cheese most of the time. One cup of skim milk has only a trace of fat, 1 cup of 2% milk has 5 g fat, and 1 cup of whole milk has 8 g fat.

Developing Good Eating Habits

Is it possible to look at a person and tell whether that person's body is well nourished? A well-nourished person usually has shiny hair, clear skin, good posture, and firm flesh. The person also appears alert and energetic. To be well nourished, people must select the correct foods. Lower forms of animals seem to have a natural body wisdom. They eat only those foods that are good for them and they do not overeat. People, however, have so many foods to choose from that they often make mistakes.

Often people living alone do not get the proper nourishment. They may not have the desire to eat, or they may not have the knowledge or energy to prepare nutritious meals.

Empty Calorie Foods

Favorite foods are often oversalted, oversweetened, or high in fat content. Examples of such favorite foods are potato chips, candy, soda, and french fries. Teenagers especially have a tendency to eat these foods. In everyday language, these foods are called junk foods but the proper descriptive name for them is **empty calorie** foods or hollow calorie foods. Empty calorie foods are high in carbohydrates and fats; they are very low in proteins, minerals, and vitamins.

WORD	DEFINITION	EXAMPLES
Carbohydrates	Sugars or starches which are made up of carbon, hydrogen, and oxygen and deliver quick energy to the body.	Found in grains, potatoes, corn, fruits, and sweets
Proteins	Compounds composed of amino acids needed for growth and tissue repair.	Found in meats, fish, milk, eggs, nuts, dried beans
Fats	Oily substances made up of glycerin and fatty acids, which provide stored energy to the body, and protect vital organs.	Present in meats, butter, milk, peanuts
Minerals	Inorganic elements essential in tissue building and in regulation of body fluids.	Iron, calcium, sodium, and zinc
Vitamins	Organic substances vital to certain metabolic functions and needed to prevent deficiency disease. Vitamins are needed only in small amounts but must be obtained from food sources since they are not produced in the body.	Vitamins A, C, B_{12}
Water	A tasteless, odorless liquid compound of hydrogen and oxygen necessary in the digestive process and to regulate body processes.	
Calorie	A measure of heat produced by the body when using a specific portion of food.	
Metabolism	Sum total of processes needed for the breakdown of food and absorption of nutrients.	

Figure 11-2   Knowing terms used in nutrition helps us to understand how the body uses food.

Overindulgence in these empty calorie foods leads to poor nutrition.

Refer to Figures 11-2 and 11-3. Figure 11-2 provides definitions of important nutritional terms. Knowing these terms will help you understand the value of meal planning for a balanced diet. Figure 11-3 lists vitamins, their imporant food sources, and their functions.

Overeating

Another dietary problem is overeating. Normally, the body can only burn or use a certain number of calories every day. Those calories that are not used are turned into fat tissue. In the United States it has been estimated that as much as 60% of the population is 10 lb or more overweight. Excess weight forces the heart to work harder and is a major cause of heart disease.

Degenerative Diseases

Many degenerative diseases can be traced directly to the kinds and amounts of food eaten.

Degenerative diseases cause tissues or organs to weaken and become diseased. Included in this category are diabetes and arteriosclerosis. The most common of all degenerative diseases is tooth decay. Strong, healthy teeth are important for the proper digestion of food. Eating too much sugar is a main cause of tooth decay.

Malnutrition

Malnutrition is poor nourishment, which most often occurs when the body does not get a full, balanced diet. Early signs of malnutrition include muscle weakness and a constant feeling of tiredness or fatigue. Later symptoms include a distended or swollen abdomen, a dull film over the eyes, hair that is dry and brittle, and bones that become deformed. A state of malnutrition may occur after a person has gone on a severe weight-reducing diet. This condition is most often found among teenage girls who diet. After a time the lack of nutrients causes serious body fluid imbalances. It can reach a

VITAMINS	BEST SOURCES	FUNCTIONS
Fat-Soluble Vitamins		
Vitamin A	Vegetables (dark green and deep yellow) Fish liver oils Liver Egg yolk Fruits (yellow)	Essential for: Growth Health of eyes Structure and functioning of the cells of the skin and mucous membranes
Vitamin D	Sunshine Fish liver oil Milk (irradiated) Egg yolk Liver	Essential for: Growth Regulating calcium and phosphorus metabolism Building and maintaining normal bones and teeth
Vitamin E	Wheat germ and wheat germ oils Vegetable oils Margarine Legumes Nuts Dark green, leafy vegetables	Not conclusively defined in humans; may affect the red blood cells Recommended for middle-aged women as it helps in the metabolism of calcium
Vitamin K	Spinach Kale Cabbage Cauliflower Pork liver	Essential for: Normal clotting of blood

Figure 11-3   Many foods contain more than one vitamin.

VITAMINS	BEST SOURCES	FUNCTIONS
Water-Soluble Vitamins		
Vitamin C (Ascorbic acid)	Citrus fruits, pineapple Melons and berries Tomatoes Broccoli Green peppers	Essential for: Maintaining strength of blood vessels Health of the teeth and gums Aids in wound healing
Thiamine (B$_1$)	Wheat germ Lean pork Yeast Legumes Whole grain and enriched cereal products Liver, other organ meats	Essential for: Carbohydrate metabolism Healthy appetite Functioning of nerves
Riboflavin (B$_2$)	Milk, cheese Enriched bread and cereals Yeast Green, leafy vegetables Eggs Liver, kidney, heart	Essential for: Health of skin, eyes and mouth Carbohydrate, fat, and protein metabolism
Niacin (Nicotinic acid)	Meats (especially organ meats) Poultry and fish Yeast Enriched breads and cereals Peanuts	Essential for: Prevention of pellagra Carbohydrate, fat, and protein metabolism
Vitamin B$_6$ (Pyridoxine)	Wheat germ Liver and kidney Meats Whole grain cereals Soybeans and peanuts	Essential for: Metabolism of proteins
Pantothenic Acid	Heart, liver, kidney Eggs Peanuts Whole grain cereals	Aids various steps in metabolism
Biotin	Organ meats Yeast Mushrooms Peanuts	Aids various steps in metabolism
Vitamin B$_{12}$ (Cobalamin)	Liver, kidney Muscle meats Milk, cheese Eggs	Essential for: Metabolism Healthy red blood cells Treatment of pernicious anemia
Folacin (Folic acid)	Dark green, leafy vegetables Liver, kidney Yeast	Essential for: The blood-forming system Metabolism

Figure 11-3   *(Continued)*

point that the dieter is unable to eat at all, and the body rejects all foods. It may be necessary to hospitalize the person and provide liquid nourishment through intravenous feedings. A long time may be needed before the body systems are again in balance.

The Importance of Water

One item that many people overlook in their daily diet is water. It is generally recommended that each individual drink 6 to 10 glasses of water daily. This is necessary for proper digestion; it also helps to maintain proper elimination. Wastes are eliminated from the body by the kidneys. This flushing process is helped by the amount of water taken into the body. Water keeps feces from becoming hardened and decreases the chances of constipation. Water also prevents dehydration.

General Guidelines for Meal Planning

There are some general rules to follow when planning nutritious meals for clients. In addition to the general rules listed, the aide should see that an emergency food supply is on hand. The home health aide should take into consideration the ethnic and regional preferences of the client when planning a menu.

Eating Patterns

Generally, people expect to have three meals a day—breakfast, lunch (dinner), dinner (supper), Figure 11-4. The midday and evening meals are a cultural choice. For example, farmers who work hard during planting and harvesting often expect and need a hot, full meal at noon. They expend so much effort in the morning that they need to replace energy at noon so they can go back to work. Office workers usually do not need nor want more than a light lunch. They usually prefer to have their main meal in the evening in the comfort of their homes. This gives them a chance to be with their families as they all enjoy a hot meal.

Some older people find that eating the main meal in the evening makes them uncom-

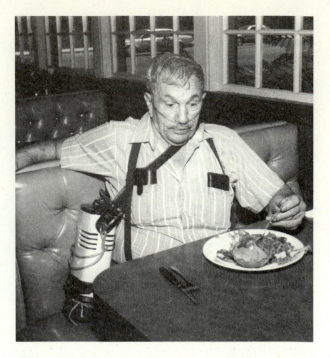

Figure 11-4   A middle-aged man eating a balanced meal in a restaurant. Note the portable oxygen equipment.

fortable. They find that they feel better having their main meal at midday and then eating a light meal in the evening. This relieves the feeling of heaviness and discomfort when they go to bed. **Meals on Wheels** (a service that brings hot meals to shut-ins and the elderly) usually provides the food at midday for this reason.

Some elderly who can ambulate prefer the companionship of a meal shared with friends at a local senior citizen center, Figure 11-5.

Some people prefer to have five or six smaller meals that can be divided into a light breakfast, an early light lunch, a midafternoon snack, a small dinner, and a late night snack. Cancer patients are often encouraged to follow this practice. The aide should also remember that persons who are ill may lose their appetites as a result of their condition.

Food Allergies

Some foods cause an allergic reaction in certain people. Some individuals cannot digest milk or milk products. Others may be unable to eat eggs, strawberries, or foods made with wheat (celiac disease). Substitute foods must be

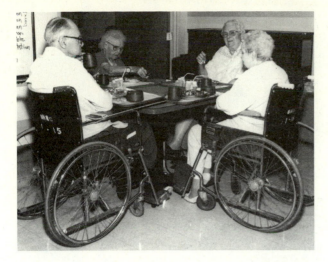

Figure 11-5   Many older individuals enjoy a daily meal at their local senior citizen center.

found to provide the nutrients normally provided by these foods. Allergies may be a result of an emotional reaction. It may not be possible to determine the emotional cause of the allergy, but substitute foods will have to be used by these persons.

Food Preparation and Appeal

Foods may be prepared in a number of ways. They may be eaten raw. Some can be broiled, baked, fried, boiled, or steamed. Overcooking causes the loss of minerals, vitamins and other nutrients. Some meats, particularly pork and chicken, must be thoroughly cooked.

When planning and preparing food the home health aide must always remember that a menu should provide proper nutrition. This is the most important rule. Foods selected must fall within the limits of those foods allowed by the client's medical condition.

When planning and preparing meals, a home health aide should keep the following in mind:

- Variety
- Appearance
- Flavor and aroma
- Satiety (hunger satisfaction)
- Individual preferences, Figure 11-6
- Food costs
- Five food groups

Variety.   Variety is necessary to avoid dulling the appetite. People become bored with the same menu day after day. This can cause a loss of interest in food. It is important for sick people to receive appealing meals. The same nutrients can usually be obtained from a variety of foods. Variety in the menu helps improve the client's interest in eating.

Appearance.   Appearance is the way food looks when it is served. Nicely arranged food adds to the pleasure and enjoyment of eating. When foods are overcooked they become mushy and unappetizing. At the same time overcooking destroys many of the nutrients. Overcooked meats become tough and lose flavor. Foods that appeal to the eye perk up the appetite. Properly cooked vegetables, for example, retain their natural color. The color enhances the appearance of the vegetables on the plate. The attractiveness of the meal can be illustrated by two examples. Imagine a plate of food consisting of a chicken breast, mashed potatoes, white bread, and cauliflower. This meal would be nutritious but it would look dull and colorless. If the potatoes or cauliflower were replaced by a garden salad and string beans, the meal would look much brighter and more appealing.

Flavor and Aroma.   Flavor and aroma set the digestive juices into action. Seasonings most often used are salt, pepper and garlic. However, there are many herbs, such as thyme, rosemary, parsley and sage, that can be added to bring out the aroma and sharpen the flavor. Often these herbs and spices can be used when a client is on a salt-free diet. Fresh lemon juice can be squeezed over meat and vegetables also. Since both sight and smell affect the appetite, proper use of seasonings can be of value in planning a menu.

Satiety.   Satisfying the pangs of hunger is another reason people eat. Some foods make the stomach feel full but not uncomfortable. This feeling is called satiety. If daily menus are well planned, the satiety value will be provided. Bulk foods such as bread, macaroni, beans, and spaghetti are good fillers.

Individual Preferences.   An important factor in meal planning is providing foods that the person likes to eat. There is no logic to explain why some people like certain foods and dislike others. Some individuals want steak served rare; others will only eat it well done. Some people dislike spinach, cabbage, beets, or mushrooms. The home health aide must try to prepare foods the client likes, cooked as the client likes them.

Food Costs.   In most homes, it is necessary to work within a budget. Therefore, it is important to check newspaper ads for daily specials, coupons, and seasonal bargains. Fresh fruits and vegetables are lower in price during the summer and fall. At other times it is more economical to purchase frozen, canned, or dried items, such as powdered milk. If money is a consideration, then planning and purchasing must

ETHNIC GROUP	BREAD AND CEREAL	EGGS, MEAT, FISH, POULTRY	DAIRY PRODUCTS	FRUITS AND VEGETABLES	SEASONINGS, ETC.
Chinese	Rice, wheat, millet, corn, noodles	Little meat and no beef, fish, including raw fish, eggs of hen, duck, pigeon	Water buffalo milk occasionally, soybean milk, cheese	Soybeans, soybean sprouts, bamboo sprouts, soy curd cooked in lime water, radish leaves, legumes, vegetables, fruits	Sesame seeds, ginger, almonds, soy sauce
African American	Hot breads, cookies, pastries, cakes, cereals, white rice, corn breads	Chicken, salt pork, ham, bacon, sausage, salted salmon, salt herring, fish	Milk and milk products, little cheese	Kale, mustard, turnip greens, cabbage, hominy grits, dandelion greens	Molasses
Jewish	Noodles, crusty white seeded rolls, rye bread, pumpernickel bread, chalah	Koshered meat (from forequarters and organs from beef, lamb, veal), milk not eaten at same meal (not a rule for all Jewish people), fish	Milk and milk products, cheese	Vegetables (sometimes cooked with meat), fruits	Salt, garlic, dill, parsley
Italian	Crusty white bread, cornmeal and rice (northern Italy), pasta (southern Italy)	Beef, veal, chicken, eggs, fish	Milk in coffee, cheese (many different kinds)	Broccoli, zucchini, other squash, eggplant, artichokes, string beans, tomatoes, peppers, asparagus, fresh fruit	Olive oil, vinegar, salt, pepper, garlic

Figure 11-6   Traditional ethnic, regional, and racial food patterns

Ethnic Group	Bread and Cereal	Eggs, Meat, Fish, Poultry	Dairy Products	Fruits and Vegetables	Seasonings, Etc.
Puerto Rican	Rice, beans, noodles, spaghetti, oatmeal, cornmeal	Dry salted codfish, meat, salt pork, sausage, chicken, beef	Coffee with hot milk	Starchy root vegetables, green bananas, plantain, legumes, tomatoes, green pepper, onion, pineapple, papaya, citrus fruits	Lard, herbs, oil, vinegar
Near Eastern	Bulgur (wheat)	Lamb, mutton, chicken, fish, eggs	Fermented milk, sour cream, yogurt, cheese	Nuts, grape leaves	Sheep's butter, olive oil
Greek	Plain wheat bread	Lamb, pork, poultry, eggs, organ meats	Yogurt, cheeses, butter	Onions, tomatoes, legumes, fresh fruit	Olive oil, parsley, lemon, vinegar
Mexican	Lime-treated corn, rice	Little meat (ground beef or pork), poultry, fish	Cheese, evaporated milk as beverage for infants	Pinto beans, tomatoes, potatoes, onions, lettuce	Chili pepper, salt, garlic, herbs

Figure 11-6   (Continued)

be worked around the prices. Careful planning makes it possible to meet nutritional needs while keeping costs at a minimum.

Diet Therapy

Certain medical conditions require special diets. The home health aide must carefully follow directions in preparing special diets. The aide should try to vary the menus and make the food look attractive. Flavor and aroma of the food should be maintained. Meals should satisfy hunger while taking into consideration the client's food preferences. However, it may not always be possible to meet all of these conditions. There may be times when the client begs the home health aide for "just a little taste" of a forbidden food. At such times, the aide should gently and kindly refuse the client's request. An answer to such a plea might be, "I know you would rather have something else, but it would not be wise to go off your special diet. See if the

dietitian will add new foods." An attractively arranged tray may stimulate the appetite of a client whose diet is limited.

Special Diets

Special diets may be ordered by the doctor to meet a client's specific health needs. A description of some special diets follows. Figure 11-7 lists recommended foods and foods to avoid for these special diets.

Low-fat (fat-controlled) Diet.   A low-fat diet is required for those with gallbladder conditions, heart disease, and hypertension.

Diabetic Diet.   A **diabetic diet** calls for using measured amounts of the foods allowed on the food pyramid. All foods must be carefully measured. Sugar or foods high in sugar such as sugar-cured ham and many sweetened, dry cereals must be limited or avoided. A special diet list is supplied by the dietitian.

Calorie-controlled Diet.   A **calorie-controlled diet** may be ordered for an obese person or a malnourished person. The calorie count is very low for the obese person and high for the person who is underweight. The individual client's needs and characteristics (age, sex, height, type of work done, and weight) determine the size of the portion served and the total intake of calories. Whatever the size of the servings or the prescribed caloric intake, proper selections

DIET	GENERAL USE	FOODS ALLOWED	FOODS TO AVOID
Low-calorie	overweight	skim milk, fresh fruits, lean meat or fish, vegetables, 1–2 servings cereal per day	fried foods, rich gravies and sauces, jams, jellies, rich desserts
High-calorie	underweight	peanut butter, eggnog, jellies, ice cream, desserts, frequent snacks, milk shakes	none
Bland	stomach or intestinal problems; ulcers	milk, cream, buttermilk, cottage cheese, cream cheese, mild cheddar cheese, butter, eggs (not fried), beef, lamb, veal, chicken, fish, liver (only tender meats, roasted, boiled or broiled), refined cereals, macaroni, white rolls, crackers (unsalted), cream soups, white potatoes, peas, tender carrots, most fruit juices, canned fruits, peaches, pears, puddings, custards	highly seasoned, fried foods, raw vegetables and fruit, whole grains and cereals
Diabetic	diabetes	canned fruits without sugar, fresh fruits, regular meat, vegetables, bread, sugarless gelatin, custards	foods containing sugar, alcoholic beverages, gravy, sauces, chocolate, carbonated beverages
Low-sodium	fluid retention; heart problems; high blood pressure	foods cooked without salt, regular meat, vegetables, fruits, salt substitute	smoked, cured, canned meats, cold cuts, cheese, potato chips, pickles, bouillon, prepared mustard, catsup, commercial salad dressings, soy sauce
Low-fat	gallbladder; liver disease; heart disease; hypertension	veal, poultry, fish, skim milk, buttermilk, yogurt, low-fat cottage cheese, fat-free soup broth, fresh fruits and vegetables, cereals, gelatin, angel cake, ices, carbonated beverages, coffee, tea, jams, jellies	fatty meats, bacon, butter, whole milk, cheese, kidney, liver, heart, fried foods, rich desserts, sauces
Clear-liquid	postoperative	tea or black coffee with sugar, apple juice, plain gelatin (no fruit), fat-free broth	solid foods
Full-liquid	intestinal problems; chewing problems	all foods in clear-liquid diet, strained juices, milk, cream, buttermilk, eggnog, strained cream soups, strained cereal, cocoa, carbonated beverages, ices, ice cream, gelatin, custard puddings, sherbets, milk shakes, bouillon, yogurt	solid foods

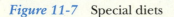

Figure 11-7   Special diets

DIET	GENERAL USE	FOODS ALLOWED	FOODS TO AVOID
Soft	gastrointestinal conditions; chewing problems	milk, cream, butter, mild cheeses (cottage, cream cheeses), eggs (not fried), soup, broth, strained cream soups, tender cooked vegetables, fruit juices, cooked fruits, bananas, grapefruit and oranges peeled with all section skins removed, white bread, cereals, cooked cereals, spaghetti, noodles, macaroni, pasta, tea, coffee, carbonated beverages, sherbets, ices, sponge cake, tender chicken, fish, ground beef or lamb, only small amounts of salt and spices	fibrous meat, coarse cereals, fried foods, raw fruits and vegetables, rich pastries
Low-residue	postoperative; colitis; diverticulitis	milk, buttermilk, butter, mild cheeses, tender chicken, fish, ground beef, ground lamb, soup broths, fruit juices, breads and cereals, macaroni, noodles, custards, sherbet, vanilla ice cream, sponge cake, plain cookies, strained and cooked vegetables	fried foods, fresh fruits and vegetables, fibrous meats, nuts
High-fiber	constipation	whole grain breads and cereals, raw and cooked vegetables, fruit juices, water, milk, protein-rich foods, bran or bran flakes	
High-potassium	potassium loss due to medication; kidney disease	fresh fruits and vegetables, especially bananas and raisins	canned tomato juice, raw clams, sardines, frozen lima beans, frozen peas, canned spinach, canned carrots

Note: This chart is a general guide to special diets. Always follow the dietitian's prescribed diet plan.

Figure 11-7   *(Continued)*

must be made from the food pyramid. It should be remembered that very active children burn more calories per day than an aging person who is confined to bed.

Bland Diet.   A person with a peptic ulcer is kept on a **bland diet.** The foods allowed are served without strong spices and usually contain milk and milk products.

Low-residue Diet.   A **low-residue diet** is one in which tough fiber foods are kept at a minimum. It is low in vitamins and is used only as long as needed to clear up a condition in the intestinal tract. Clients with colitis or diverticulitis may be on low-residue diets. There is very little waste product in this diet. Examples of food allowed in the low-residue diet are strained and cooked vegetables, custards, mild cheeses, and tender meats.

High-potassium Diet.   Persons with high blood pressure are treated with a drug called a **diuretic.** A diuretic helps to lower blood pressure by washing salt from the body. However, it also causes potassium to be flushed from the body. The loss of potassium may cause muscle cramps and muscular weakness. Some older persons not taking diuretics, persons with kidney disease, or persons taking the drug digitalis may also need added potassium in their diets. Very often this can be provided by eating foods high in potassium.

Most fruits are high in potassium; bananas and raisins are especially high in potassium. Fresh vegetables, raw or cooked, are also good sources of natural potassium and are included in a high-potassium diet.

Liquid Diets.   A person recovering from an illness, injury, or a surgical operation may require a light, easily digested diet. Especially after surgery, the body needs to be treated very carefully. Postsurgical patients are usually put on a **clear liquid diet.** Liquids which are light and easy to digest such as broth, tea, and apple juice are given. As the client becomes better, a **full-liquid diet** is prescribed. Milk, pudding and strained cream soups are added to the clear liquid diet.

Soft Diet.   After the client is able to tolerate a full liquid diet, the **soft diet** is prescribed. Soft boiled eggs, toast and other easily digested foods are added. As the body heals, the client can gradually return to eating a regular diet. Clients with chewing problems or gastrointestinal conditions may also be on a soft diet.

High-fiber Diet.   Another special diet is the **high-fiber diet.** Elderly clients or clients on bed rest are often prescribed high-fiber diets. Fiber is helpful for providing good bowel elimination.

Vegetarian Diet.   **Vegetarians** (people who eat only vegetables, fruit, grains, eggs, dairy products, and nuts) are increasing in number in the United States, especially among the young adults. (Another group may omit dairy products, others just red meats.) People become vegetarians usually because of religious, ethical, cultural, and financial reasons. If you have a client who requires this type of diet, more time will be required for meal planning and preparation than for a regular diet.

AIDS Diet.   Clients with AIDS generally need a diet high in protein, high in calories, and nutrient-dense. An extra liquid nutritional supplement (special concentrated drink that contains all the essential nutrients) is often included. Using liquid nutritional products to supplement regular food intake can offset the client's

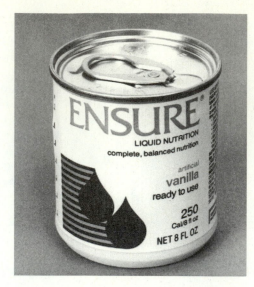

Figure 11-8   Extra nourishment can be obtained by the use of special nutrient drinks.

decreased intake of calories, Figure 11-8. The AIDS client will need more frequent meals and regular snacks. As a home health aide, you will need to be aware of the client's likes and dislikes. In general, highly seasoned and spicy foods and very hot or very cold foods should be avoided. In some cases, bland or dry food may be more readily tolerated. A few AIDS clients may request low-fat foods rather than foods high in fat content. Fad diets should be discouraged. The goal is to provide a balanced, nutrient-packed diet that allows for individual food preferences with an adequate intake of protein and calories for the body needs.

Low-sodium (sodium-restricted) Diet.   **Low-sodium diets** are prepared without salt. They may be prescribed when the client has a heart condition, kidney disease, or hypertension. Some clients on a low-sodium diets are able to use salt substitutes.

Experts recommend that the daily intake of sodium (salt) be limited to 2400 mg.

Salt Use*

Table salt contains sodium and chloride—both are essential in the diet. However, most Americans eat more salt and sodium than they need. Food and beverages containing salt provide most of the sodium in our diets, much of it added during processing and manufacturing.

*Courtesy of U.S. Department of Agriculture

In populations with diets low in salt, high blood pressure is less common than in populations with diets high in salt. Other factors that affect blood pressure are heredity, obesity, and excessive drinking of alcoholic beverages.

In the United States, about 1 in 3 adults has high blood pressure. If these people restrict their salt and sodium, usually their blood pressure will fall.

Some people who do not have high blood pressure may reduce their risk of getting it by eating a diet with less salt and other sources of sodium. At present there is no way to predict who might develop high blood pressure and who will benefit from reducing dietary salt and sodium. However, it is wise for most people to eat less salt and sodium because they need much less than they eat and reduction will benefit those people whose blood pressure rises with salt intake.

To Moderate Use of Salt and Sodium

- Use salt sparingly, if at all, in cooking and at the table.
- When planning meals, consider that—
  - fresh and plain frozen vegetables prepared without salt are lower in sodium than canned ones.
  - cereals, pasta, and rice cooked without salt are lower in sodium than ready-to-eat cereals.
  - milk and yogurt are lower in sodium than most cheeses.
  - fresh meat, poultry, and fish are lower in sodium than most canned and processed ones.
  - most frozen dinners and combination dishes, packaged mixes, canned soups, and salad dressings contain a considerable amount of sodium. So do condiments, such as soy and other sauces, pickles, olives, catsup, and mustard.
- Use salted snacks, such as chips, crackers, pretzels, and nuts, sparingly.
- Check labels for the amount of sodium in foods. Choose those lower in sodium most of the time.

SUMMARY

....

- Food is a major part of recreation and is sometimes the main feature of a social occasion. However, the true purpose of food is to provide the fuel needed by the body to keep the body machinery working.
- A practicing home health aide must be aware of the client's need for suitable nutrition.
- The aide must be able to prepare and serve those foods best for each client.
- Aides should also understand the importance of maintaining the right kind of nutrition needed by their own bodies. The kind of foods eaten determine how well the body systems function.
- A home health aide can provide better care for clients by making sure that the necessary nutrients are being provided.
- The aide must also know the special diets that may be ordered by the doctor.
- The diet for an AIDS client is a well-balanced, nutrient-packed diet that is individualized to the client's preferences and contains adequate amounts of protein and calories.

REVIEW

1. List the six groups of food on the food guide pyramid.

2. Name four considerations for making the client's meals appealing.

3. Name six special diets that may be ordered to meet a client's specific health need.

4. A client with a gallbladder problem may be placed on what type of special diet?

5. Foods cooked without salt are to be included in what type of special diet?

6. What type of foods should be omitted in a diet for a client with hypertension?

7. A client's appetite may be increased when (s)he is:
    a. served food (s)he likes
    b. eating alone
    c. smelling bad odors
    d. inactive
    e. experiencing pain

8. One guide for adequate nutrition is the food pyramid plan. The type of foods included in the six groups are:
    a. milk, meat, vegetables-fruit, and bread-cereals
    b. bread-cereal, fruit, vegetables, milk-cheese, meat-poultry, oils-sweets
    c. bread-cereal, milk, protein, vegetables, and fruits
    d. milk, bread, cereal, meat, and vegetables

9. Identify, by circling, the two items on each tray that should not be on the listed special diet:

    Low Cholesterol
    batter fried fish fillets
    baked potatoes with sour cream
    steamed green beans
    angelfood cake with fresh raspberries

    Clear Liquid
    apricot nectar
    beef broth
    cherry gelatin cubes
    grape juice
    coffee with cream and sugar

10. Clients with heart problems are usually placed on:
    a. low-sugar diet
    b. low-salt diet
    c. low-protein diet
    d. none of the above

11. Clients with AIDS need to be on a diet that is _____ and
    _____.

12. Place a letter, which best represents the nutrient function in Column II, with the appropriate nutrient name in Column I.

    Column I
    ___1. Vitamin B$_{12}$
    ___2. Vitamin K
    ___3. Vitamin C
    ___4. Vitamin D
    ___5. Vitamin B$_1$

    Column II
    a. essential for normal blood clotting
    b. regulates calcium and phosphorus metabolism
    c. use in treatment of pernicious anemia
    d. essential to maintain strength of blood vessels
    e. essential for carbohydrate metabolism

Unit *12* Principles of Safety and Body Mechanics

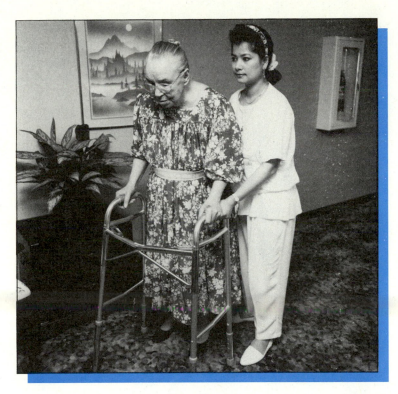

KEY TERMS
....

body mechanics	extinguish	peripheral vision
cyanosis	hazard	transfer belt
evacuate	immobilize	

LEARNING OBJECTIVES
....

After studying this unit, you should be able to:

- Identify five causes of accidents around the home.
- Name two conditions in aging which may contribute to the incidence of accidents.
- State the basic rules to follow in the event of a home fire.
- Define and demonstrate good body mechanics.
- List ten rules of good body mechanics.
- Briefly describe physical restraint.

According to the National Safety Council, at least 4 million persons are injured each year in home accidents. This means that about 1 person in 50 suffers some kind of injury as a result of an accident that takes place in the person's home. As many as 8000 people die each year because of falls.

AGE	ACCIDENTS
Infants up to 1 year are physically active and willing to touch or taste most anything.	Falls from a bed or table Burns from stoves or heaters Swallowing small objects Small objects stuffed in ears Smothering in bedding/pillows Cuts from sharp pointed toys Choking on candies or food, toys or coins
Preschool children are curious and extremely active. They explore most everything by looking, tasting, and touching. They have few fears and no judgment.	Scalding from pulling pot handles on stove Electrocution from playing with electrical cords and outlets Burns from stove or radiators or playing with matches Poisoning from pesticides or cleaning supplies, lead-based paint chips, medicines Falls from chairs, tables, countertops, open windows or falls into deep holes in ground Drowning in unattended pools Smothering in discarded refrigerators, freezers, and plastic bags Cuts from kitchen knives
Preteen children are adventurous and not aware of dangers. They become involved in play and do not watch for hazards.	Injuries from bicycle and auto accidents. Hit by car when darting into street or between parked cars Poisoning Drowning
Teenagers like to experiment and are influenced by their peers (others in their age group). They like to show off and are careless.	Injuries from auto, motorbike, or bicycle accidents because of carelessness, drunkenness, or drug abuse Wounds from accidents with guns Burns from careless smoking habits Injuries from carelessness with tools and machinery Drug overdose
Adults have fewer accidents since learning is based on experiences. Self-control and judgment are better developed, but overconfidence, negligence, and carelessness may cause accidents.	Burns from careless use of outside fire, and inside fireplace; from overloading electrical circuits; from smoking in bed Electrical shock from attempting to repair home appliances Using table or chair for climbing instead of sturdy ladder Automobile accidents from carelessness or drunkenness Poisoning or drug abuse from failure to read labels
Old age causes many changes within the body; bones are brittle, eyesight and hearing may fail. Minor accidents may cause great bodily harm.	Falls Burns Cuts and bruises Poisoning because labels can't be seen due to poor eyesight

Figure 12-1   Age group-related accidents

Common Hazards

In addition to actual physical **hazards,** human factors are directly related to many home accidents. Statistics show that certain kinds of accidents happen most often in some age groups. Most of the accidents identified in Figure 12-1 could be prevented. Young children must be carefully watched at all times. Parents should be aware of the actions of teenagers. Adults should use good judgment and not attempt to do too many things at one time. Carelessness and accidents go hand-in-hand. Since home health aides are caring for clients in the home, they should be aware of potential hazards in this environment.

An aide should be aware of the effects of medication on the client. Sometimes muscle relaxants or tranquilizers can cause the client to become unsteady so that they may fall if they get up from a chair or bed without assistance. If an aide observes that a client becomes disoriented and loses balance easily after taking medication, the aide should inform the supervisor immediately. Sometimes clients have such reactions because of the interactions between several medications or too high a dose of a single medication. It is important that the doctor become aware of these abnormal signs.

The aide should be on the alert for a client who takes additional medication. Clients who are confused will not remember if they have taken a particular medication. For this reason, it is best to keep medications out of such clients' rooms, Figure 12-2. Overmedication can be just as bad as undermedication, Figure 12-3.

Falls

As the human body ages, the bones become brittle and break easily. Broken hips are a common injury of the elderly.

Many clients may need canes, walkers, or wheelchairs. There are a number of accidents that may happen to persons using these aids. Before allowing the client to use a cane, walker, crutches, or other device make certain that each rubber tip is firmly in place and has not worn through.

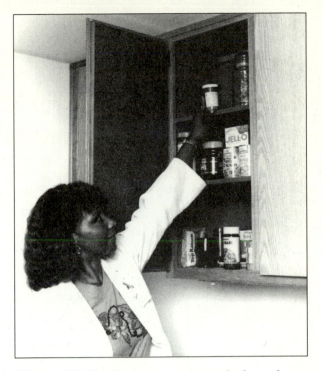

Figure 12-2   It is recommended to keep medication in a safe place if the client is either forgetful or confused.

Some hazards may be avoided by providing a safer environment. Stairways and landings should be kept uncluttered, Figure 12-4. Children's toys, such as skateboards, balls, blocks, and roller skates, must be put away after use. Waxed and polished floors and stairways can be

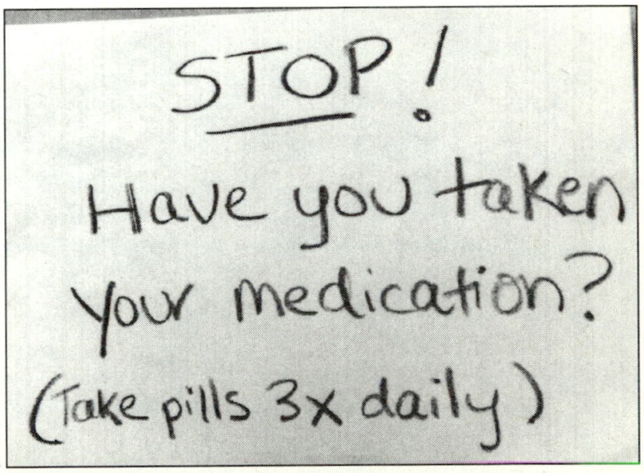

STOP!
Have you taken your medication?
(Take pills 3x daily)

Figure 12-3   Reminder signs may be posted in various places in a client's home reminding the client to take medications.

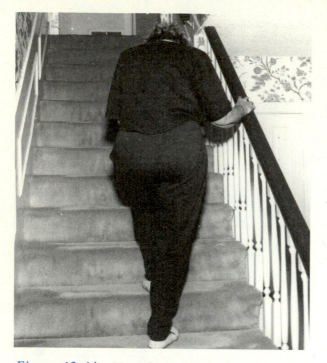

Figure 12-4A Uncluttered hallways and stairs can prevent falls and other accidents.

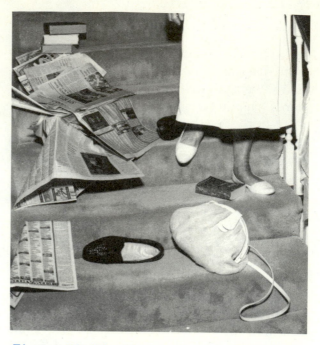

Figure 12-4B Cluttered stairway can be hazardous for the elderly client who has vision or balance problems.

very dangerous. Scatter rugs in hallways should have a skid-proof backing or be removed if older people are in the home. Spills on kitchen and bathroom floors should be wiped up at once so that falls may be avoided.

Do not permit the client to walk about with untied shoelaces. Tripping over the laces can result in serious injury in the elderly. If the client cannot reach the laces to tie them, even with

the use of aids designed for this purpose, the home health aide should tie the laces so they do not present a hazard.

The bathroom is one of the most dangerous rooms in the house as far as accidents are concerned. Bath mats should have a rubber backing so they won't skid. Bathtubs should be

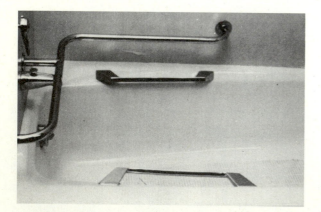

Figure 12-5A Safety features for the tub may include several types of bars and nonskid strips to allow the client to get into and out of the tub safely.

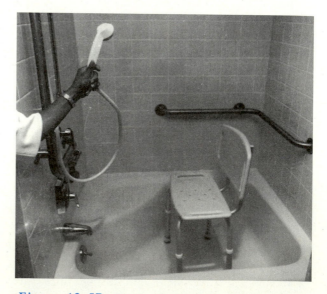

Figure 12-5B Bath chairs are often used to assist the client to get into and out of the tub safely.

equipped with nonskid rubber strips to decrease the danger of slipping when getting in and out of the bath. For older persons, special handrails should be installed to assist them as they use the tub or shower, Figure 12-5A. A bath chair should be provided for some elderly clients, Figure 12-5B. Faucets for hot water should be clearly marked so that accidental scalding will not occur. Special elevated toilet seats and handrails make it easier for clients to use the toilet safely, Figures 12-6A and 12-6B.

When transferring a client from bed to wheelchair, the home health aide must remember to lock the wheels, Figure 12-7. The client is less likely to fall if the chair remains still. It is a good idea if the client is unsteady to use a gait belt while transferring the client. Be sure to get the proper training before using the lift belt, Figure 12-8. Another reason clients may fall is due to poor lighting. When elderly clients get up in the middle of the night, it takes their eyes a few more seconds to adjust from the dark to the lightness of the room. It is advisable to keep

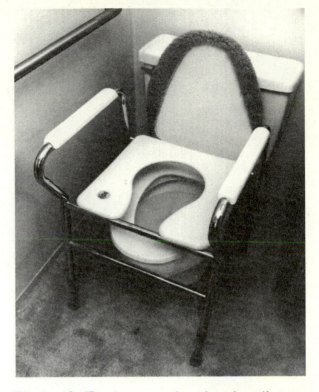

Figure 12-6B   Seats can be placed easily over toilet.

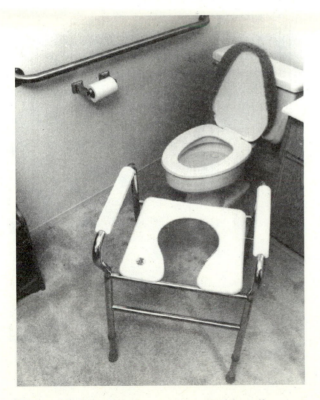

Figure 12-6A   Special raised portable toilet seats allow the client easier transferring onto and off the toilet.

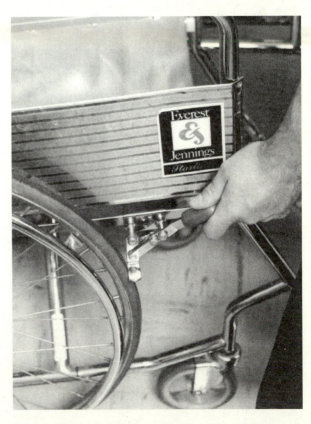

Figure 12-7   Lock the wheels of the wheelchair before transferring the client to the chair.

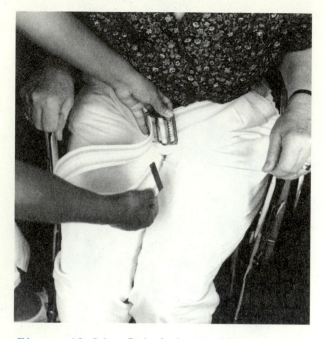

Figure 12-8A   Gait belts or lift belts are commonly used to ambulate or transfer a client.

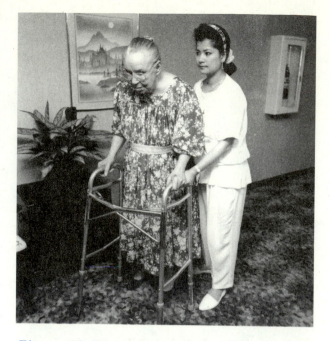

Figure 12-8B   A gait belt is often used to ambulate a client who is unsteady on her feet. If the client starts to fall, the aide can safely ease the client to the floor by holding on to the gait belt.

a night light on in the bedroom at night so the adjustment from dark to light is minimal. A common reason for elderly persons to get up in the middle of the night is to go to the bathroom. Clients are usually in a hurry to do this and forget to wait a few seconds for their eyes to adjust to the light. Another reason for falls in the elderly is due to the loss of **peripheral vision** (side vision), which means they can see only things straight ahead and not on the sides.

If a client does suffer a fall and if a cast is used to **immobilize** the broken bones, the home health aide should check the skin around the cast frequently for signs of irritation such as redness or swelling. Skin areas below the cast must be observed for signs of **cyanosis,** unusual coldness, or any unusual odor, which may indicate a serious problem. These signs and any complaints of numbness should be reported to the supervisor.

Elderly or disabled clients may need assistance in sitting safely in chairs or wheelchairs or to keep from falling out of bed. The home health aide must be aware, however, that the physician or case manager must order the use of the safety product. The care plan for the client will indicate if the use of safety products has been approved. If you recognize any unsafe

conditions, Figure 12-9, or if you have suggestions to make the client's home more safe, please relay this information to the case manager. Special training from a nurse or physical therapist is usually recommended for clients

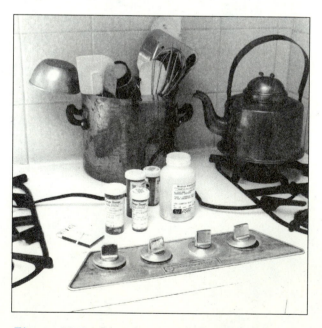

Figure 12-9   List the potential hazards in this picture for a client with mild confusion.

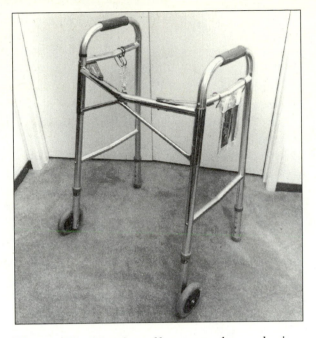

Figure 12-10 A walker may have devices attached to assist the client in carrying often-used equipment.

using safety equipment such as walkers and grab bars for the first time. When using a walker, the client's hands must be free to guide the walker. Figure 12-10 shows how the walker can be adapted to carry often-used items. Under no circumstances is the home health aide to initiate the use of such items.

Fire

Few words are more frightening to hear than, "fire, fire!" The smell of smoke or the flash of flames from the kitchen stove can cause panic. Some people are stunned and unable to function. Others rush around wildly trying to save their belongings. The home health aide should advise the client and the client's family whenever a fire safety problem is noticed. If necessary, report your concerns to your supervisor so the family can be notified. All homes should be equipped with ceiling or wall smoke alarms, Figure 12-11. They can run by electricity or batteries. If they run by batteries, the aide should check them periodically to see if they need new batteries.

As a home health aide, there are basic rules to follow in case a client's home, or something

in it, catches on fire. *Remaining calm* is the first and most important rule. Lives can be saved if an emergency plan has been made beforehand. A home health aide, on entering a client's home, should make note of the nearest exit from each room. The telephone number of the fire department should be placed close to the telephone, Figure 12-12.

The aide must consider the client's condition and decide the best way to move the client in case of a fire. At the time of the fire, other decisions must also be made:

1. Decide if the client or family members are in immediate danger. If so, **evacuate** them at once.
2. If the client cannot be safely moved, place a damp towel over the client's mouth and nose to lessen the danger of smoke inhalation. If there is heavy smoke, try to move the client's bed to a less smoky area, or move the client to the floor where the smoke is less concentrated. Remember, smoke rises, and if it is inhaled for a long period, it can cause death.
3. Determine if the fire is major. If it is minor, put it out at once, following the directions given in Figure 12-13.
4. Decide if there is time to call the fire department before evacuating the client. If there is no time, move the client and call the fire department from a phone outside the house.

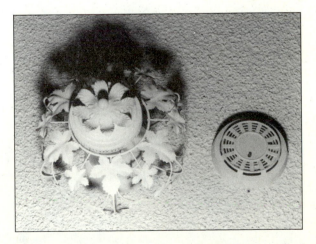

Figure 12-11 Smoke alarms should be standard equipment in the clients' homes.

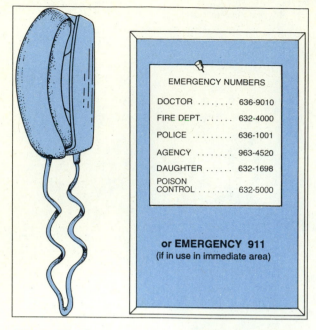

EMERGENCY NUMBERS

DOCTOR 636-9010

FIRE DEPT. 632-4000

POLICE 636-1001

AGENCY 963-4520

DAUGHTER 632-1698

POISON
CONTROL 632-5000

or EMERGENCY 911
(if in use in immediate area)

Figure 12-12   Important phone numbers posted next to the phone may save precious moments at the time of an emergency. Check your local directory for the correct numbers.

Waiting for the fire department to arrive is difficult for the aide and family members. Under no circumstances should the home health aide return to the burning building. Family members and neighbors should also be stopped from returning to the building. No personal possession is valuable enough to risk a human life.

Fire Extinguishers.   Small fires may be extinguished by using a fire extinguisher. There are four main types of fire extinguishers, each of which is used for a specific type of fire.

1. **Class A extinguishers** contain water that is under pressure. They are used to douse fires involving paper, wood, or cloth.
2. **Class B extinguishers** contain carbon dioxide. They are used to put out fires caused by igniting gasoline, oil, paints or other liquids, and cooking fats. These types of fires would spread if water were used to extinguish them. The carbon dioxide smothers

---

BASIC RULES IN CASE OF FIRE

1. Know the location of the nearest fire alarm box in the area.
2. Know how to phone for the fire department.
3. Remember the location of the nearest exits.
4. Close any door that will tend to confine the fire.
5. See that everyone is out of danger.
6. Know where a fire extinguisher is located and how to operate it. Check batteries of smoke alarms regularly.
7. Never try to fight a fire in a room filled with smoke; the fumes and lack of air are dangerous.
8. Never try to enter a room where much fire is in evidence.
9. Remember that a woolen blanket or other heavy covering will help to smother a small fire.
10. Keep boxes of inexpensive baking soda handy to extinguish kitchen fires. The boxes can be kept in the refrigerator so you will always be able to find them.
11. Use baking soda instead of water to extinguish small grease, oil, paint, varnish, and similar fires because water spreads such a fire. Dust the flames with baking soda; this smothers the flames physically and chemically with carbon dioxide gas.
12. Smother small grease fires in cooking utensils by covering them with a lid or long-handled pan or by throwing baking soda on the blaze.
13. Extinguish small broiling pan fires by first turning off oven and then throwing handfuls of baking soda on the blaze.
14. Throw baking soda on small fires in ashtrays, wastebaskets, or upholstered furniture.
15. Do not try to be a hero. If the small fire does not respond to your efforts to extinguish it immediately, remove the client and yourself from the house as quickly as possible. Call the fire department from a neighbor's house or flag down passing motorists and ask them to call.

Figure 12-13   Basic rules for the home health aide to follow in case of fire in the client's home.

the fire, leaving a snowy residue. These extinguishers should be used with caution, since the residue they leave may irritate the skin and eyes. Fumes may also be dangerous to inhale.

3. **Class C extinguishers** contain dry chemicals and are used on electrical fires.

4. **Class ABC** or **combination extinguishers** contain a graphitelike chemical. They can be used on any type of fire. The residue that results from their use can cause irritation of the skin and eyes.

If an aide uses a fire extinguisher on a minor fire, the manufacturer's operating instructions must be carefully followed. Most extinguishers have a lock on the handle which must be unlocked before use. The extinguisher should be held firmly and the nozzle aimed at the near edge of the fire, Figure 12-14. **Caution:** Do not aim toward the center of the fire. Discharge the extinguisher, using a slow, side-to-side motion, until the fire has been extinguished. Avoid contact with the chemical residues from the extinguisher. To prevent personal injury, the aide should always stay a safe distance from the fire.

Once an extinguisher has been used in a fire, it must be replaced or recharged. Notify your agency of the need for replacement.

To review the prevention of common household hazards in every room of the house, see Figures 12-15 through 12-22.

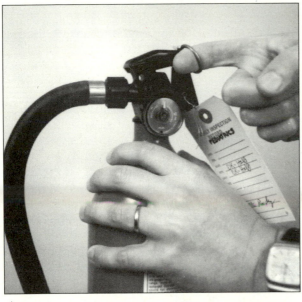

A

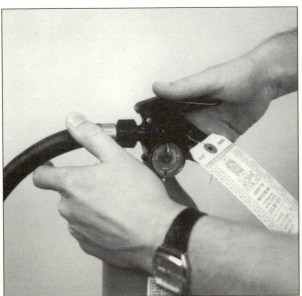

B

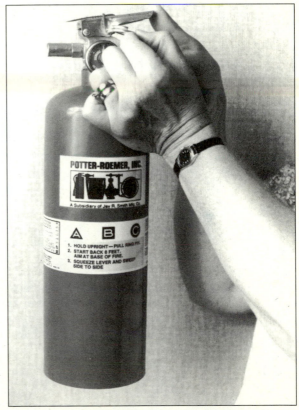

C

Figure 12-14 Use of the fire extinguisher. *A.* Remove pin. *B.* Push top handle down. *C.* Aim at fire. (From Hegner and Caldwell, *Nursing Assistant, A Nursing Process Approach,* 6E, copyright 1992 by Delmar Publishers Inc.)

Here's how to be
BURN WISE!

The majority of burns *can* be prevented. Being *burn wise* is the best way to avoid serious burns. Burn prevention is the most effective way to be *burn wise* but knowing what to do if you are burned is also important. The National Fire Protection Association suggests three ways to protect your client:

1. correct any household hazards you find
2. practice client escape planning
3. teach your client fire-safe behavior

Here are some information and activities to make you *burn wise*.

Safety Tips to Tell Your Client

The Kitchen

- Never leave small appliances with the cords hanging over the edge or within sight of a child.
- Never leave heat-producing appliances (such as a toaster oven) plugged in. If the starter button is accidentally hit, it could start a fire. This is especially dangerous if it is covered with a decorative cover.
- Pot handles should always be turned inward so that they cannot be pulled down by a child or knocked off by an adult.

- Never use the stove when wearing loose-fitting clothing. Always tie back long hair.
- Salt, pepper, and other spices should not be stored on top of the stove where someone must reach across a flame for them.
- Always cover a frying pan with a frying screen to prevent a burn from spattered grease.
- When lighting a gas stove: always stand to the side; use long matches, if possible, to light the stove; when frying, always keep a lid cover and baking soda close at hand.
- If grease catches on fire and the flame is minimal, cover the frying pan with a lid and smother the flame. If the flame becomes bigger, throw baking soda on it, evacuate, and call for help!
- Always use pot holders to remove pots and pans. Do not store them over the stove where they may catch on fire.
- When cooking with only 1 or 2 burners on the stove, always use the back ones.
- Put a *child safety lock* on all cabinets which are used to store chemicals such as cleaning agents. *Chemicals can cause severe burns!*
- Hot water can cause very serious burns. If infants and small children are bathed in the sink: obtain all necessary equipment before beginning; test the temperature of the water before placing the child in it; and *do not leave the child alone for any amount of time.* If you must leave the sink, take the child with you. Left alone, children may burn themselves.
- With small children around, use placemats instead of table cloths.

The kitchen is an important and busy workplace in the home. Children should not be allowed to play in the kitchen. It only takes a second to trip over a small child.

Figure 12-15   Preventing burns (Reprinted by permission of The Burn Center at New York Hospital–Cornell Medical Center, 535 East 68th Street, New York, NY)

Living Room

- Wires should not be left running under a rug. Walking on the rug will eventually fray the wire and possibly cause the rug to catch on fire.
- Replace frayed wires immediately.
- Attachments added to an outlet to increase the number of plugs are potentially very hazardous.
- Outlets not in use should be covered with child safety covers to prevent children from putting their fingers in the openings.
- Fireplaces must be covered by a protective screen at all times. Magazines and newspapers should never be left near the fireplace as a spark can ignite them.
- Never allow small children to be left unattended in a room where a fireplace is in use.
- DO NOT CONSUME HOT LIQUIDS WHILE HOLDING A CHILD!
  Keep children at a safe distance from all hot liquids—they make very quick movements.

Bedroom

- NEVER SMOKE IN BED!
- If you must use a space heater be sure that it is a safety-approved model and in good working order. Do not leave small children or pets unattended in the room with a heater in use, and never place a space heater on a rug or near curtains or other flammable materials.
- Never drape clothing over lamps.

Holidays

Increased activity and excitement often make people less careful just when they should be most cautious. Please take care all the time, but *especially* during holidays.

- Remember that Christmas trees are cut early in the season and quickly dry out to become fire hazards. Never put the Christmas tree in front of *any* exit.
- Never decorate Christmas trees with candles even if you do not intend to light them. Don't tempt someone else.
- Only buy Christmas tree lights which have been inspected by the Underwriters Laboratory. Inspect and test them each year before putting them on the tree.
- Never leave the Christmas tree lights on when you go out at night. If a wire should short out you might return to find your home on fire!
- Never place a Christmas tree near a fireplace. If there is no other place to put it, do not use the fireplace until the tree has been removed and the needles cleaned up.
- Never leave religious or holiday candles burning while unattended.
- When using a barbeque, *never* apply additional lighter fluid once the fire has been lit.

Miscellaneous Hints

- All children become curious about fire and should be taught about matches and fire safety. Teach children that matches are tools, not toys. They should be instructed in the proper way to strike a match and told not to do so except under the supervision of an adult. Matches should be stored in unattractive containers out of children's sight or reach.
- Water heaters should be lowered to 120–130°F. Thermostatically-controlled faucets and shower heads should be installed particularly in the homes of elderly or handicapped people.
- Smoke detectors are a vital part of being *burn wise*. Experts recommend one per floor in every home or office.

Figure 12-15   (Continued)

Continued on the following page.

First Aid—What to Do

If you catch on fire:
DON'T PANIC. DON'T RUN—RUNNING WILL INCREASE THE FLAMES. *Instead:*
1. **Stop**
2. **Drop** to the ground.
3. **Roll.** Continue to roll until you have completely put out the fire.
4. Remove clothing from the affected area. *Do not* attempt to remove clothing that sticks.
5. Flush area with cool water.
6. Cover with a sterile pad or a clean sheet.
7. *Seek immediate medical attention.*

If the burn is from a chemical:
1. Follow steps 4–7 and be sure to flush with cool water for 20–30 minutes.
2. If the eyes are involved, flush the eyes for at least 20 minutes or until medical attention arrives.
3. Remove contact lenses.

If the burn is electrical:
1. Turn off electrical source before touching victim.
2. Check for breathing and pulse. If absent, start Cardiopulmonary Resuscitation (C.P.R.), if qualified.
3. Follow steps 4–7.

Home Fire Escape Plan
- Develop a Family Escape Plan
- Include 2 exits from each room
- Plan a meeting place outside the home
- Practice the plan

Plan of Escape:
Evacuate!
Do not attempt to fight the fire.
1. If in bed, roll off onto floor.
2. Stay low! Crawl if necessary. Smoke rises, and oxygen will remain near the floor.
3. Cover your mouth and nose with some clothing or material to aid in breathing.
4. Place your hands on any closed door before opening it. If it is hot *do not open!* Find another exit. If it is not hot, open it slowly, standing to the side. *Do not use elevators.*
5. *If you are trapped in a room:*
   a. Roll a rug or other materials and place across the bottom of the door
   b. Open a window, both top and bottom, to allow air to enter and smoke to escape.
   c. Telephone for help, if possible.
   d. Attract attention and call for help.
(For further information call 212-472-6890)

Figure 12-15   *(Continued)*

Clearing an Obstructed Airway (Heimlich Maneuver)

Sometimes an individual can choke on a piece of food or a piece of candy can lodge in the throat, making it impossible for the person to breathe. If the person is unable to speak or breathe, that might be a sign that the airway is obstructed. The procedure for clearing an obstructed airway is described below.

1. Ask the client if he or she is choking. "Are you choking?"
2. Determine if the client can breathe or speak. "Can you speak?"
3. Stand behind the client if sitting or standing, Figure 12-23.
4. Make a fist with one hand. Place the thumb side of the fist against the abdomen. The fist is below the end of the sternum and above the navel.
5. Grasp your fist with your other hand.
6. Press your fist and hand into the client's abdomen with several quick, upward thrusts.
7. Repeat the abdominal thrusts until the object has been expelled or the client becomes unconscious.

SAFETY IN THE LIVING AND DINING ROOMS

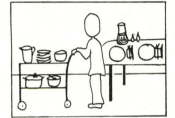

- Arrange furniture so that sharp edges are out of the way and the passageway is unobstructed.

- Do not use wheels under *any* piece of furniture.

- If furniture is to be rearranged, plans should be discussed with you beforehand so that you do not lose familiarity with your surroundings.

- Floors should be free of clutter and small objects, such as footstools, magazine racks, plants, etc.

- Door sills should be removed by a carpenter.

- Wipe dry any spilled water, grease or food.

- Keep all rugs and carpets in good repair. Scatter rugs should be either taped down or removed.

- Rough edges of carpeting should be taped in the same manner or tacked down. Frayed edges and loose strings could catch on toes or heels and cause a fall.

- Tack down telephone and electrical wires. Keep electrical equipment away from walking areas. Don't run electric cords under rugs or doors.

- Carry dishes on a tray or utility cart to and from the table. Always keep vision clear when carrying things.

- Keep the trash basket and garbage pail away from areas where people walk.

- Keep mops, brooms, vacuum cleaner and hoses, etc, stored in a closet.

- Always eat at the table.

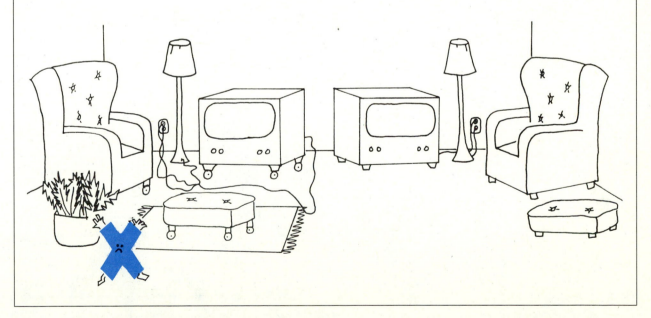

Figure 12-16   Safety in the living and dining rooms (Courtesy of The Burke Rehabilitation Center, White Plains, NY, the Auxiliary and Sylvia Watkins, Ph.D.)

SAFETY IN THE KITCHEN

- Do not stand on chairs to reach objects on shelves. Always ask someone to reach for you or use reachers if the object is not heavy. Reachers, with magnets on the tips, should be kept in the kitchen to help pick up objects that fall to the floor.

- The kitchen should be kept well organized and uncluttered, especially if it is small. Frequently used items must be kept where they can be easily reached so that you need not bend.

- Do not wax your floors. Waxed floors are slippery, and the shine of the wax may cause glare.

- Always wipe up water, grease and food spills. A fall in a kitchen can be very bad. There is an added danger of burns and cuts happening during the fall.

- Keep floor tiles and linoleum repaired.

- Keep drawers and closet doors closed.

- Keep electric appliance cords up away from the edge of the counter.

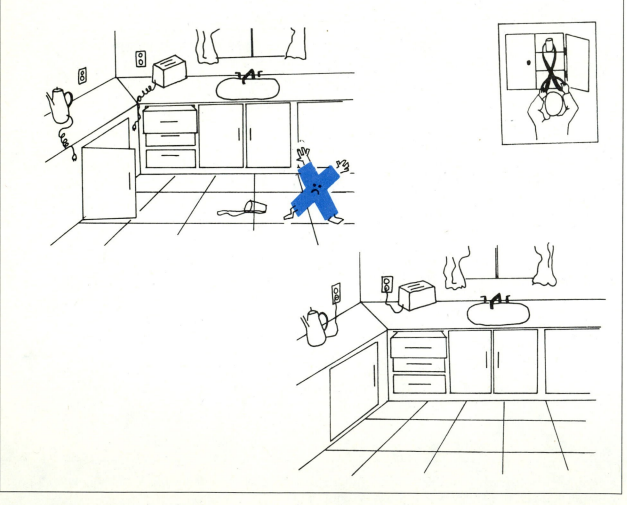

Figure 12-17   Safety in the kitchen (Courtesy of The Burke Rehabilitation Center, the Auxiliary and Sylvia Watkins, Ph.D.)

SAFETY IN
THE BEDROOM

- A chair with armrests and a firm seat should be part of the bedroom furniture. Dressing should be accomplished while seated in the chair, eliminating the risk of falling.

- Your bed must be low enough to allow you to get in and out with ease but should be no lower than knee height. If your bed is too high, a carpenter can adjust the height by cutting off part of the legs.

- Night lights should be installed in wall sockets near the bedroom door, in the hallway leading to the bathroom and in the bathroom. They help you avoid accidents.

- A urinal or bed pan may be kept within reach on the bed table, or commode placed by the bed for nighttime use to eliminate walks to the bathroom.

- Never get out of bed in the dark. Make sure that you have a night light or light switch within easy reach of your bed. Also keep a flashlight handy.

- Keep a clear path between the bed and the door.

- Do not wear loose-fitting slippers, night clothes and clothing. Always tie your robe and clothing with belts attached. Loose garments can cause a fall by catching on drawers, door knobs and other objects. Keep cuffs of trousers at proper length to avoid catching heel and tripping.

- Keep drawers and closets closed to avoid bumping into them.

- Before getting out of bed or standing, check your legs for numbness.

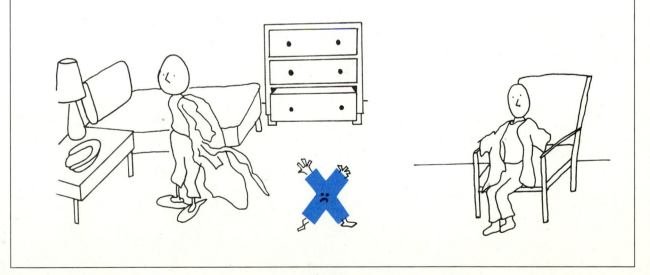

Figure 12-18   Safety in the bedroom (Courtesy of The Burke Rehabilitation Center, the Auxiliary and Sylvia Watkins, Ph.D.)

SAFETY IN
THE BATHROOM

- Do not use small bathroom scatter rugs on the floor. A large rug that covers all of the floor is best.

- Place non-skid decals, strips or rubber mats on the floor of the shower or tub to help eliminate falls.

- Do not use glass tumblers for drinking water in the bathroom. Paper or plastic cups are safe, inexpensive and disposable.

- Place grab bars in strategic locations around the bathtub, shower and toilet. Never support yourself on towel racks or wall soap holders, as they are not designed to bear weight and may break away from the wall under pressure. If standing tires you, a tub bench or bath chair may be useful.

- A raised toilet seat can be purchased from a surgical supply house and attached to the toilet. The raised seat increases the height of the toilet from the floor and it helps to make it easier to sit down and to rise from the toilet.

- Always step over the edge of the tub when getting in and out. You can easily lose your balance or slip on the edge of the tub.

- Do not keep clothes lines in the bathroom. Clothes may drop on the floor, and you might trip over them. Have a clothes hamper or basket for dirty clothes.

- Never use an electric appliance while in the bathtub or shower.

- Hang up towels and wash cloths. Place hooks clearly above or well below eye level.

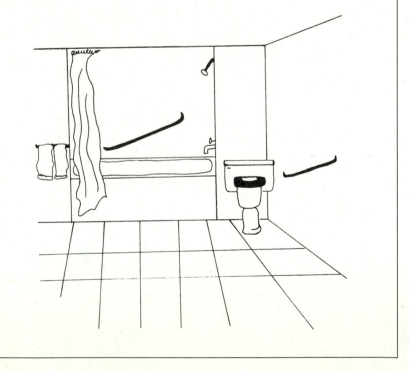

Figure 12-19   Safety in the bathroom (Courtesy of The Burke Rehabilitation Center, the Auxiliary and Sylvia Watkins, Ph.D.)

SAFETY OUTSIDE

- Avoid using steps whenever possible. When steps must be used, make sure there are sturdy railings and USE THEM.

- When using an elevator, wait until it has leveled completely before stepping on.

- On the curbs, be aware of holes. Do use appliances prescribed. Do not attempt to cross the streets unless the "WALK" sign is lighted and you have checked for cars in both directions.

- If your vision is poor, do not hesitate to ask for help when crossing the street.

- If weather is inclement, consider postponing your outing until better weather. When you go out, wear supportive walking shoes with non-slippery leather soles. Tie shoes are more supportive than slip ons. Avoid wearing heels.

- When you go shopping, use the pushcart to hold your groceries and walking equipment. Do not attempt to hold a cane with one hand and a shopping bag with the other hand. You may lose your balance and fall. Ask for assistance when putting groceries in the car.

- Consider using catalogs for department store items and clothing, i.e., J.C. Penney or Sears Stores.

- Avoid going out at night; you may not see a dangerous spot.

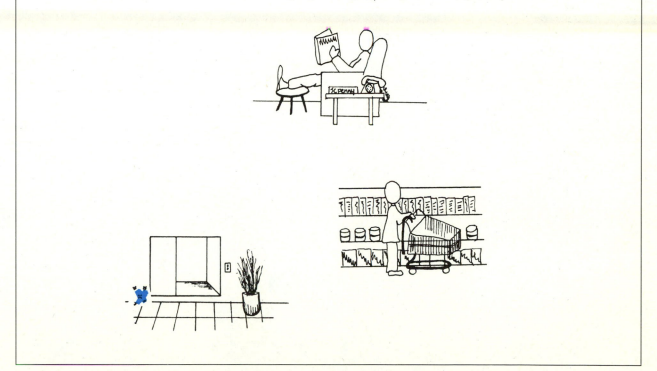

Figure 12-20   Safety outside (Courtesy of The Burke Rehabilitation Center, the Auxiliary and Sylvia Watkins, Ph.D.)

SAFETY IN THE BASEMENT

- Keep the passageway unobstructed.

- Do not carry heavy or large piles of loose laundry. You may drop some of the clothes and trip over them.

- Keep clothes lines above head height.

- Do not use basement steps for storing things. Keep steps clean.

- Never accumulate junk in the basement. Get rid of trash, boxes, old newspapers, and anything else you don't need. In addition to causing falls, junk is responsible for spreading fires.

- Keep all tools put away when not in use.

Figure 12-21   Safety in the basement (Courtesy of The Burke Rehabilitation Center, the Auxiliary and Sylvia Watkins, Ph.D.)

SAFETY AT STAIRWAYS

- Stairways and hallways should be equipped with handrails on both sides.

- Keep stairways well lighted. There should be a light switch at the top and the bottom of stairs.

- Keep all objects off the stairs.

- Don't put scatter rugs at the bottom or top of the stairs.

- Wipe dry immediately all spilled water, food, etc.

- Watch your step when wearing loose-fitting slippers or shoes.

- Put a gate at the top and bottom of stairs to protect a confused or wandering family member.

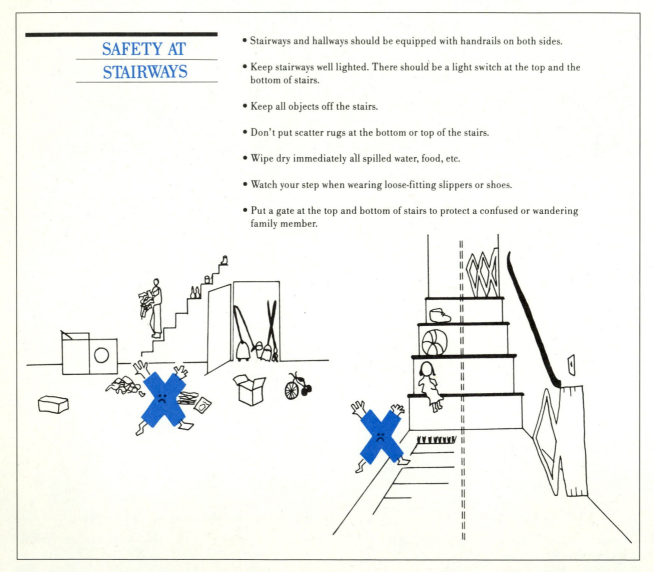

Figure 12-22   Safety at stairways (Courtesy of The Burke Rehabilitation Center, the Auxiliary and Sylvia Watkins, Ph.D.)

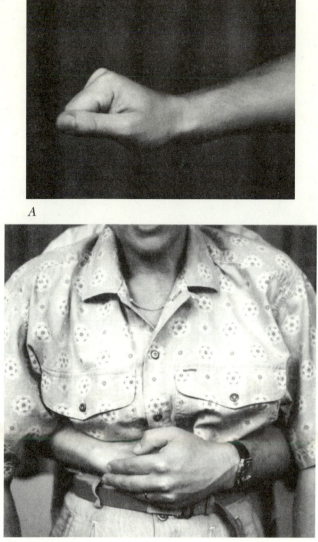

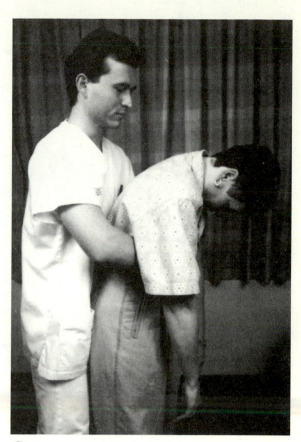

Figure 12-23   Abdominal thrust (From Hegner and Caldwell, *Nursing Assistant, A Nursing Process Approach,* 6E, copyright 1992 by Delmar Publishers Inc.)

Principles of Good Body Mechanics

The way in which the body moves and keeps its balance through the use of all its parts is referred to as **body mechanics.** When the human body is used incorrectly, the bones, muscles, and organs are thrown out of alignment. Use of body mechanics means that each part of the body works together. Some muscles are better at pushing then pulling. The body organs are held in their cavities by the muscles surrounding them. When one part of the body is under strain, it may affect other parts of the body.

Much of your work as a home health aide requires physical effort. To avoid injury to yourself, good body mechanics are required when you lift a client, transfer a client from bed to wheelchair, cook meals, do laundry, or even stand, sit, and walk. All of these tasks require physical effort. All require correct, careful, and efficient use of your muscles to prevent injury and reduce fatigue. Each year hundreds of home caregivers jeopardize their career and ability to work because they use their muscles incorrectly and use inappropriate techniques for lifting.

Each year, because of incorrect body and muscle use, millions of dollars are lost in wages and millions of dollars are spent on treatment of unnecessary injuries and disability payments. The most common injuries for the home health aide involve the muscles, ligaments, and joints of the lower back. These injuries are caused by lifting, bending, pulling, twisting, and pushing incorrectly.

Your spine is like a flexible, bendable rod with a crossbar near the top where the shoulders and arms are attached. The muscles of the spine are small straps that run up and down the spine. They are designed to hold the spine steady and to bend in different directions. They are not designed to lift heavy loads. The strong muscles of the hips and of the shoulders and arms are there to do the heavy work. When you lift, push, or pull, be aware of the positions of the different parts of your body. Keep your back straight and steady. Bend your knees and use the muscles of the thighs and shoulders to do the work. When you carry an object, hold it close to your body. Good body mechanics start with proper posture—the way you hold and position each part of your body. Correct posture means that there is a balance between your muscle groups and that the different parts of your body are in good alignment—in the correct position relative to each other, Figure 12-24.

Correct posture makes lifting, pulling, and pushing easier. Correct posture is important at all times—standing, sitting, walking, and lying. A good standing posture begins with having feet flat on the floor, separated by about 12 inches, knees slightly bent, arms at the sides, abdominal muscles tight. Ten basic rules will help your body and muscles work well for you, prevent injury, and reduce fatigue.

1. Keep your back straight—don't twist or bend.
2. Keep your feet apart, to provide a good base of support, Figure 12-25.
3. Bend from the knees, particularly when lifting—don't bend from the waist or spine, Figure 12-26.
4. Use the weight of your body to help pull or push an object, Figure 12-27.

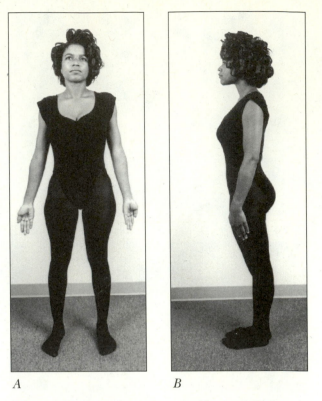

A   *B*

Figure 12-24 Correct standing position. *A.* Front view. *B.* Side view.

5. Use the strong muscles of your thighs and shoulders to do the work, Figure 12-28.
6. Hold objects close to your body. This allows your strong shoulder and thigh muscles to work most efficiently, Figure 12-29.

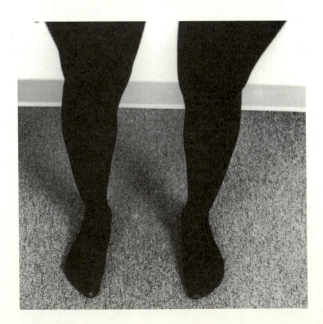

Figure 12-25 Keep your feet apart.

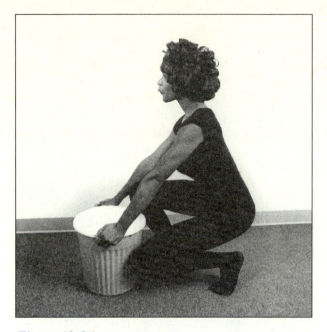

Figure 12-26 Bend your knees, not your back.

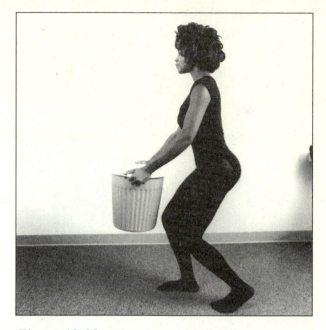

Figure 12-28 Use the strong muscles of your thighs and shoulders when lifting.

7. Avoid twisting your body as you work and bend. Pivot the whole body, Figure 12-30.
8. Push or pull, rather than lift.
9. Always get help if you feel you cannot do the lifting or moving on your own, Figure 12-31.
10. Synchronize movements with client or others, count 1 . . . 2 . . . 3 . . . and do the job together.

Remember, it's your body, they are your muscles, and you are responsible for the way you use them to ensure that you can work tomorrow.

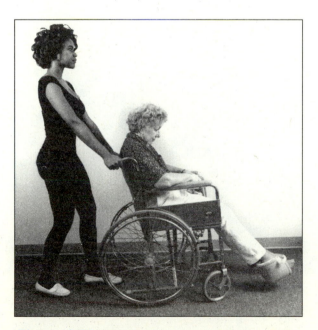

Figure 12-27 Push an object rather than lift it.

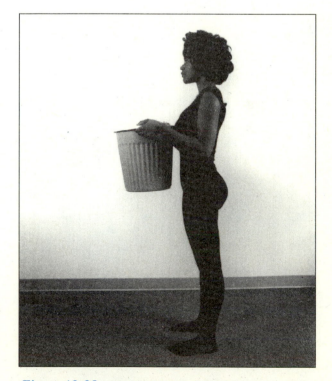

Figure 12-29 Hold objects close.

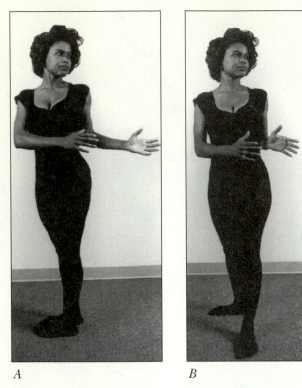

A   B

Figure 12-30   A. Avoid twisting your body. B. Pivot instead of twisting.

Applications of Good Body Mechanics to Client Care

Many client care procedures require moving and turning the client. To ensure the safety of the client and to avoid self-injury or injury to the client, the home health aide should apply the techniques of good body mechanics to the work situation. This means that the aide should do the following:

- Stand straight rather than slouch. Keep the back and shoulder muscles in a straight line.
- Push, pull, slide, or roll the client whenever possible. Try to avoid lifting the client.
- When turning the client, try to make the movement smooth and fluid so that the entire body shifts at the same time.
- When repositioning the client in bed, turn the client toward you rather than away from

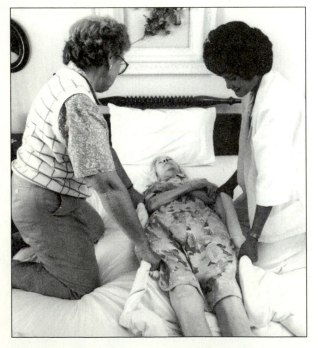

Figure 12-31   Size up your load and get help if needed.

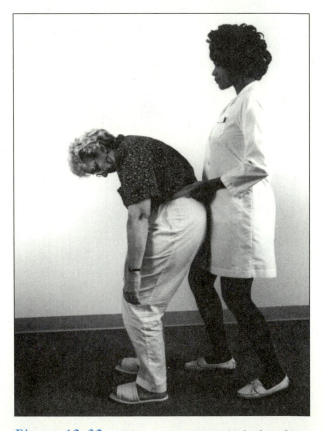

Figure 12-32   Always use a gait belt when ambulating a client who is unsteady on her feet. If the client starts to fall, you can slowly lower her to the floor with the belt.

you. This lessens the danger of the client falling out of bed and keeps your weight more evenly distributed.

- When walking with the client remain on the client's weak side. Try to stay near chairs or a couch so you can quickly seat the client if the client tires.
- If the client becomes faint while walking, help the client to sit in a chair. If there is no chair nearby, help the client slide slowly to the floor. Call for assistance.
- When walking or transferring a client remember to use a gait or transfer belt. A **transfer belt** is a wide canvas belt that is placed around the client's waist for the home health aide to hold on to when transferring or walking a client, Figure 12-32.

Physical Restraints

A physical restraint is any device applied to an individual for the purpose of limiting physical movement. These can include vests, belts, arm and ankle restraints, handmitts and geri-chairs with locking trays. Also included are the use of bindings, sheets, and other materials that may be used to prevent free movement. Restraints are used primarily on three types of clients—the wanderers, the unsteady, and the combative.

Restraint use in this country became accepted because the legal system determined that it was the caregiver's responsibility to prevent injury to those in their care. This has resulted in the loss of dignity, decreased quality of life, and physical and mental deterioration of the client. New federal guidelines have now set definite restrictions on the use of restraints. A few of these restrictions are that the doctor must order the specific restraint; the restraint must be the proper size and kind; and the restraint must be released and the client repositioned every 2 hours. Another requirement is that an alternative living environment be investigated to decrease the need for a restraint. A few suggestions that may overcome the need for restraints are to keep the bed at the lowest level; place the client in a rocking chair to work out some of his or her energy; or install a buzzer system on outside doors. At times restraints are necessary, but other times a few changes in the environment might be all that is needed. In a few states, the use of restraints is illegal.

SUMMARY

- A practicing home health aide should do everything possible to ensure a safe environment.
- Hazardous items or conditions should be identified and measures taken to correct the situation.
- The home health aide should be aware of the types of accidents to which the client's age group is prone.
- The aide should make sure that emergency phone numbers are visible and are posted near the phone.
- It is also important for the aide to know what procedures to follow in the event of a fire.
- In performing all tasks, the aide should use proper body mechanics to avoid self-injury or injury to the client.
- An aide knows what action to take when a client has an obstructed airway (cardiopulmonary resuscitation certification is highly recommended).

REVIEW

1. Name two ways to extinguish grease fires in cooking utensils.

2. How should a fire in an ashtray or upholstered furniture be extinguished?

3. Name five common home accidents.

4. Name two physical conditions of the elderly that contribute to accidents.

5. What does the term *body mechanics* mean?

6. List ten basic rules of good body mechanics.

7. List three rules regarding the use of restraints.

8. You have identified a fire hazard in the client's room. What should you do?
   a. call 911
   b. notify the doctor
   c. notify your case manager
   d. all of the above

9. The Heimlich maneuver is used to relieve an obstructed airway. Which statement is not true?
   a. The victim can be sitting or standing.
   b. A fist is made in one hand.
   c. The thrusts are given inward and upward at the upper end of the sternum.

10. Some hazards that may jeopardize the safety of clients include:
    a. poor lighting at night
    b. cluttered walkways and corridors
    c. defective electrical cords
    d. scatter rugs in hallways
    e. all of the above

11. You are going to pick up the laundry basket from the floor. You should:
    a. use only one hand for lifting
    b. flex your knees
    c. bend over at the waist
    d. keep your feet close together

12. When lifting a client, you should keep your _____ straight.
    a. back
    b. hips
    c. knees
    d. thighs

Unit **13** Understanding Illness

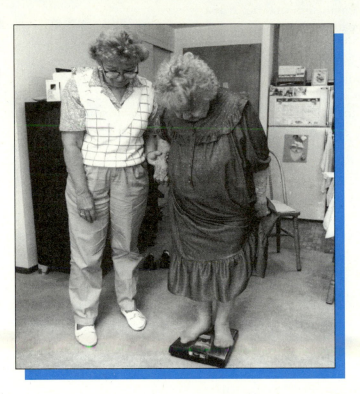

KEY TERMS

acute

apnea

blood pressure

bradycardia

cardinal signs

Cheyne-Stokes

chronic

contracture

diastolic

dyspnea

pulse

rales

range of motion exercises

rehabilitation

respiration

sign

sphygmomanometer

symptoms

systolic

tachycardia

LEARNING OBJECTIVES

After studying this unit, you should be able to:

- Identify the four cardinal signs and their normal values.
- Name three body sites where temperature is taken.
- Identify four signs that a client may be ill.
- Define rehabilitation.
- Explain the difference between a sign and a symptom.
- Describe the care given to the unconscious client.

Wellness is the normal state of the human body. Illness occurs when the body machinery is not working properly. This may be caused by external factors or it may result from an internal disorder (abnormality). Internal problems occur when some part of the body is not working correctly. Accidents and environmental hazards are examples of external causes of illness.

Some external environmental factors that may affect people's health are air and water. Particles or organisms present in the air and water can enter the body and cause illness. People who have asthma and lung disorders have great difficulty breathing when the air quality is poor. Men who work in coal mines may breathe in coal dust, which harms the lungs. These particles can seriously damage the respiratory system. Viruses are external organisms carried through the air in water droplets. When they enter the nose or mouth they can cause infectious diseases. Flu, the common cold, and measles are examples of virus infections.

Illnesses may be either acute or chronic. An **acute** illness is one that begins suddenly and usually is severe. A **chronic** illness is one that continues to affect a person for a long period of time.

Illness, an accidental injury, or a birth defect may be the cause of a disability (a physical, emotional, or mental handicap). Usually, a disability involves an impaired body function, such as eyesight or ambulation (walking).

Because the home health aide will be caring for clients who are ill or disabled or who are recovering from an illness, it is important for the aide to understand the basic principles and terms related to disorders and diseases and to their treatment.

Internal Disorders

Internal disorders may happen at any age. However, they are more likely to occur as the body grows older and becomes more prone to break down. Usually young people recover more quickly from accidents and diseases because their body tissues and cells repair and grow at a faster rate. It takes longer for recovery in older persons because the growth rate of new cells is slower. The circulatory system often becomes less efficient as people age. Heart diseases, strokes, diabetes, and hypertension are major physical disorders of the aged.

Mental Disorder

An internal disorder that can happen at any age is mental or emotional breakdown. Some mental disorders are so severe that the client must be hospitalized. Many times, a person who normally functions well suffers an emotional breakdown when external stress becomes too great. Mental illness in the aged usually has other causes, however. Chronic brain disorder and Alzheimer's disease are caused by a change in the brain tissue. The client loses memory of recent events and is often confused. Another mental condition of the aged is caused by arteriosclerosis. In this condition, the blood vessels become narrow and do not permit enough blood flow into the brain. The resulting lack of oxygen going to the brain causes periods of confusion and irritable behavior from time to time. In either condition, clients often cannot remember when they have had their last meal. They may forget that they just had a visit from close relatives. Often, early childhood memories are more real to them than the present. A home health aide must show patience with aged persons having these conditions. The aide must recognize that mentally ill clients, young or old, need just as much care and consideration as the ones with heart conditions or other physical disorders.

Emotional illness may sometimes cause a physical illness. For example, a client who believes that there is poison in the food will refuse to eat. This can lead to severe malnutrition. Physical illness can bring on emotional problems, too. Some clients seem more able to cope with illness than others. One person may become emotionally disturbed because of illness; another is able to take illness in stride. A home health aide must be able to recognize and deal with the emotional and psychological effects of an illness on both the client and the client's family.

Observing Signs and Symptoms

In later chapters, individual medical conditions will be discussed. For each condition, the home health aide will be told the signs and symptoms that may arise during the illness. The aide must be able to recognize, record, and report significant signs and symptoms. A **sign** is a change that can be observed or measured. Signs of emotional stress might include wringing of the hands and unusual or sudden changes in behavior. Signs of a physical change include changes in the client's appearance. For example, the client may become flushed, turn pale, break into a heavy sweat, or turn blue (cyanotic). With experience, the home health aide learns which signs should be reported to the supervisor. Irregular eating patterns, swelling of lower limbs (edema), and a deep yellow complexion (jaundice) are also physical signs which may be observed. **Caution:** Medical signs that should be reported at once are bleeding, vomiting, unusual coldness, flushing and heavy perspiration, loss of consciousness, severe shortness of breath.

A home health aide should also be alert to the client's symptoms. **Symptoms** are changes that cannot be observed but are experienced by the client. Examples of symptoms are pain and discomfort. A pain can be described as dull or sharp. It may be localized (in one area) or generalized (all over). The aide should have the client describe how the pain feels so that the pain can be reported accurately to the supervisor. As a home health aide becomes more familiar with a client, the aide can better observe signs of stress and recognize symptoms. After the aide has seen the normal reactions of the client, deviations (change), which could be serious, can be recognized.

Cardinal Signs

Cardinal signs are signs obtained by use of an instrument; they indicate the status of a person's life functions. They include temperature, pulse, respiration rate, and blood pressure. Cardinal signs must be measured accurately and regularly. Changes out of the normal range must be reported to the supervisor. The home health aide will be given exact instructions as to when to take these measurements for each assigned case.

Temperature

The difference between the heat produced and the heat lost is the body temperature. Temperature is measured with a thermometer. An oral thermometer is used to take oral and axillary temperatures. When the temperature must be taken in the rectum, a rectal thermometer with a rounded end is used. Today the glass thermometer is often replaced with an electronic thermometer. Figure 13-1 shows the normal body temperatures taken by various methods. The detailed procedure for taking temperatures is presented in a later unit. Each home health aide must be able to take and record temperature accurately.

Pulse and Respiration Rates

Two other cardinal signs that a home health aide is required to take and record are the pulse and respiration rates. These two readings are usually taken one after the other. After taking the pulse, the client's arm is held in the same position and the respirations are counted. It is better if the client does not realize that respirations are being counted. The results are more accurate if the client thinks that only the pulse rate is being checked.

	ORAL	AXILLARY	RECTAL
Average Temperature	98.6°F	97.6°F	99.6°F
Range	97.6–99.6°F (36.5–37.5°C)	96.6–98.6°F (36–37°C)	98.6–100.6°F (37–38.1°C)

Figure 13-1   Temperature variations in the same person (From Hegner and Caldwell, *Nursing Assistant, A Nursing Process Approach,* 6E, copyright 1992 by Delmar Publishers Inc.)

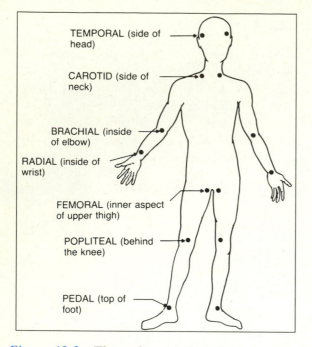

Figure 13-2   The pulse may be taken at any of the places shown.

The **pulse** is the artery contracting. Arterial contractions are initiated by the heart. Thus, the pulse rate should be the same as the heart rate. The pulse may be felt at any of the sites shown in Figure 13-2. The most common site for checking the pulse is the radial artery, which can be felt inside the wrist on the thumb side,

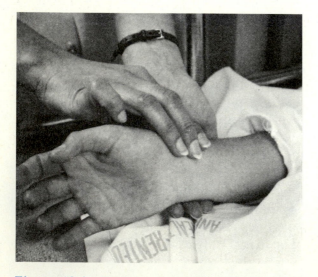

Figure 13-3   Position for taking client's pulse (From Hegner and Caldwell, *Nursing Assistant, A Nursing Process Approach*, 6E, copyright 1992 by Delmar Publishers Inc.)

Figure 13-3. Pulse rates differ depending on age, sex, size and physical condition of the client, Figure 13-4. An extremely slow heartbeat is called **bradycardia.** An extremely rapid heartbeat is called tachycardia. A sudden change to either condition must be reported immediately to the supervisor. Pulse readings show the rate, rhythm, and volume of blood pulsing through the artery. Rate is the times per minute. Rhythm is the evenness or regularity of the beat. Volume is the fullness of the beat. An example of how a normal pulse would be recorded is 70 (rate), regular (rhythm), and full (volume). An abnormal pulse for an adult might be 90 (rate), irregular (rhythm), and weak or thready (volume).

Respiration is the sum total of processes that exchange oxygen and carbon dioxide in the body. However, respiration is most commonly known as breathing. The act of inhaling and exhaling once is counted as one respiration. Difficult or labored breathing is called **dyspnea.** Sometimes respirations stop for a few moments. This absence of breathing is called **apnea.** A bubbling sound may be heard when fluid or mucus gets caught in the air passages. This condition is called **rales,** and can often be heard in clients with pneumonia or emphysema. The normal rate of respirations for adults is 16 to 20 per minute. In adults, respiration rates of 25 or more are called accelerated. Weak respirations, which are characterized by only slight chest movements, are described as being shallow. Breathing characterized by many large breaths is described as being deep. **Cheyne-Stokes** is a term used to describe respirations that are very rapid and then stop and then start again. This type of breathing pattern occurs prior to the client's death.

Adult men	60–70 beats per minute
Adult women	65–80 beats per minute
Children over 7 years	75–100 beats per minute
Preschoolers	80–110 beats per minute
Infants	120–160 beats per minute

Figure 13-4   Average pulse rates (From Hegner and Caldwell, *Nursing Assistant, A Nursing Process Approach*, 6E, copyright 1992 by Delmar Publishers Inc.)

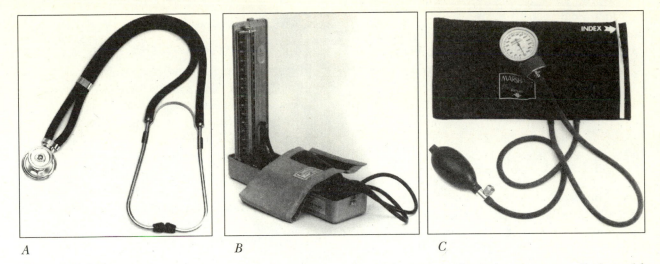

A   B   C

Figure 13-5   Blood pressure equipment. *A.* Stethoscope. *B.* Mercury sphygmomanometer. *C.* Aneroid sphygmomanometer.

Blood Pressure

Blood pressure is measured in two parts—systolic and diastolic—by using an instrument called a **sphygmomanometer,** Figure 13-5. Blood pressure is the amount of force the blood exerts against the walls of the arteries as it flows through them. It is expressed in numbers, with the higher number (**systolic**) representing the pressure while the heart is beating, and the lower number (**diastolic**) representing the pressure when the heart is resting between beats. The systolic number is always stated first and the diastolic second, for example: 134/72 (134 over 72); systolic = 134, diastolic = 72. Although this procedure requires concentration and demands accuracy, the home health aide should become familiar with the technique.

Unusually high blood pressure readings can be extremely dangerous and are often life threatening. Studies to date link obesity and hypertension (high blood pressure) as common physiologic problems. Careful attention must be given to this growing health condition. High blood pressure can lead to serious medical problems. Blood pressure varies with age, sex, race, altitude, muscular development, and the state of mind or tiredness. It is usually lower among women than men. It is also generally low in childhood, becoming higher with advancing age, Figure 13-6. African Americans and Native Americans have a greater incidence of high blood pressure than Caucasians.

In some areas of the country, taking and recording blood pressure is considered to be

AGE	SYSTOLIC	DIASTOLIC	BLOOD PRESSURE
18–59	< 140 mm Hg	< 90 mm Hg	Normal
18–59	≥ 140 mm Hg	≥ 90 mm Hg	Elevated
60 or over	< 160 mm Hg	< 90 mm Hg	Normal
60 or over	≥ 160 mm Hg	≥ 90 mm Hg	Elevated
All adults		86–88 mm Hg	High normal
All adults	≥ 200 mm Hg	≥ 115 mm Hg	Elevated (seek medical care immediately)

Figure 13-6   Blood pressure guidelines (American Heart Association)

too technical for the home health aide to perform. Other areas expect home health aides to be able to take and record blood pressure accurately. Home health aides should check with their particular agencies to determine if they are permitted or expected to obtain blood pressure readings.

Height and Weight

Occasionally it is necessary to obtain a client's height. You will need a tape measure to do this. You have the client stand to do it. Be sure the client is standing as straight as possible and that the client is not wearing shoes. Another task that may need to be done monthly, weekly, or daily is weighing a client, Figure 13-7. This is often required if the client is on a diuretic, has kidney problems, or has a nutritional problem. Some rules to follow to ensure accuracy are:

1. Weigh client on the same scale.
2. Weigh client at same time of day—preferably in the morning.
3. Weigh client with the same amount of clothing on each time.

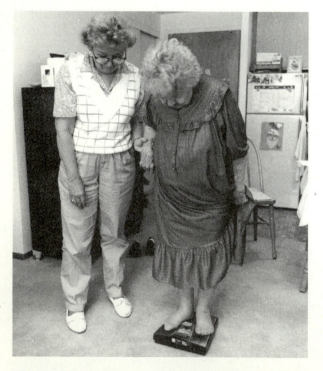

Figure 13-7   The home health aide checking the client's weight

Conscious and Unconscious Clients

In most cases, a home health aide will be assigned to care for clients who are conscious. Consciousness is the normal state of awareness. Conscious people are responsive and know who and where they are. Normal consciousness varies in intensity throughout the day.

Have you had the experience of going to look for an item only to forget what it was when you got into the room? Have you ever been talking to someone and at some point lost the purpose of the conversation? These examples show that different levels of consciousness exist. While doing routine work, thoughts may wander and daydreaming may occur. At other times, a person may be extremely aware and sensitive of surroundings and events.

Just as there are varying levels of awareness or consciousness, there are different levels of unconsciousness, Figure 13-8. Sleep is a temporary state of unconsciousness. Other types of unconsciousness are due to a body malfunction or an injury. Fainting is an example of a temporary loss of consciousness. The blood supply to the brain is decreased; the person feels dizzy and may black out. When the head is lowered, the blood rushes back to the brain and the faintness disappears.

The deeply unconscious client is totally helpless and the home health aide must follow supervisor's instructions carefully. The client's bed should be comfortable and kept clean and dry. The client should also be given frequent mouth care. Two of the greatest potential problems for an unconscious client are pressure sores and contractures. **Contracture** is the abnormal shortening of muscle tissue. When contractures occur, the muscles become inelastic and fixed. The hands may curl into tight fists and become locked into that position. The arms and legs also become stiff. In some cases, the entire body curls into the fetal position. Exercising the client's limbs can help prevent contractures. Exercises done to prevent contractures and the loss of motion in the joints are called **range of motion exercises.**

An unconscious client must have special care. Figure 13-9 indicates the special needs

LEVEL	PHYSICAL SIGNS AND CLIENT REACTIONS
Somnolence	Client can answer questions but is confused and fades in and out of sleep.
Stupor	Client is restless and can only be aroused by continuous stimulation. Must be protected from falling out of bed. Responds to bright lights, loud sounds and can locate painful site.
Semicoma	Client can only be aroused with difficulty. May groan or mutter, reacts to painful stimuli (when pinched or stuck with needle). Usually loses control of bowel and bladder (is incontinent).
Coma	Responds only to painful stimuli if at all. In a deep coma, all responses are lost. Must be turned and repositioned or will remain in one position. Client is incontinent.

Figure 13-8   Levels of unconsciousness

of the unconscious client and how to meet those needs.

Need for Rehabilitation

Part of the care plan for a client may include **rehabilitation,** which is the restoring of physical abilities to the highest level possible. Most rehabilitation is planned and carried out by a specialist such as the physical or occupational therapist. When physical ability or skill has been lost, the client must relearn it or adjust to coping without it. A blind client must be taught self-feeding and learn how to become more independent. A stroke victim must learn again to use parts of the body which may be paralyzed. Range of motion exercises, speech therapy and other kinds of rehabilitation may be needed. In some cases the home health aide will be able to assist in the rehabilitation program.

While recovering from an illness, clients sometimes become discouraged and depressed and fear they will never feel better. A home health aide must encourage the client, but not raise the client's expectations beyond a reasonable level. It is better to emphasize the client's "abilities" rather than "disabilities." It is important to set realistic daily goals while at the same time working toward a long-term level of physical rehabilitation that can be reasonably expected. If, for instance, a client is relearning to walk after an accident or stroke, the client should be praised and consistently given positive strokes for being able to take one more step

than the client took the day before. The aide and client could set a goal of walking from the chair to the door by the end of the week, for example. If that goal is reached, the client will be very happy. If, on the other hand, the goal is not quite reached, the aide can point out how much closer the client is than the client had been the week before. This is an example of positive reinforcement.

If an aide were working with a young person recovering from a fractured leg and the client claimed the exercises planned by the physical therapist were too painful and refused to do them, what would the aide do? A home health aide's job is to encourage the client and explain that although there is pain, it is best to follow a daily plan. Let the client know that he or she is responsible for his or her own recovery. Suggest that a little pain now is better than permanent stiffness, which can lead to permanent disability. The aide should, of course, report to the physical therapist or case manager that the client is avoiding doing the prescribed exercises.

The important fact to know about rehabilitation is that the client's condition will determine the extent of rehabilitation possible, Figure 13-10. A blind person will probably never be able to see again. A client with crippling arthritis will probably never have the full use of the hands or feet. The aide's job is to assist clients to regain as much use of their body as is possible under a given set of circumstances. The aide should remember to give honest praise when a client is making progress and encourage a client who is reluctant to even try to help him-

CARE REQUIRED	FREQUENCY	WHAT TO DO
Mouth care	Every 2 hr	Wipe tongue, lips, gums, and teeth with gauze pad or cotton swab moistened with water or mouthwash. Lubricate and moisten mouth tissues with glycerin or vegetable oil. Wipe away saliva as it dribbles from the mouth.
	When client vomits	Turn client to side at first sign of vomiting. Catch vomitus in a bowl or basin held to the side of the mouth. Wipe mouth with gauze pads or clean damp cloth.
Eye care	Wipe clean in AM and PM	Cover eyelids with soft cloth moistened in water. (Prevents eye cavity from becoming dry, since eyes may not close or blink).
Repositioning	At least every 2 hr	Turn from back to side, and side to front, etc. (This prevents pressure sores from forming).
Range of motion (ROM) exercises	As ordered by doctor	Exercise all client's body parts if permitted. (Keeps blood circulating, prevents contractures, and prevents loss of motion in joints.)
Body massage with lotion	At least daily	Rub skin firmly but gently. Rub in a circular motion around bony prominences.
Care of bowel and bladder drainage	At least every hour	Check perineal area and bed linens to see if they are clean and dry. If client has not voided for 8 hr, report it to the supervisor. If client has not had bowel movement for 2 days, report it to the supervisor.
Accident prevention	At all times	Put up guard rails or place chairs beside bed to prevent falls. Observe for signs of vomiting and keep saliva wiped away; client may choke or inhale fluids into the lungs. Keep blankets and pillows away from the client's nose and mouth to avoid smothering.
Easy access to client	At all times	Safety and ease of working with client. Place the bed away from the wall so both sides of the bed are accessible.
Room ventilation	Open windows or vent daily	Keep temperature between 66-70°, keep drafts from client. Open windows or vents to circulate air.
Tender loving care (TLC)	At all times	Talk to the client as if the client were conscious. Client may be able to hear and understand. (Communication gives client link with reality). Use gentle touch often; if time allows, hold the client's hands and run fingers across forehead.

Figure 13-9   Meeting the special needs of the unconscious client

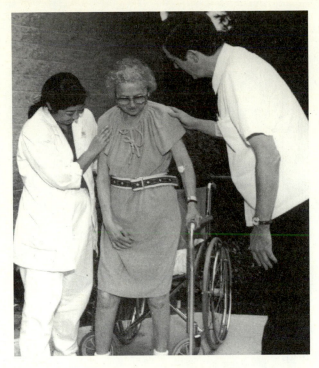

Figure 13-10   The physical therapist and aide assisting the client to walk with a cane

self. In this case, the aide needs to be firm but not harsh with the client.

Diversion and Recreation

A care plan is developed to make the ill client comfortable and to bring about recovery. Several factors influence the care that is planned. The home health aide must consider the sex and age of the client and the type and severity of the illness. The personal habits and the client's personality also enter into the total care plan. Suitable foods must be given to the client and the physical environment must be maintained. In addition, the client must have diversion and some kind of recreation. The client's thoughts need to be taken off the illness. Illness often confines the client and this is rarely pleasant. The home health aide should make special efforts to give the client outside interests. It is not hard to plan small pleasures to ease the boredom of illness. Some clients like to read; books can be borrowed from the local library. If the client is well enough, visits from friends may be enjoyable. A home health aide can suggest activities to a client. Even moving the bed so the client can look out the window and watch the sky and trees can be a diversion for the client. The client who is able should be taken out of doors in nice weather. This provides a change of scenery and makes the client feel better. Reading to the client may also be a pleasant diversion. The activities the client can participate in depend on past interests, age, and present condition. The possibilities for activities are unlimited. A recreational therapist can recommend activities geared to the abilities and interests of the client, including:

bingo and playing cards
writing/taping oral history
clay sculpture
water colors
sketching
dictating poetry to a home health aide, or letters to family and friends
finger paints
handcrafts
needlecrafts
simple to advanced crossword puzzles
planting seeds for a window garden
making scrapbooks
couponing
bird watching and recording birds sighted

Diversion and recreation play an important part in lifting the spirits of a sick person.

SUMMARY

••••••••••••••••••••••

- The home health aide must learn to understand both the emotional and physical aspects of illness.
- Routine care requires the aide to accurately measure and record the cardinal signs: temperature, pulse, respiration, and blood pressure.
- An important duty is to report to the supervisor any unusual or significant changes in the client's appearance or behavior.

- The aide must also give the special care required by the unconscious client.
- A client's care plan includes diversion for the client as well as recreation and rehabilitation.
- A home health aide should help the client become as independent as possible. The aide is an important member of the rehabilitation team.

REVIEW

1. a. List the four cardinal signs.
    b. Indicate the normal values of each cardinal sign.

2. What is the difference between a sign and a symptom?

3. a. Describe the mouth care given to an unconscious client.
    b. How often is mouth care given to the unconscious client?

4. How often should an unconscious client be repositioned?

5. Explain rehabilitation.

6. List three sites where a person's temperature can be taken.

7. List four signs that a client may be ill.

8. Explain the role of a home health aide in restoring skills lost by disease or accidents.

9. When counting a client's pulse rate:
    a. place your thumb over the client's artery
    b. with your fingers, use light pressure on the wrist on the thumb side
    c. count the beats over any vein
    d. check the artery on the right side of the wrist

10. When recording blood pressure you should write it as 130/72. The bottom number stands for the:
    a. systolic pressure   c. mercury pressure
    b. diastolic pressure   d. pulse deficit

11. The top number of a recorded blood pressure stands for the:
    a. systolic pressure   c. mercury pressure
    b. diastolic pressure   d. pulse deficit

12. Blood pressure above normal is called:
    a. hypotension   c. dyspnea
    b. rales   d. hypertension

13. Mrs. Tan's nursing care plan states that her vital signs are to be taken twice a day. Another commonly accepted meaning of vital signs is:
    a. cardinal signs   c. graphic signs
    b. essential signs   d. objective signs

Unit **14** Preventing the Spread of Disease

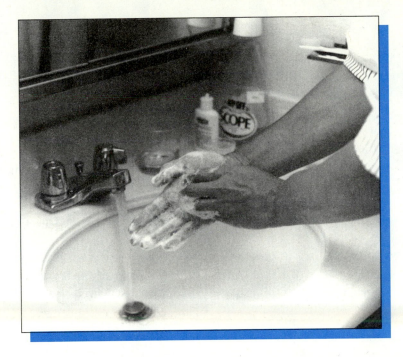

KEY TERMS
....

asepsis
bacteria
contagious
contaminated
disinfected
fungi

germs
incubation period
infection control
isolation
microorganisms
pathogens

protozoa
rickettsiae
sterile
universal precautions
virus

LEARNING OBJECTIVES
....

After studying this unit, you should be able to:

- Name three different types of microorganisms.
- Identify three universal precaution techniques.
- Give three examples of ways germs can spread from one person to another.

- Give three examples of situations requiring universal precautions.
- Name the single most effective precaution to prevent spread of infections.
- List five times when aides must wash their hands.

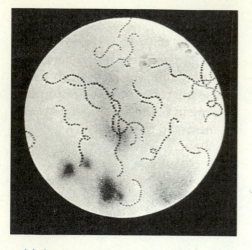

Figure 14-1   *Streptococcus hemolyticus* (Courtesy of the Centers for Disease Control, Atlanta, GA; from Hegner and Caldwell, *Nursing Assistant, A Nursing Process Approach,* 6E, copyright 1992 by Delmar Publishers Inc.)

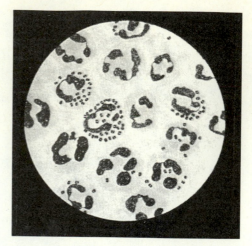

Figure 14-3   *Neisseria gonorrheae* (Courtesy of the Centers for Disease Control, Atlanta, GA; from Hegner and Caldwell, *Nursing Assistant, A Nursing Process Approach,* 6E, copyright 1992 by Delmar Publishers Inc.)

Microorganisms

Microorganisms are so small that they can be seem only under a high-power microscope. There are good microorganisms and also a few bad microorganisms that can cause disease. The bad microorganisms that are capable of causing disease are called **germs** or **pathogens.** Most of the pathogens like dark, damp, warm, and dirty places to live and multiply. The time between the entry of germs into the body and the appearance of the first sign of disease is called the **incubation period.** Infections only occur when the body cannot control the growth of germs. Strong, healthy people are more able to fight off pathogens than weak or unhealthy people.

There are many different types of microorganisms, Figures 14-1 through 14-4. **Bacteria** are microscopic organisms that multiply rapidly. **Protozoa** are tiny one-cell animals.

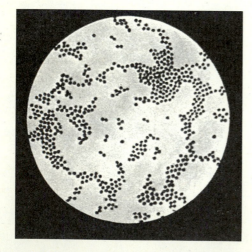

Figure 14-2   *Staphylococcus aureus* (Courtesy of the Centers for Disease Control, Atlanta, GA; from Hegner and Caldwell, *Nursing Assistant, A Nursing Process Approach,* 6E, copyright 1992 by Delmar Publishers Inc.)

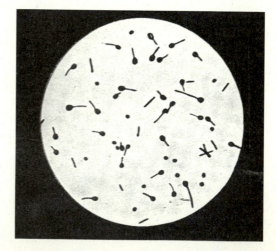

Figure 14-4   *Clostridium tetani* (Courtesy of the Centers for Disease Control, Atlanta, GA; from Hegner and Caldwell, *Nursing Assistant, A Nursing Process Approach,* 6E, copyright 1992 by Delmar Publishers Inc.)

Bacteria and protozoa can live for a long time and continue to multiply in air and water. Many types of bacteria and protozoa exist, but only a few cause disease. **Viruses** are microorganisms that can live only by feeding on living cells. Most viruses are capable of causing infections. Diseases caused by viruses are flu, colds, and acquired immunodeficiency syndrome (AIDS). **Fungi** include two groups of organisms—yeast and molds—that live normally in the body. Under optimum conditions they can cause diseases such as athlete's foot (tinea pedis), ringworm (tinea capitis), thrush, or vaginitis (*Candida albicans*). Another example of a microorganism that can cause a disease and lives on lice, ticks, fleas, mites, and other insects is called **rickettsiae.** Figure 14-5 lists the ways in which organisms causing various diseases are carried.

Most germs grow and reproduce very rapidly. They spread disease from one part of the body to another. They also may spread disease from one person to another. A home health aide must learn how to keep pathogens from spreading.

Practicing good infection control techniques is the best defense against the spread of germs, Figure 14-6. If there is a possibility of the presence of germs on an article, the article is considered contaminated. Articles that are free of all living organisms are sterile. The process of sterilization completely destroys microorganisms on objects. Aseptic techniques are used to handle sterile articles in the client's home. Many sterile supplies such as gauze dressings, applicators, and instruments come prepackaged in paper for convenience. They must be opened, handled, and used in a special way so that they will not become contaminated. Disinfection is the process of destroying disease-producing organisms by using chemicals. Chemical disinfectants do not kill

AIRBORNE	ANIMAL CARRIED	INSECT CARRIED
Colds Flu (influenza) Measles Chicken pox Smallpox	Rabies; occurs from bite of infected dog, squirrel, bat Trichinosis; occurs from eating poorly cooked pork of an infected pig Tularemia (rabbit fever); occurs from touching or eating contaminated rabbit	Lyme disease; Deer tick Malaria; occurs from bite of Anopheles mosquito Sleeping sickness (narcolepsy); occurs from bite of a tsetse fly Encephalis; mosquito
CONTACT	**HUMAN CARRIED**	**PRENATAL**
Mononucleosis Venereal diseases (syphilis, gonorrhea, and AIDS) Infectious hepatitis Tuberculosis Conjunctivitis Poliomyelitis	Typhoid fever Mumps Impetigo Whooping cough (pertussis) Diphtheria Poliomyelitis Syphilis and gonorrhea	Syphilis may cause fetal blindness, deafness, malformation, or retardation Rubella (German measles); may lead to fetal blindness, deafness, or malformation
FOOD CARRIED	**WATER CARRIED**	**SOIL CARRIED**
Dysentery Botulism Worms Salmonella	Typhoid fever Dysentery Poliomyelitis	Tetanus (lockjaw) Dysentery Worms

Figure 14-5 Methods by which diseases are carried

WAYS TO KILL GERMS	DESCRIPTION	USE
Disinfection:	The use of chemical products to kill pathogens. Mouthwash, green soap, borax, commercial disinfectants, alcohol, boric acid, chlorine, chlorhexidine. Follow instructions.	Household items Clothes Hands Wounds Thermometers
Sterilization:	The application of dry or steam heat under controlled conditions. (Boiled or steamed in pressure cooker or covered pot at 212°—in oven 2–3 hr at 165–170°—aired in sunlight for 6–8 hr)	Baby bottles Dishes and utensils Hypodermic needles Contaminated clothing Bed linens
Incineration:	Burning contaminated items such as tissues, etc.	Used tissues Soiled dressings Disposable paper products
Pest control:	Use of chemicals and other means to rid area of pests. (Follow instructions carefully to avoid danger of accidental poisoning.)	Rats, mice Flies, roaches Fleas, mosquitos

WAYS TO RESTRICT GERMS	DESCRIPTION	USE
Waste disposal:	Daily removal of nonburnable waste products, double bagging and discarding in covered garbage cans.	Food scraps Tin cans, bottles Contaminated dressings or tissues
Isolation techniques:	Keeping client in controlled environment so germs won't spread or new ones enter. Especially important if client has highly contagious disease, or is weakened and unable to resist added infections. Using special equipment and supplies such as rubber gloves, apron or coveralls, cap, mask and disposable paper products.	Restrict client's mobility Contaminated dishes Contaminated linen Body discharges Personal and household items
Damp cloth dusting and mopping:	Use of wet cloth or sponge to remove germs and dust from surfaces. Prevents raising germs into the air where they can be spread easier.	Furniture surfaces Floors Walls and window sills

Figure 14-6 Germs can be destroyed or restricted by applying aseptic techniques.

all organisms that may be present on an article. If an aide is using a stethoscope other aides use, the aide must disinfect the ear pieces with alcohol before using the stethoscope to prevent transmission of germs from one person to another.

Cleanliness in the Home

"Cleanliness is next to godliness," "Dirt breeds germs, and germs can make you sickly and weak," "Her house is so clean you could eat off the floor." These are all old sayings about cleanliness. Of course, one does not expect to eat off the floor. However, cleanliness can help stop the spread of germs and, therefore, limit the spread of disease. This is why it is so important to keep the environment clean.

In many homes, the kitchen is the center of family life. Most families eat three meals a day, and may raid the refrigerator for between meal snacks. This means that the traffic in and out of the kitchen is heavier than in any other room in the house. The kitchen probably offers the home health aide more challenge than any other room. Keeping the kitchen clean can be a time-consuming job. Good organization can lighten the work load a great deal. In some kitchens, the aide will see piles of dirty dishes and garbage. Floors may also be dirty and sticky. When dishes are washed as they are dirtied, spills wiped up at once, the garbage taken out regularly, this messy condition does not develop. Equipment should be kept clean and supplies properly stored immediately after use. Kitchen tasks that are left until the end of the day cause unsanitary and unhealthy conditions. Hours are added to the work load because the dirt has hardened.

Much of the home health aide's job is to clean the kitchen and prepare meals. However, other important housekeeping duties are to clean the bathrooms and the client's room. The same need for cleanliness applies to these rooms as to the kitchen.

Controlling the Spread of Illness

Most everyone practices aseptic techniques for **infection control** in daily living. Some of the most common practices are:

- Handwashing
- Bathing, brushing teeth
- Changing clothing regularly
- Using fresh towels and washcloths
- Sterilizing baby bottles
- Cleaning bathroom sink, tub, bowl, and floor
- Cleaning kitchen, washing dishes
- Vacuuming and mopping floors
- Laundering clothing and linens

When illness is present, added care must be taken to prevent the spread of germs. An ill person's body is producing pathogens. At the same time, the person is weak and cannot resist other germs. The person's body is so busy fighting one illness that it cannot fight off other germs. The home health aide is responsible for controlling the spread of the client's germs so others in the home will not be harmed. The aide must also help protect the client from the germs carried into the home.

Germs can enter the body in many ways. However, they are harmful or pathogenic only when they enter and settle in the particular part of the body that is most suited to their growth. For example, a germ that causes the common cold will not cause a cold if that germ enters the skin. If the germ enters the respiratory system (the nose, the lungs, etc.) the person would develop a cold because the respiratory system provides just the right climate for the cold germ to grow.

Germs can be spread when others touch contaminated objects or surfaces. Tissues used by the client should be placed in a paper bag at the client's bedside. Dressings or bandages from open cuts or wounds must be double-bagged in paper and then discarded. Careful cleaning of the client's room is very important in stopping indirect spread of germs.

Infectious or **contagious** diseases are those which spread rapidly and easily from person to person or place to place. Many contagious diseases that once caused many deaths have been largely controlled. Today there are vaccines given to prevent hepatitis, polio, diphtheria, whooping cough, mumps, and measles. Gamma globulin shots may be given to persons exposed to diseases such as hepatitis, measles, and mumps. Although these shots do not always prevent the disease, they cause the client's reaction to be milder.

Universal Precautions

Universal precautions is a system of infectious disease control which assumes that every direct contact with body fluids is infectious and requires every health care worker exposed to di-

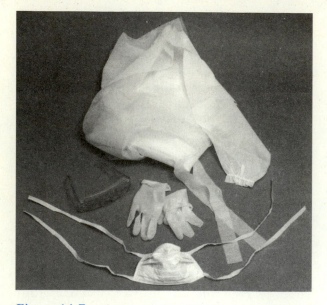

Figure 14-7   Protective barriers used in universal precautions—gloves, disposable gown, goggles, and disposable mask

rect contact with body fluids or body substances to be protected. Universal precautions are intended to prevent home health aides from exposure to these pathogens from whatever source possible. Body fluids to which universal precautions apply include: blood, semen, blood products, and vaginal secretions. Other body substances that home health aides

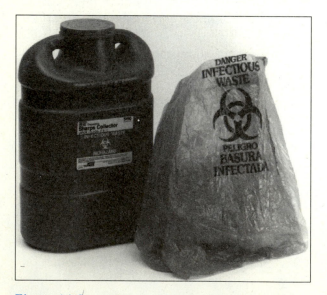

Figure 14-8   Specially marked container and bag for biohazardous wastes

must protect themselves from are stool-feces, urine, sputum, saliva, perspiration, and drainage from any break in the skin. Universal precautions are based on the use of barriers. A barrier is a gown, glove, masks, sometimes goggles, or a plastic face shield, Figure 14-7. Different combinations of these barriers are worn to prevent contact with blood and body fluids, which may carry the germs that cause serious infections or diseases.

These precautions for preventing the spread of infectious diseases such as AIDS, hepatitis B and their blood-borne pathogens are recommended by the Centers of Disease Control (CDC), US Department of Health and Human Services. Your employer will provide you with this additional equipment if you are caring for a client whose medical condition requires you to wear protective barriers. Equipment will also be provided for the safe disposal of hazardous waste, Figure 14-8.

Isolation

The client with communicable disease may be placed in **isolation.** This means that the client is kept away from others in the household. Isolation helps prevent family members from getting the client's germs. In such cases home health aides will have to be especially careful in maintaining aseptic conditions. Isolation is more difficult to arrange in the home than it is in a hospital. Isolated clients should, ideally, have a bathroom that only they may use. However, when this is not possible, the home health aide will have to clean the sink and toilet area each time the client uses it. The aide's hands and the client's hands should be washed often. Hand-washing destroys many germs. Disposable dishes, equipment or tissues should be used whenever possible. The client should use a separate set of dishes and utensils than is used by the family. Combs, brushes, toilet articles, towels, and washcloths used by the client should not be used by others. Keeping these items separate helps prevent indirect spread of infection.

Aides should wear a bib apron or smock over the uniform while in the client's room. Before leaving the room, the cover garment should be placed into a laundry bag or hung inside the door of the client's room. When changing the bed linens, the soiled linens should be held away from the aide's garment. Disposable gloves should be used to pick up soiled linens and place them into a laundry bag. If blood is spilled on the floor, a preparation of 1 part bleach and 10 parts water must be used to clean it up, Figure 14-9.

All contaminated materials from the client's room must be discarded by placing in a special paper or plastic bag and burned or placed in a covered garbage container. Disposable tissues, dishes or equipment should be burned. In some cases, linens must be boiled but most often hot water and soap is adequate. The client's linens and clothing must be washed separately from other family laundry. The client's dishes must be washed separately in hot, soapy water, rinsed, and air dried. After the isolation period is ended, any items used by the client should be sterilized or **disinfected** completely. It is important to destroy all germs on the items used before returning to general family use.

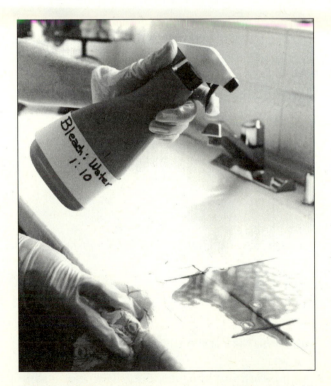

Figure 14-9 Solution to clean up blood is 1:10 bleach to water. This solution must be mixed every 24 hours.

Infection Control Measures

A home health aide has a duty to protect clients from unnecessary harm. In addition to keeping the home environment clean and following everyday aseptic practices, the aide should also be in good physical health. An aide who is ill risks carrying germs into the client's environment.

The home health aide's hands are the most common means of carrying infection. To control the spread of germs and to protect the aide and client, the aide's hands must be washed frequently. Just a quick rinse is not acceptable. The aide should use plenty of warm water and soap, and wash for 2 minutes. If, for any reason, there is no water available, commercially prepared washing pads may be used. To dry the hands, use of disposable paper towels is best. Cloth towels can spread germs when reused. If the hands are dry and chapped, lotion may be used after washing. Hands should be washed:

- Before and after each client contact
- Before preparing food
- Before and after each meal
- After blowing the nose or sneezing
- After using the bathroom
- After handling soiled items such as linens, clothing, or garbage
- Before putting on gloves and after using gloves
- After contact with items contaminated with blood, feces, or other body fluids

THE AIDE SHOULD KEEP IN MIND THAT HANDWASHING IS THE MOST IMPORTANT PROCEDURE INVOLVED IN CONTROLLING THE SPREAD OF DISEASE.

Other infection control measures a home health aide should use include the following:

- Rinse off the top of cans before opening. After being stored in a grocery shelf or pantry, the top of the cans may have been contaminated. Wash pots, pans, or dishes that have been unused for a long time. They may have been contaminated by roaches, ants, flies, or mice.

• Wash fruits and vegetables before eating or before storing them. If they are stored, rinse again just before use. Cook pork and chicken thoroughly. Animal-carried pathogens are killed by proper cooking.

• If sterile water is needed, boil water for 20 minutes. Sterile water which is stored in the refrigerator in a sterile container usually remains sterile for a 36-hour period.

SUMMARY

• Many types of microorganisms exist but only a few cause disease.
• It is the aide's duty to help prevent the spread of disease.
• The body has natural defenses against disease. However, the aide must help the client maintain these natural defenses.

• Universal precautions usage applies to all aspects of the client's care.
• Good handwashing is important in the control of infectious diseases.
• When handling body fluids or substances always wear gloves.

REVIEW

1. What is the best defense against germs?

2. Name three infection control procedures commonly practiced in daily living.

3. List the times when the home health aide's hands should be washed.

4. List five ways that disease can be transferred from one person to another.

5. Name three different types of germs that can cause diseases.

6. Describe three techniques for universal precautions.

7. Give three examples of situations where universal precautions must be followed.

8. A disease-producing microorganism is called:
   a. virus
   b. germs
   c. vector
   d. pathogen

9. All home health aides should use universal precautions when caring for all clients. The term means:
   a. wearing gloves when handling body substances
   b. wiping up blood spills with a solution of bleach and water
   c. wearing goggles and gloves if required to prevent contact with client's infectious substances
   d. all are correct

10. Most germs require _____ to grow and multiply.
    a. oxygen-free environment
    b. sunlight
    c. cool temperature
    d. source of food

11. An effective method of preventing the spread of infectious diseases in the home is:
    a. isolating client from family
    b. soaking clothes in bleach
    c. handwashing
    d. hanging clothing of clients outside on clothesline

12. Before using a stethoscope, the aide wipes the ear pieces with alcohol—this is an example of
    a. disinfection
    b. sterilization
    c. cross-infection
    d. contamination

Unit 15 Caring for the Client with an Infectious Disease

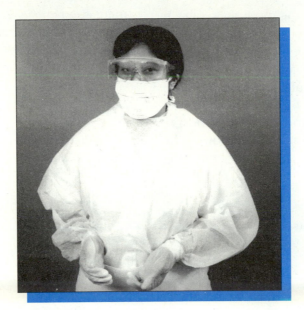

KEY TERMS

AIDS
AZT
contagious
empathy
hepatitis A

hepatitis B
HIV
homosexual
immune deficiency
infection

infectious disease
invasion
jaundice
tuberculosis

LEARNING OBJECTIVES

After studying this unit, you should be able to:

- Recognize, define, and use key terms appropriately.
- List two contagious/infectious diseases.
- Explain the signs and symptoms and nursing care for a client with tuberculosis.
- Explain the signs and symptoms and nursing care for a client with hepatitis B.
- Recognize and discuss ethical problems regarding the client with acquired immunodeficiency syndrome (AIDS).

- Describe the common signs and symptoms of AIDS.
- Discuss the emotional needs of an AIDS client.
- List six rules to follow when caring for a client with an infectious disease.
- List six precautions or guidelines to follow when caring for an AIDS client.

199

Infectious Diseases

An **infection** is the **invasion** of body tissue by disease-producing organisms. An **infectious disease** is one which is readily communicable or easily passed on to others (contagious), Figure 15-1.

Hepatitis B

Infectious **hepatitis B** affects the liver mainly. It is caused by a virus, Figure 15-2, and is transmitted by blood or blood transfusion or by use of contaminated needles or contaminated items. The disease comes on quite suddenly and can be severe and result in a chronic illness. The disease can cause a fever and tiredness, and the client's skin becomes **jaundiced** (yellow). The client may be nauseated and have breathing problems; the liver may become enlarged. A vaccination is available to prevent this disease. All home health aides should have this vaccination. Your employer should provide you with this vaccination at no cost to you. One never knows when he/she will be exposed to the virus that causes hepatitis B.

Clients with hepatitis B need excellent skin and mouth care. You will also need to supplement their meals with highly nutritious liquid drinks. These clients usually have no appetite and have problems eating. They need a great deal of emotional support.

Tuberculosis

Tuberculosis (TB) is an airborne disease, which means that it is spread by droplets in the air re-

DISEASE	HOW IT ENTERS BODY	HOW IT LEAVES BODY	HOW IT IS TRANSFERRED
Hepatitis A	mouth/intestine	feces	direct contact, contaminated water, contaminated food
Hepatitis B	blood contact	blood	blood transfusion, contaminated needles or instrument
Pneumonia	mouth to lungs	sputum, nasal discharge	direct contact, articles used by and around patient, hands
Influenza	mouth/nose to lungs	as above	as above
Tuberculosis	mouth/lungs/intestines/lymph system	sputum, lesions, feces	kissing, coughing, sputum, soiled dressings, hands
Poliomyelitis	mouth/nose	nasal and throat discharges	direct contact, hands
Measles (Rubella)	mouth/nose	nasal/throat discharges	direct contact, articles used by and around patients, hands
Gonorrhea	mucous membrane	body discharges, lesions	sexual intercourse, towels, linens, toilets, hands
Syphilis	blood and tissues through skin breaks	infected tissues, lesions placenta to fetus	direct contact, kissing, sexual intercourse
AIDS	mucous membrane, blood, any discharge containing blood	placenta to fetus, transfusion, body discharges, blood	sexual intercourse (anal, oral, and vaginal) needles and syringes

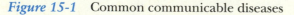

Figure 15-1   Common communicable diseases

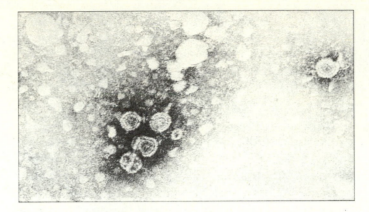

Figure 15-2   Electron micrograph of hepatitis B virus (Courtesy of the Centers for Disease Control, Atlanta, GA; from Hegner and Caldwell, *Nursing Assistant, A Nursing Process Approach*, 6E, copyright 1992 by Delmar Publishers Inc.)

leased from deep within the lungs when a TB sufferer coughs. Anyone sharing a poorly ventilated room with a cough sufferer can contract the disease. Since 1985, the incidence of TB has risen significantly. By 1990, the number of Americans suffering from the disease had increased by 16%. Individuals who live in crowded spaces, have poor nutrition, are substance abusers, under a high amount of stress, and lack medical care are good candidates for this disease.

When an aide is assigned to care for a client with TB, the aide will need to use universal precautions, especially when handling the client's sputum and nasal secretions. Another important aspect of care is making sure to remind the client to take medication as prescribed. The medication must be taken on schedule, otherwise the effects of the drugs will be decreased. TB can be cured if caught in the early stages and if the client takes the medication as ordered. If the client does not take the medications as prescribed, be sure to notify your case manager.

The home health aide will also need to be checked yearly by having a TB skin test or a chest x-ray. The signs and symptoms of TB come on rather slowly. It is common for an individual to have TB for a long time before the signs and symptoms become evident or full blown. The first signs of TB are usually chest pains, tiredness, loss of appetite, and weight loss. Night sweats, shortness of breath, spitting up large amount of pus-colored sputum de-

velop as the disease progresses. Treatment usually is with medications and rest.

There are many children's diseases that are communicable and that most individuals have experienced personally. Among these are measles, German measles, mumps, chicken pox, smallpox, and whooping cough. Most children are given immunizations so that they will not get these diseases.

Special Precautions

Here are some precautions a home health aide should take to prevent transmission of an infection.

1. A gown should be worn if there is a possibility of the aide handling bloody discharges or body fluids.
2. Disposable gloves should be worn when handling blood or body fluids.
3. Particular care should be given to handwashing procedures both before and after client contact for the protection of the aide as well as the client. (Even when gloves are used, hands must be thoroughly washed.)
4. Disposable items contaminated with blood or body fluids should be discarded and placed in a carefully sealed plastic bag or specially marked container. Sheets, towels, pillowcases, client's clothing, and gowns should be placed in a special laundry bag

and washed separately from other laundry in hot water, disinfectant, and soap.

5. If the client is given medication by hypodermic needle and the aide is responsible for disposing of that needle, or if a swab stick or syringe has been used, care should be taken to avoid needle-stick injuries to the aide. Such items should be placed in a hard specially marked container provided.

6. If there is a chance of the client's body substance getting into the home health aide's eyes, plastic goggles must be worn by the caregiver.

Immune Deficiencies

AIDS is classified as an autoimmune disease. In this disease, the body's immune system becomes severely depressed and unable to fight off any type of infection. The disease is caused by a virus called human immunodeficiency virus (**HIV**). This virus lives in the infected person's blood, semen, and other body fluids. It can be transmitted by intimate contact—oral, vaginal, rectal—or by direct contact with body fluids or blood. One does not get AIDS by casual contact such as shaking hands, kissing, coughing, drinking from glasses, or sharing dishes. Many studies have been done within the homes of AIDS

clients and no instance of AIDS was noted in the families with casual contact. In most cases, AIDS is transferred through contaminated blood transfusions (prior to 1985), sexual contact, drug users sharing needles, and babies infected with the virus before birth.

When AIDS was first diagnosed (1980), it was found mainly among **homosexuals** and intravenous drug users. Later, it was discovered that it was also transmitted by contaminated blood transfusions. At this time it is considered to be the most dangerous of the sexually transmitted diseases (STD). It has been found in persons of both sexes and in homosexuals and heterosexuals from all walks of life. Many times whole families are infected. It has spread to more than 100 countries. It has also been estimated that worldwide HIV has infected 8 to 10 million adults and a million children.

Once an individual has been diagnosed with AIDS, the client may display swollen lymph glands, diarrhea, skin lesions, Figure 15-3, fever, chills and night sweats, nausea and vomiting, mouth sores, Figure 15-4, difficulty breathing, cough, hair loss, tiredness, difficulty in walking, memory loss, and confusion. Your nursing care will be designed around these problems. Remember no two clients will be alike. Some may be confused, whereas others

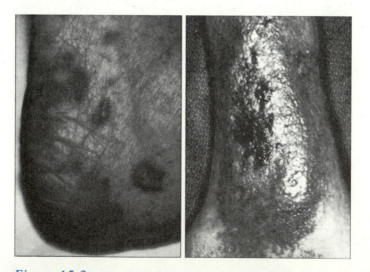

Figure 15-3   Typical skin lesions of Kaposi's sarcoma (Photo courtesy of the Centers for Disease Control, Atlanta, GA; from Hegner and Caldwell, *Nursing Assistant, A Nursing Process Approach,* 6E, copyright 1992 by Delmar Publishers Inc.)

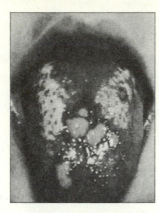

Figure 15-4   White patches on the tongue are evidence of the infectious process called thrush. (From Hegner and Caldwell, *Nursing Assistant, A Nursing Process Approach,* 6E, copyright 1992 by Delmar Publishers Inc.)

will be alert and oriented. Every client's care plan will need to be individualized to meet the physical and emotional needs of the client, Figure 15-5.

There is a great deal of fear as well as a lot of misinformation about this disease. With all of the publicity about the disease and the fact that a number of famous people have died from it, many people have become unreasonably fearful. In a town near Kokomo, Indiana,

a large number of citizens grew alarmed because it was learned that a young boy suffering from hemophilia had developed AIDS from blood transfusions given to him at the hospital. They demanded that he not be allowed to go to the public school because he would spread the disease. For several months he was denied the right to attend school and some teachers refused to go to his home to give home-bound classes.

It has been found that AIDS can also be transmitted to newborn babies during delivery or through the mother's milk. A new mother infected by a blood transfusion can also pass the disease by breast-feeding her infant. However, diagnosis of an infant with AIDS is difficult during the first year of life. Nonetheless, every effort is being made to make an immediate diagnosis of the newborn since it is hoped that experimental drugs, **AZT** and DDZ, may arrest the disease if given immediately after birth. Children with AIDS need special attention and care, Figure 15-6.

The incubation time for the virus varies, but can be as long as 7 to 15 years. Thus, it is possible that individuals who received blood transfusions as far back as 1977 may be at risk for AIDS. Anyone who feels that he or she has been exposed because of sexual contact, transfusion, or

1. Be with the client. Listen to him/her. Do not lie or give false encouragement. Empathize rather than sympathize.
2. Get the client to participate in care plan. Allow him/her to be dependent, but encourage as much independence as possible.
3. Assist as necessary but allow the client to do as much as possible for himself/herself.
4. Encourage participation in social, recreational, and occupational activities.
5. Encourage client to talk, but discourage self-pity or self-blame.
6. Do not start working with an AIDS client if you think you may not be able to handle it. If you take an AIDS client, work with your supervisor and plan a regular rotation so that the client has consistent care.
7. Don't try to become the client's "best friend," but do try to establish a good relationship and develop mutual trust.
8. Allow your client to feel anger and frustration and recognize that he may take it out on you. Let the client vent the anger or frustration—but don't take it personally.
9. Do not condemn or blame yourself if you feel fear, anxiety, or discomfort. Working with terminally ill clients is very difficult. Such feelings are natural. Discuss your feelings with your supervisor. Learn as much as you can about the illness. Facts can fight fears!

Figure 15-5   Working with the AIDS client

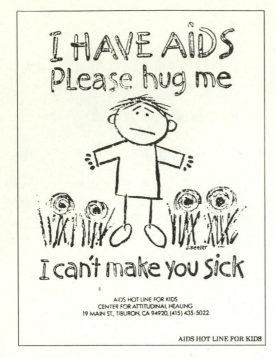

Figure 15-6 Love might be the hardest thing to get. (Courtesy of the Center for Attitudinal Healing, 19 Main St., Tiburon, CA 94920; 415-435-5022)

drug use can be tested for AIDS. The results of such tests must be kept confidential.

As more information has come to light about this dread disease, the public is more aware of what is and what is not true. According to Dr. C. Everett Koop, former Surgeon General of the United States, we must come to terms with the fact that we are fighting a disease, not the people who have AIDS. He also said that those who are already afflicted are sick people who need to be cared for like any other sick individuals.

How to Protect against AIDS

At this time there is no vaccine to prevent AIDS and there is no cure for AIDS. There are experimental drugs being used for AIDS victims and a great deal of research is underway to isolate the virus and discover effective treatments.

The only way to lessen the impact of the AIDS virus is to avoid situations that are dangerous. For example, careful choice of sex partners, practicing safer sex by using condoms, establishing a monogamous relationship (staying with one partner), practicing abstinence, not "shooting" drugs intravenously, not using a "dirty" needle (best of all, not getting involved in drug use of any kind), making sure that blood used for transfusions is free from the AIDS virus, and using precautions when caring for an AIDS client. Such precautions include wearing gloves when cleaning up vomitus or when changing a soiled bed.

By 1993, it is predicted that of the 300,000 to 480,000 people who develop AIDS, most will require hospitalization at least once and between 285,000 and 340,000 will die of AIDS. This means that home health aides will probably be involved in caring for AIDS clients between hospital visits. The Surgeon General states that quarantine has no role in the management of AIDS because AIDS is not spread by casual contact, unless the AIDS victim deliberately exposes others by sexual contact and sharing drug equipment.

Caring for the AIDS Client

What does this information mean to a health care worker? One of the major concerns of the Department of Health is to provide proper care for the AIDS client while protecting the health care workers. At this time the CDC and Human Services indicate that one cannot get AIDS from casual social contact (shaking hands, hugging, coughing, sneezing, or kissing), contact with tears of an AIDS individual, or from their perspiration. AIDS probably is not spread by swimming in pools, bathing in hot tubs, or from eating food prepared or served by an AIDS victim, or from health team members working with AIDS clients. You will not get AIDS from handling bed linens, towels, cups, straws, dishes, or other eating utensils. You do not get AIDS from toilet seats, telephones, or household furnishings. However, until definitive answers are found, it is strongly recommended that health care workers always follow universal precautions.

What an Aide Can and Should Do

Your employer must provide you with basic training on AIDS. The training program must

SIGN/SYMPTOM	CARE TO PROVIDE	PURPOSE
Weakness/tiredness	High calorie diet with in-between meal high protein snacks	To provide protein nutrition and to slow muscle deterioration
Fever	Sponge baths, give additional fluids by mouth; cover with blankets during chill periods	To lower the temperature and to prevent complications. To get client comfortable
Night sweats	Sponge baths, frequent linen changes, give additional fluids to avoid dehydration	To provide comfort and to return skin to normal condition
Cough	Observe and record patterns and changes and report findings. Offer cough medicine if prescribed. Gloves required when working.	To make the client comfortable and to obtain relief from strain
Dyspnea	Note patterns and changes—record and report. Calm client and avoid exertion by client and help with breathing exercises	To provide breath control and relaxation
Skin lesions	Keep client from scratching—be sure nails are properly cut by nurse—wear gloves when working with client with lesions and wash hands carefully after contact with client	To prevent infections
Dry hair and hair loss	Avoid too frequent shampooing—use mild shampoo containing no alcohol. Use hair conditioner	To prevent further hair loss and to avoid scalp irritation
Mouth lesions	Provide saline or anesthetic mouthwashes; brush teeth gently. Check to be sure client can swallow without difficulty—observe, record and report to supervisor. Avoid spicy, acid foods and carbonated beverages. Gloves are required when giving mouth care.	To provide infection control, client comfort, and maintain adequate nutrition
Diarrhea	Encourage fluid intake; change linens as needed; apply brief if required; observe, record and report; gloves required	To maintain nutrition and fluid balance. To prevent pressure sore formation
Impaired immune system (when client picks up any infection around)	Give daily shower or bath; both client and aide wash hands frequently; request nurse to apply sterile dressings as needed with gloves; do not allow visitors who have infections, such as colds; do not come to give client care if you are suffering from any infection.	To prevent infection and to assist in client protection
Unstable emotional responses	Be aware of client's feelings as well as your own. Be honest with client and accept him as a person not as an AIDS victim. Offer emotional support, kindness. Communicate by touching client's hand, pat on back, etc.	To create an atmosphere of mutual trust

Figure 15-7   Sample care plan for client with AIDS

Continued on the following page.

THE FOLLOWING RULES ARE DESIGNATED TO PREVENT TRANSMISSION OF THE INFECTION:

1. Wear a gown if there is a possibility of soiling your clothing with blood or body secretions of client.
2. Wear gloves when touching blood or body secretions.
3. Wash hands before and after client contact and immediately if they are potentially contaminated with blood or body secretions.
4. Discard articles contaminated with blood or body secretions and secure in plastic bag or specially marked container.
5. IF YOU HAVE AN OPEN CUT OR WOUND, DO NOT CONTAMINATE THE WOUND WITH CLIENT'S BODY SECRETIONS.
6. Follow any additional instructions by your supervisor or case manager.

Figure 15-7   *(Continued)*

cover topics such as how it is spread, signs and symptoms, and necessary precautions to be aware of while caring for the client. If this is your first case with an AIDS client, your employer may pair you with another more experienced aide for a day in the field. The first day you may be an "observer." The experienced aide will share his or her own feelings and fears and also discuss with you how he or she handles friends and family members. He or she will also share the daily routine of care for the client, Figure 15-7. This arrangement is often called "the buddy system."

For the safety of oneself, a home health aide who is assigned to work with an AIDS client will be told to follow universal precautions.

A home health aide MUST NOT reveal to friends, neighbors, or anyone else the nature of a client's illness. That is considered an invasion of privacy and the client can file a complaint with the State Department of Human Rights if such information is revealed by the agency or the aide.

Ethical Questions

Lawmakers have suggested that all health care workers should be tested for AIDS. If the test is positive, they should not be allowed to work. However, that takes away an individual's privacy and denies one the right to earn a living. In addition, since the AIDS virus can lie dormant and not show up on tests for 7 months up to a year or 2, what would the test prove?

One consideration an infected health care worker might ponder is the personal risk if exposed to a client with an infectious disease such as tuberculosis or hepatitis. If transmitted to the health care worker with AIDS, disease could cause serious complications.

Special Precautions

1. Wash hands properly before and after client's care, before and after food preparation, before and after using the bathroom. If the client's home has no provision for handwashing, your employer must provide either antiseptic hand cleanser with paper towels or antiseptic towelettes.
2. Wear disposable gloves when handling blood or body fluids. A gown needs to be worn only if the client has severe diarrhea or if there is a chance of blood or body fluids being splashed. Masks or goggles will not need to be worn unless one expects to be splashed with blood or body fluids, such as when the client has a wet cough and cannot cover his mouth.
3. Discard any sharp item such as needles and razor blades in puncture-resistant, closable, leak-proof containers. These containers must be labeled and color-coded.
4. It is recommended that the primary cleaning product be household bleach. At the beginning of each visit, the home health aide should prepare a solution of 1:10 bleach and water. Gloves should be worn when

using this bleach solution as it may be very harsh on the skin. Do not mix bleach with anything other than water. Be careful not to splash in the eyes. This solution can be used to clean the bathroom, counters, and floors.

5. Laundry can be done in the home, making sure you wear gloves if the laundry is soiled with urine or blood. If the laundry is to be sent out, you will either have to **double bag** it or place it in strong plastic bag and mark the linens "contaminated."

6. A home health aide who has an infection or illness should follow reverse isolation procedures—putting on gloves, gown, and mask before giving client care, and removing those items after completing client care. However, in the interest of the client, it is best for the aide to stay away from work until the aide is well again. This is especially true in the case of an AIDS client because such individuals have a damaged immune system unable to fight off germs or infections carried by the aide.

7. If the home health aide has open cuts or skin sores oozing fluid (weeping dermatitis), he or she should not give direct client care. This is for the safety and health of both the aide and client.

8. The aide is not allowed to tell anyone of the client's diagnosis unless a special release form has been signed by the client.

AIDS clients should also be educated about prevention of the transmission of the disease. It is their responsibility to practice commonsense hygienic measures to protect others with whom they live in close contact.

SUMMARY

- There are any number of infections and contagious diseases.
- Tuberculosis is increasing in our country. All home health aides should be tested yearly for tuberculosis. It is very important that the client with tuberculosis take all medications, as ordered.
- Hepatitis B can be prevented by a series of vaccinations. It is recommended that all home health aides have this vaccination.
- A few of the common signs and symptoms of AIDS are cough, night sweats, fever, diarrhea, skin lesions, and sores in the mouth.
- Of all the infectious diseases, AIDS is the most serious. Death may occur within a year of diagnosis.
- Some of the rules an aide must follow when caring for an AIDS client include:

1. Wear disposable gloves when handling blood or other bloody body secretions—urine, vomitus, sputum, or fecal mater
2. If you have open cuts on your hands or face, make sure they do not come in contact with the client's blood or body fluids
3. Wash your hands thoroughly before and after all client care procedures and contact

- Probably the most important rule to follow with an AIDS client is to treat him or her with respect and dignity. Do not make judgments about how the disease was transmitted.
- Many people are so fearful of getting AIDS that they will not go near an AIDS patient. This causes the victim to feel even more isolated. More than anything, an AIDS client needs to know that someone cares!

REVIEW

1. Define the terms infection and communicable.

2. List two signs or symptoms of hepatitis B.

3. List two signs or symptoms of tuberculosis.

4. List six contagious or infectious diseases.

5. List two ways AIDS can be transmitted from one person to another.

6. List three signs and symptoms of AIDS.

7. Describe the care an aide would give to a client with AIDS.

8. List six guidelines or rules to follow when caring for a client with AIDS.

9. List six rules to follow for the prevention of the spread of infections.

10. AIDS is not spread by:
    a. sexual contact with a client with AIDS
    b. sharing needles of infected client
    c. holding a baby that is infected by the AIDS virus
    d. having infected blood from an AIDS client enter an open sore on the aide's body

11. Tuberculosis is spread through sexual contact.
    a. true
    b. false

12. Signs and symptoms of AIDS is/are:
    a. swollen lymph glands   c. skin lesions
    b. diarrhea   d. all are correct

13. Hepatitis can cause a client to become jaundiced.
    a. true
    b. false

14. The incubation time for the AIDS virus can be as long as 7 years.
    a. true
    b. false

Section 5

Caring for Clients with Acute and Chronic Disorders

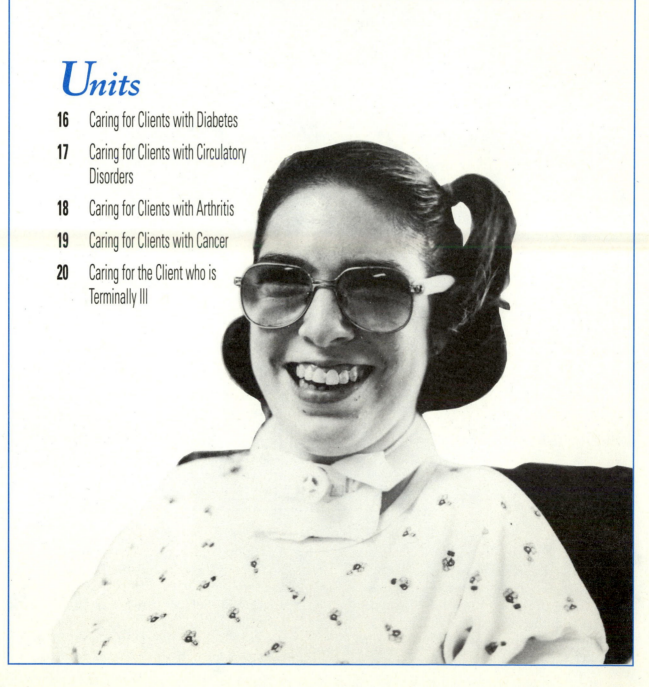

Units

16 Caring for Clients with Diabetes

17 Caring for Clients with Circulatory Disorders

18 Caring for Clients with Arthritis

19 Caring for Clients with Cancer

20 Caring for the Client who is Terminally Ill

Unit **16** Caring for Clients with Diabetes

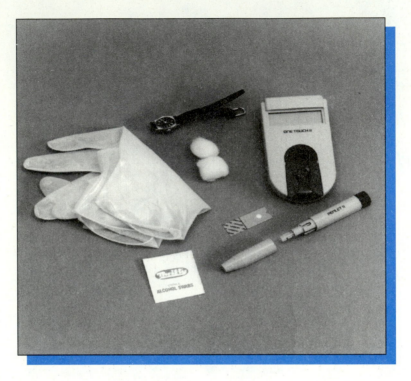

KEY TERMS
· · · · · · · · · · · · · · · · · · · ·

blood lancet	gestational	insulin
cyanotic	glucometer	hyperglycemia
diabetes	glucose	hypoglycemic
gangrene	hormone	subcutaneously

LEARNING OBJECTIVES
· ·

After studying this unit, you should be able to:

- Name four signs and symptoms of diabetes.
- List four types of diabetes.
- Name three ways of controlling diabetes.
- Describe the procedure for testing blood sugar with the use of a glucometer.
- Name three long-term complications of diabetes.

- List signs and symptoms for insulin shock and diabetic coma and the immediate care for each.
- Explain special foot care given to the diabetic client.
- Describe special techniques used in caring for a client who has vision impairment.

Diabetes Mellitus

Diabetes mellitus is a disease of the endocrine system. It is a chronic disease with no cure. The disease is primarily managed through diet, exercise, and drug therapy. The pancreas either does not produce any or produces an inadequate amount of a hormone called **insulin. Hormones** are natural chemicals that the body secretes directly into the bloodstream. The hormones are carried through the bloodstream to regulate and control specific body functions. Hormones are very powerful substances; only a small amount of a hormone is needed to trigger body reactions. The brain sends messages to the endocrine glands, which are then stimulated to secrete the hormones needed by the body.

The functions of insulin are to enable the body to use glucose, to aid in the storage of nutrients, and to make possible the metabolism of carbohydrates and protein. When insulin is not manufactured or cannot be used correctly, a condition called **diabetes** develops. In diabetes, the person's blood sugar level is elevated because the sugar remains in the blood instead of being absorbed into the tissues and used for food. The buildup of sugar in the blood is unhealthy for a number of reasons. It disturbs the fluid balance in the body because it causes kidney problems. Diabetes suppresses the immune system and this allows infections to flourish. Sugar buildup in the blood vessels results in restricted circulation. The lack of adequate blood supply to certain body areas causes many problems in the brain, extremities, eyes, kidney, and heart.

Facts and Figures*

- More than 11 million Americans have some form of diabetes—and 5 million of them do not know it.
- Diabetes is the third leading cause of death by disease in the United States.
- Each year, more than 150,000 people die from diabetes or its complications such as kidney failure.
- In the 45-to-65-year-old age group, twice as many African Americans have diabetes as white Americans.

*American Diabetes Association

- Native Americans have a higher rate of type II (noninsulin-dependent) diabetes than any other population in the world.
- Among Japanese Americans in the West Coast cities, the rate of type II diabetes is two to three times higher than anywhere else in the United States.
- Japanese children living in Japan have a lower risk of developing type I (insulin-dependent) diabetes than do children in any other country.

Classifications

Diabetes mellitus can be classified into four main types and named according to the age of onset and need for insulin.

- Insulin-dependent (IDDM)—type I—often called juvenile diabetes because it affects the young and most often before the age of 36. Other names for this type are brittle or familial. The body does not produce any insulin and the person needs daily insulin injections to stay alive.
- Noninsulin-dependent (NIDMM)—type II—often called maturity-onset diabetes because it comes on after the age of 36. A person usually produces some insulin, but cannot use this insulin effectively to convert **glucose** (sugar) into energy. More than 80% of all persons with diabetes have this kind of diabetes.
- **Gestational**—type III—occurs only temporarily while a woman is pregnant. After she delivers the blood sugar level returns to normal ranges.
- Other types—type IV—come on for various reasons. One cause might be treatment with high doses of steroids or hormones. This type is only temporary because once the drug is discontinued the individual's blood sugar level returns to normal ranges.

Signs and Symptoms

Clinical manifestations of diabetes can come on slowly and sometimes can only be detected during an annual physical examination. Occasionally the disease comes on suddenly. Some of the signs and symptoms to watch for are:

- weakness
- sudden weight loss
- unusual thirst
- frequent need to urinate
- crankiness
- itching
- sores that do not heal

Testing

Routine testing for diabetes during an annual physical examination is important for early diagnosis and detection. The common tests used to diagnose diabetes are:

- Blood sample—usually taken from the arm; tested for the level of blood glucose (type of sugar)—normal being between 80 and 120 mg
- Urinalysis—sample of urine is tested with a chemically treated dip stick
- Glucose tolerance test—series of tests done on urine and blood within the designated time period

Once diagnosed with diabetes, the clients are taught how to test their blood or urine at home. In recent years, technology for testing blood at home has improved tremendously. Doctors prefer that clients test their blood versus their urine because it is a more accurate evaluation. Testing the blood gives a reading of what the blood sugar value is at present. This is not true with urine testing because urine may have been produced in the body hours before an individual voids.

Common urine testing equipment is available at any drugstore. These kits (Ketodiastix and Diastix) include specially treated sticks to be dipped in a urine sample and read according to the directions. This testing is rarely done today. Blood testing equipment has been greatly improved in the last few years, although the initial cost of such equipment is higher than that for urine kits. Many different kits are available on the market (such as Accu-Chek-Easy, Answer, Glucometer5, Tracer II), which are readily available in a local drug store, Figure 16-1.

A few machines have the ability to "talk" you or the client through the procedure. It is important that you know when the reading is normal and when it is high or low. Most physicians say that the "normal range for diabetics should be between 70 and 140 mg/dL." Your nurse supervisor will advise you when to call to report abnormal readings for your client. Each diabetic client needs to have individualized care. For a few clients, a reading of 200 mg is normal, whereas for others it is abnormal. It is the responsibility of your nurse supervisor to interpret the reading. Be sure to check the expiration date on the blood strips. Store the strips in the original vial in a cool dry place. Do not store in a humid area such as a bathroom. Always keep the vial capped tightly. Dispose of the blood lancet in a "sharp" container. Be sure to wash your hands before you start with the procedure and also at completion of the task.

Emergency Treatment

A home health aide needs to be alert for signs and symptoms of diabetic coma or insulin reaction and follow the emergency plan of care for your client. As mentioned, the blood sugar level must be kept in a certain range or problems will occur in the diabetic body. If the blood sugar

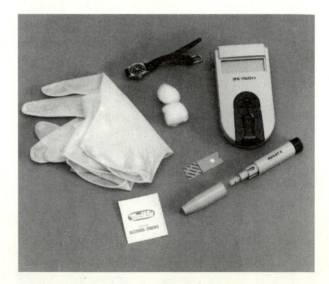

Figure 16-1A Diabetic blood testing equipment: glucose meter, cotton balls, lancet, alcohol, blood testing strips, gloves, and watch

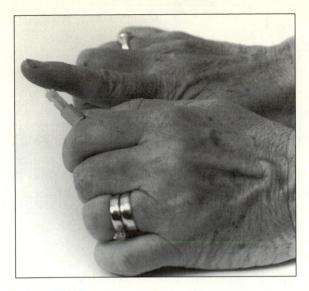

Figure 16-1B   Client pricking finger

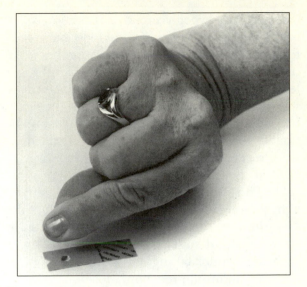

Figure 16-1C   Drop of blood from client's finger on blood testing strip

Client Care Procedure 1:
Testing Blood

Purpose

Testing procedures for blood sugar vary according to the type of **glucometer** the client has purchased. The instructions must be followed carefully to avoid an inaccurate reading. It is also important if you assist with the procedure that you follow universal precaution guidelines. *Always check with your agency to see if you are allowed to do this task.*

Procedure

1. Gather necessary equipment, see Figure 16-1A:

   glucose meter apparatus
   blood lancet (sharp prick)
   gloves
   alcohol swab and cotton ball
   watch with second hand
   blood strips—be sure you have blood
       strips that correspond with your glu-

cometer. Also check to see that the blood strips are not outdated.

2. Cleanse the side of a distal finger with alcohol, then squeeze the finger and prick the finger with the lancet, Figure 16-1B. Wipe away the first drop of blood. You may also use a special apparatus to prick the finger. Rotate fingers if doing this procedure daily.

3. With palm facing down, firmly apply pressure to the pricked finger until a large drop of hanging blood forms. Bring the blood strip to the finger and touch the blood strip to the drop of blood. Completely cover the test zone of the strip with the blood. Wear gloves when doing the testing for infection control purposes, Figure 16-1C.

4. Insert blood strip into machine and observe read-out.

5. Record reading and discard blood strip in proper container.

goes too low (**hypoglycemia**), a condition called insulin reaction occurs; if the blood sugar goes too high (**hyperglycemia**), a condition known as diabetic coma occurs. If a client's blood sugar level is low, the client might experience excessive sweating, headache, pounding of the heart, hunger, irritability, a personality change, and be unable to awaken. This condition is called insulin reaction. It is usually caused by a lack of food in the body and an overabundance of insulin. The client most likely might have skipped a meal, overexercised, or taken too much of the drug, insulin. You can confirm this condition by doing a blood sugar test. If the blood sugar reading is under 60 mg, most likely your client is having an insulin reaction. Most long-term diabetics can tell you if they are in an insulin reaction and if awake will ask you to give them some hard candy or foods containing sugar immediately. If you cannot awaken them, you will need to call an emergency number.

If a client's blood sugar level is high, the person might experience increased thirst and urination, weakness, abdominal pains, generalized aches, heavy breathing, nausea, and vomiting. This condition is called diabetic coma. This is just the opposite of an insulin reaction. This client lacks an adequate supply of insulin in the body, but has an adequate supply of food. It is usually caused by failure to follow the prescribed diet, drinking alcoholic beverages, infections or fever, emotional stress, or too little of the drug, insulin. You also can confirm this condition by doing a blood sugar check. If the blood sugar level is over 200 mg, your client may be going into diabetic coma. You will need to contact your nurse supervisor or follow the plan outlined. If either insulin reaction or diabetic coma is not corrected immediately, coma or death can occur.

A few older clients with diabetes may have vision problems and are unable to read directions to do blood sugar testing or read the numbers on the insulin syringe. Because of these vision problems, you may need to read the directions to them and also double-check their readings. The majority of the clients you will be working with will be able to do their own insulin injections and own blood testing. Loss of vision is a common complication of diabetes.

Diet

Diet is the cornerstone to the management of diabetes. The diet should contain necessary elements of good nutrition, maintain blood sugar levels, and be acceptable to the client's preferences. The diet needs to contain a defined number of calories and consist of 50% to 60% carbohydrates, 12% to 20% protein and 30% to 36% fat. The food intake should be distributed throughout the day and accommodate the client's life-style, activity, and diabetic medication. Because 80% of diabetics are classified as type II diabetics, they will also need to have their calories limited to maintain their ideal weight. The American Diabetes Association has developed exchange lists of foods that can assist the aide and the client in meal planning.

An important duty of the aide is to prepare meals using the dietitian-prescribed diet and exchange list. The aide must be sure the food selected for the meals includes items on the food pyramid and are allowable on the exchange list and diet. The aide needs to encourage and reinforce the importance of abiding by this diet. Occasionally the client will try to deny the disease and not follow the prescribed diet. There is little you can do in the client's own home to force the individual to eat the correct foods. Many times the client will eat the correct foods when you are there, but when you leave he or she might eat a dozen cookies. If this happens, you need to report this to your nurse supervisor.

Obesity and poor nutrition are two common problems in diabetes. Using the prescribed diet can limit these problems. Most diabetics who stick to a diet, take medication, and exercise moderately have fewer health problems. The diabetic client who does not follow the doctor's orders risks serious problems.

Can you imagine how difficult it would be for children to have diabetes and not eat candy bars, cookies, and potato chips like their peers? It is so easy for them (and also adults) to go off the prescribed diet and eat some form of concentrated sugar—like pie or cake. A diabetic client also needs to remember to eat meals and snacks at the same time every day. This is not easy to do. As a home health aide, you need to be supportive and give your client constant encouragement to follow the prescribed diet.

Exercise

Regular exercises are often recommended in the daily routine of clients with diabetes. The benefits of exercise are many. Exercise can improve the client's circulation, assist in maintaining ideal weight, increase a person's well-being, and improve control of glucose in the body (in type II diabetes). A home health aide should encourage and assist the client in doing the prescribed exercise. There will be a wide range of exercises that you might become involved in depending on the mobility and the environment the client lives in. If the client is unable to walk or do the exercises, you will need to do the prescribed passive range of motion exercises for the client, Figure 16-2. If your client is able to do the exercises with little assistance, you will need to encourage the client to do exercises on a regular basis. Your nurse supervisor will assist you in setting up an appropriate exercise plan for your client.

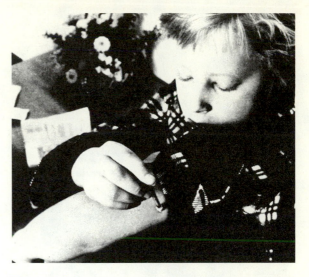

Figure 16-3   This young diabetic is self-injecting insulin into the upper arm. (Courtesy of Diabetes Education Center, Minneapolis)

Drug Therapy

Type I Diabetes

Type I diabetes is always treated with a drug called insulin, which needs to be injected **subcutaneously** (under the skin). It cannot be taken orally because the stomach juices will dissolve the drug. The person with diabetes is taught where, when, and how to inject the medication, Figure 16-3. If a diabetic person is unable to self-inject, another member of the family might be taught to give the injections. Some diabetics are too young to give themselves injections; other clients with diabetes may have poor eyesight or be uncoordinated. Most diabetic clients, if instructed properly, are able to inject their own insulin. **Caution:** A home health aide is NOT permitted to inject insulin. The aide's responsibility is limited to bringing the medication and necessary supplies to the client, Figure 16-4. You should always check the expiration date on the insulin bottle. The insulin should not be used if it is past the expiration date because it might not be effective any longer. It is not necessary to refrigerate insulin, but it should be kept in a cool place and where the temperature stays the same. Most clients prefer to keep their insulin in the refrigerator. Once insulin is prescribed, it will have to be used for the rest of a diabetic

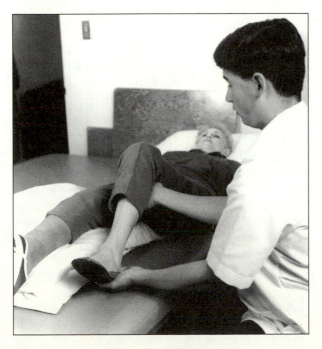

Figure 16-2   The home health aide assists the client with range of motion exercises.

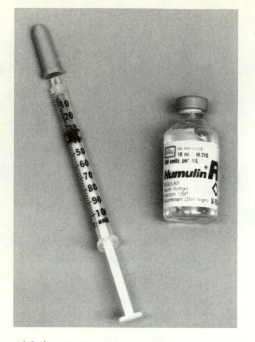

Figure 16-4   Bottle of insulin and insulin syringe

client's life. The three most important factors to remember about insulin are:

1. Measurement must be ACCURATE.
2. The drug must be taken at the same time every day.
3. Sterile technique must be maintained when injecting the drug.

The physician may prescribe different kinds of insulin. Some insulins are fast acting and some are slow acting. The physician will prescribe the type of insulin needed, the frequency, time, and amount of insulin.

Sites recommended for injections include the abdomen, upper arms, and thighs. Most clients are encouraged to rotate injection sites on a daily or weekly basis to avoid changes in the skin tissues, which can alter the rate of absorption of the drug. It is a good idea to keep a record of where the injection was given to assist the client in rotating sites.

The insulin pump is a recent development, but use is limited because of the cost of the equipment and the vigorous participation that is required by the client for safe maintenance and monitoring. A small needle is inserted in the abdomen. The needle is connected to a pump worn on the waist, which holds the insulin supply. This device administers insulin continuously. A control button or a switch allows the client to adjust the release of insulin. In the future, this device may be implanted in diabetic clients just as pacemakers are now implanted into heart clients.

Experiments are now being conducted with pancreatic transplants. The purpose of the transplant is to replace noninsulin-producing cells with insulin-producing cells.

Type II Diabetes

Type II diabetes can be treated in three ways. One way is by diet alone. Once individuals have reached their ideal weight and eat the proper foods, they can maintain their blood sugar level without drugs. The second way is by taking oral hypoglycemic drugs daily. These drugs stimulate the pancreas to make more insulin available. A few hypoglycemic drugs are:

Generic Name	Brand Name
Tolbutamide	Orinase
Acetohexamide	Dymelor
Tolazamide	Tolinase
Chlorpropamide	Diabinese
Glyburide	Diabeta

As a home health aide you need to remember to encourage your client to take the prescribed drug as ordered. Generally, the drug is taken once a day, but it is not uncommon for a physician to order them two (BID) or three (TID) times a day. You need to reinforce to your client the importance of taking the drug as ordered and have an adequate supply of drugs on hand. These drugs are costly and occasionally, a client will want to save money and stop taking the medication. If this does happen, be sure to notify your nurse supervisor. The third way of treating type II diabetes is with insulin injections.

Long-term Complications

Untreated or improperly treated diabetes can lead to many physical problems. Abnormal conditions that occur after a person develops dia-

LONG-TERM DISORDERS	CAUSE	SYMPTOMS	TREATMENT	AIDE'S CARE
1. Blindness	Cataracts, glaucoma, hemorrhage	Partial or total loss of sight, client drops items, stumbles or falls; develops tunnel vision	Surgery can remove cataracts; medication or surgery for glaucoma	Assist in activities of daily living
2. Gas gangrene	Poor circulation; skin breakdown; invasion of tissue by bacteria	Heat in area, skin reddened, formation of ulcers which don't clear up; foul odor and spread of infection and tissue destruction	Medication under physician's order; may require amputation of limb	Assist with dressing changes and rehabilitation
3. Kidney disease	Too much sugar free in urine; filtering system works inefficiently	Frequency, pain, burning while voiding; retention of urine may occur	Diet modification and medication	Observe and record intake/ output; note color and composition of urine
4. Vascular disease and nerve degeneration	High sugar level; poor fat metabolism; poor tissue repair; poor circulation	Open lesions form on skin tissue as vascular degeneration occurs; nervous system functions at decreased level—sight, sound, taste, touch, smell may be affected	Bed rest, moist heat/dressings, diet and medication	Give proper foot care; assist in activities of daily living

Figure 16-5   Complications of diabetes

betes are called diabetic complications. In some cases, even a well-cared-for diabetic may develop serious complications. The most common complications are vascular disease and a high risk of infections. The most common long-term complications are described in Figure 16-5. Although many long-term disorders cannot be avoided, the home health aide can help the client deal with them.

Special Nursing Care

Neuropathy in the Diabetic

Neuropathy is defined as a destructive disorder of the nerves. Diabetic neuropathy is the loss of sensation in nerves. These individuals may be unable to feel pain or differentiate between hot and cold temperature. This can be extremely

dangerous. For example, a diabetic injures a foot or leg and because no pain is felt, continues to use the limb. An infection can occur and the diabetic does not even realize there is a problem. Cuts or wounds not felt and thus not cared for can become infected. A home health aide carefully and routinely must check the client's feet and legs for any sign of redness, any "warm" area, any swelling, or any open cuts. Many diabetics have poor eyesight and are unable to see to check their feet and rely on you to do the checking.

Foot Care

The home health aide should give special attention to the diabetic's feet every day. Client's feet and legs need to be examined daily for signs of dry, scaly, itching or cracked skin; blisters; corns;

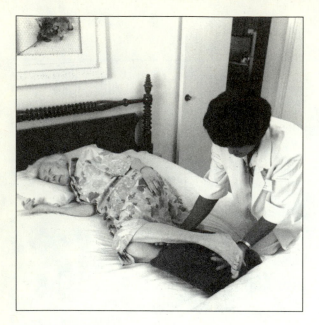

Figure 16-6 A home health aide observing the client's feet for any skin breaks or reddened areas

infections; blueness and swelling of the ankles; and discolored nails, Figure 16-6.

Any abnormality must be reported to the nurse supervisor. Feet are bathed and soaked in warm water with mild soap and then dried with a soft towel. A good lanolin-based lotion is then applied starting at the client's toes and working toward the ankles. This helps stimulate the blood circulation to the feet. If the areas between the toes are moist due to perspiration, a very small piece of lambs' wool or cotton can be placed between the toes. Bunions and corns should be treated by a podiatrist (foot doctor).

In the aged, the nails become thick and difficult to cut. Nail care (both fingernails and toenails) must be carefully done by a registered nurse or someone who has been taught to do it correctly. **Caution:** The aide may NOT cut the diabetic client's nails. There is danger of infection from skin cuts around the nails. In addition, improper cutting may cause ingrown toenails, which easily can lead to infection. If the client's feet are well cared for and examined daily, infection is unlikely to develop. The following foot care guide will help reduce injury to the feet:

- Bathe the feet daily in warm, not hot, water.
- Pat the feet dry with a soft towel, especially between the toes.

- Massage the feet to increase circulation.
- Wear clean white cotton socks and change daily.
- Do not apply iodine or carbolic acid to cuts on feet.
- Avoid walking barefoot.
- Wear comfortable, well-fitting shoes.
- Do not use commercial corn pads.

Prevention of Infections

Clients with diabetes are very susceptible to any type of infection. If they do get the flu or a cold, their blood sugar levels usually decrease and increase erratically. Diabetic clients need to have their blood sugar monitored closely if they have even a mild cold or fever.

Diabetic persons also have problems with small cuts or abrasions healing. Special attention by the aide to keep the cut or abrasion as clean as possible will assist in the healing process. Slow healing is due in part to poor circulation. Breakdown of the blood vessels prevents nutrients from being carried to the injured tissue; this delays the healing process. The slow healing process leaves the skin open to infection. The risk of infection is also increased because of the extra sugar in the tissues. The extra sugar creates an ideal environment for bacteria to grow. Bacteria can multiply quickly before the body is able to defend itself. Poor circulation delays the transport of substances needed to fight off the bacteria. It is of the utmost importance to report any sign of infection early to your nurse supervisor.

Good skin care is vital in preventing the skin from developing pressure sores and other skin lesions and is an especially important safety precaution for the diabetic client. Remember to use only a mild soap sparingly when bathing the client and use a good lanolin-based lotion on the client's body. Keep bed linens dry, clean, and wrinkle free, and turn and reposition your client every 2 hours (q2h) to avoid pressure spots.

When blood vessels are injured or diseased, the surrounding cells die from lack of nutrition and oxygen. A large area of dead tissue is called **gangrene.** Gangrene is a serious condition because it is easily infected with certain bacteria. Gangrene is a form of an infection. The bacteria causing gangrene thrive in dead tissue. The

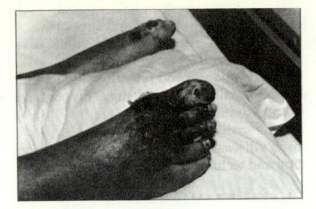

Figure 16-7   Gangrene of the toes and foot often requires eventual amputation. (From Hegner and Caldwell, *Geriatrics: A Study of Maturity,* copyright 1991 by Delmar Publishers Inc.)

bacteria spread quickly, causing severe pain and greater tissue damage.

The aide should check the client's feet and broken skin areas for signs of gangrene, Figure 16-7. The first sign is a hot and reddened skin area. This area quickly becomes cold and bluish (**cyanotic**). After the tissues are dead, they turn black and flake off. Drainage from the area may be bubbly and will emit a strong, foul odor.

Identification Tag

All diabetics should wear a Medic Alert identification tag. The ID is a labeled tag worn as a bracelet or necklace, Figure 16-8. The ID tag should be worn by the diabetic individual at all times. The label indicates the person's:

* name
* address
* telephone number
* medical condition
* physician's name

In emergencies, the Medic Alert ID informs emergency personnel, police, health care providers, and others of the diabetic's medical condition. A diabetic who develops acidosis or insulin shock needs immediate help. The ID tag notifies health personnel that the person's emergency is possibly a diabetic condition. If the person is unconscious, the tag may provide information necessary to save the person's life. Medic Alert tags are also worn by persons with epilepsy and with allergies to certain drugs.

For further information or to acquire a Medic Alert ID tag, write to: Medic Alert Foundation International, Turlock, CA 95380; phone (209)632-2371.

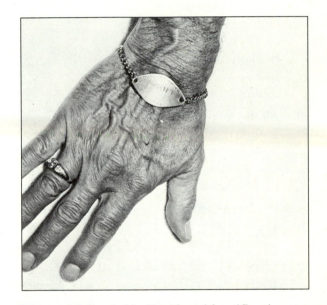

Figure 16-8   A Medic Alert identification tag provides essential information in case of an emergency.

SUMMARY

* Diabetes is treated with diet and exercise regimens, monitoring glucose levels, and drug therapy.
* As many as 11 million Americans may have diabetes and yet half of them do not know they have the disease.
* Emergency situations that need immediate attention are insulin shock and diabetic coma.
* Major long-term complications of diabetics are blindness, circulatory problems, and gangrene.
* Preventive health care can save the client needless pain and suffering.

REVIEW

1. List five signs or symptoms of diabetes.

2. What three treatments are used to control diabetes?

3. Explain the steps involved in testing a client's blood for a blood sugar reading. When is the reading abnormal?

4. What are the symptoms of insulin shock? What is the immediate care given?

5. What are the signs and symptoms of diabetic coma? What should the aide do if these symptoms appear in the client?

6. Why is good foot care important when caring for a client with diabetes?

7. Why is it important to have a client with diabetes exercise on a routine basis?

8. List three complications of diabetes.

9. Name two signs/symptoms of high blood sugar and two of low blood sugar that a home health aide may observe if a diabetic client is experiencing either of these conditions.
    a. Low blood sugar
       1.
       2.
    b. High blood sugar
       1.
       2.

10. All the following are true statements regarding foot care for the diabetic client except:
    a. toenails should be cut frequently by the home health aide
    b. feet should be soaked in warm water daily
    c. have client wear shoes or slippers
    d. feet should be rubbed with lotion to keep skin in good condition

11. Which of the following is not a common complication of diabetes?
    a. blindness   c. high risk of infections
    b. vascular diseases   d. loss of memory

12. Diabetes can be treated by:
    a. special diet   c. insulin injections
    b. oral medication   d. all are correct

13. In a client with diabetes the _____ is not producing adequate amount of a hormone called insulin.
    a. thyroid   c. adrenal gland
    b. pancreas   d. liver

Unit *17* Caring for Clients with Circulatory Disorders

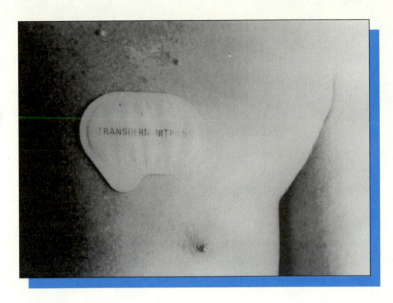

KEY TERMS

aneurysm
angina pectoris
anticoagulants
aphasia
arteriogram
arteriosclerosis
artery
atherosclerosis
cardiac arrest

catheterization
cerebral hemorrhage
cerebral vascular accident (CVA)
collateral circulation
congestive heart failure
edema
embolus
expressive aphasia
ischemia

myocardial infarction
myocardium
nitroglycerin
occupational therapist
receptive aphasia
spasticity
sublingually
thrombus
transient ischemic attack (TIA)

LEARNING OBJECTIVES

After studying this unit, you should be able to:

- Identify symptoms of four heart conditions.
- Describe care given for clients with heart conditions.
- Explain the effect nitroglycerin has on the blood vessels.
- Give two other names for a CVA.
- List six risk factors for heart attacks and strokes.

- List three signs a client might display if suffering from a heart attack.
- List four warning signs of stroke.
- List three causes of stroke.
- List two types of aphasia.
- List three physical defects a client may have following a stroke.
- Explain the role of the aide in assisting a client recovering from a stroke.

Risk Factors

Because of the many deaths due to heart problems, many research studies have been conducted on individuals with heart problems. Research has documented the following as major risk factors in heart disease.

- Heredity—Children of parents with heart problems have a greater risk of developing heart conditions.
- Male sex—Men have greater risk than women and have attacks earlier in life.
- Increasing age—Fifty-five percent of all heart attack individuals are age 64 or older.
- Cigarette smoking—Smokers have twice as many heart attacks as nonsmokers.
- High blood pressure—High blood pressure increases the heart's workload and weakens the heart and also the blood vessels in the brain, which eventually can cause either a heart attack or stroke.
- High cholesterol levels—As cholesterol levels increase, the risk of having a heart attack increases.
- Diabetes—People with diabetes have a greater incidence of heart attacks and strokes.
- Obesity—Individuals who are 30% overweight have a greater incidence of strokes and heart attacks.
- Physical inactivity—Lack of exercise combined with obesity and high cholesterol levels will definitely increase the person's chances of having a heart attack or stroke.
- Stress—There is an increased risk of heart problems in people who are under continuous stress in their life.

Disorders of the Heart and Circulatory System

The number one killer of individuals in the United States is cardiovascular disease. In 1990 more than 1 million Americans died as a result of some form of cardiovascular disease. Circulatory problems affect people of all ages. If an infant is born with a heart defect, it is called a congenital heart problem. Five percent of heart attacks occur in people under age 40, and 45% occur in people over age 65. The majority of individuals who survive after a heart attack or stroke will need some type of medical care and also assistance with activities of daily living (ADL). A home health aide has a very important role to play in the recovery of these clients. Some of these clients will need assistance with ADL for the rest of their lives.

In many cases, disorders of the heart and circulatory system force people to change their life-styles. Many people become very frightened when a heart or circulatory condition is diagnosed. The psychological effects can be almost as crippling as the illness itself. People may think they will be permanently disabled or wonder how they can support themselves and their families. People who have had one heart attack may be afraid of having another heart attack. As a result, they often avoid moving about or doing any exercise. Inactivity usually leads to boredom, irritability, and depression.

The aide may be assigned to help clients with heart problems. Certain conditions require clients to reduce their activity. Clients may need assistance with household duties or child care. The aide may need to remind clients to avoid vigorous exercise or heavy lifting. The physician's orders explain a safe range of activity. Helping the client adjust to the necessary changes may be the focus of the aide's care plan.

Angina Pectoris

Angina pectoris is a symptom of a condition called myocardial ischemia, which occurs when the heart muscle (**myocardium**) does not get an adequate supply of blood and oxygen to do its work. Lack of blood supply is called **ischemia.** Angina pectoris is a mild pain in the chest radiating to the left arm and up through the neck area. This condition results from lack of oxygen in the heart muscle due to constricted blood vessels. Angina pectoris generally strikes men of middle age. An attack can last from a few seconds to several minutes. It may occur after physical exertion or during times of stress and anxiety. The person becomes pale and ashen and the body stiffens. Blood pressure increases dramatically (hypertension). The client becomes flushed and perspires heavily.

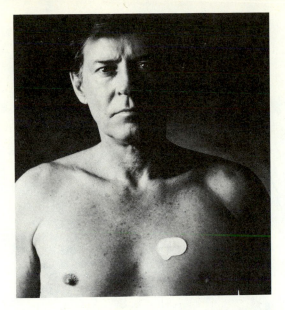

Figure 17-1   The client may receive nitroglycerin through the skin by means of a transdermal patch. (Courtesy of CIBA Pharmaceutical Co., Division of CIBA GEIGY, Summit, NJ)

Immediate treatment for angina is physical rest. If this is not the first angina attack, the client is likely to have medication on hand. A common emergency medication used for angina is **nitroglycerin.** Nitroglycerin may be taken **sublingually,** in which case the tablet is placed under the tongue. It can also be applied topically in the form of a nitro-patch placed on the skin, Figure 17-1. The nitroglycerin is absorbed through the skin; a patch provides 24 hours of medication.

Nitroglycerin opens the blood vessels to increase the blood flow. The effects of the drug occur within 2 to 3 minutes. The pain from the angina is usually relieved in 5 to 10 minutes. Nitroglycerin is one of the medications that can only be used for a specified period of time because it loses its potency and effectiveness. The aide should check the expiration date carefully to be sure the medicine is still effective. This drug must be kept in a brown bottle as exposure to light decreases its potency.

When angina pectoris has been diagnosed, the client should avoid emotional stress, exercise after heavy meals, exposure to sudden cold, and overexertion. Medication should be placed near the client for immediate use during an attack. The client often has a headache after tak-

ing the medication due to vasodilation of the blood vessels in the brain. Frequent periods of rest with restricted activities, no smoking, medications such as a nitro-patch, and a special diet are commonly ordered by the physician. If the client does not obtain relief from the nitroglycerin in 15 minutes, emergency care is required. Call an ambulance, physician, family members and case manager.

Myocardial Infarction

Myocardial infarction is more commonly known as a coronary or a heart attack. A myocardial infarction is a condition in which a blood vessel of the heart muscle closes or is blocked by a blood clot. The size and location of the incident determines the seriousness of the attack. There can be permanent damage to the heart. In the case of permanent damage, parts of the heart muscle die and **collateral circulation** may develop. This means that other small blood vessels take over the job of bringing blood to the heart muscle. These smaller vessels actually become enlarged so they can carry the required amount of fresh, oxygenated blood to the heart muscle. The symptoms of a heart attack are shown in Figure 17-2.

The person may go into shock and collapse. Prompt emergency treatment is needed and is begun in the ambulance and continued in the hospital. In the hospital the client will be treated for a heart attack. The need for specialized treatment or surgery will be determined. A **catheterization** is often done to assist in diagnosing the client's problem. During cardiac catheterization a catheter (thin tube) is introduced into a vein or **artery** and passed through the heart so that any abnormalities of the heart can be detected. One common operation is called coronary artery bypass grafting, or CABG. After release from the hospital, treatment at home may include increased activity with continuing periods of rest and a special diet.

Anticoagulants and other drugs may be part of the treatment when a person has had a coronary attack. **Anticoagulants** are drugs that reduce the ability of the blood to clot. A home health aide should observe and report any signs of side effects from the use of anticoagulants. These may include bleeding from the gums or

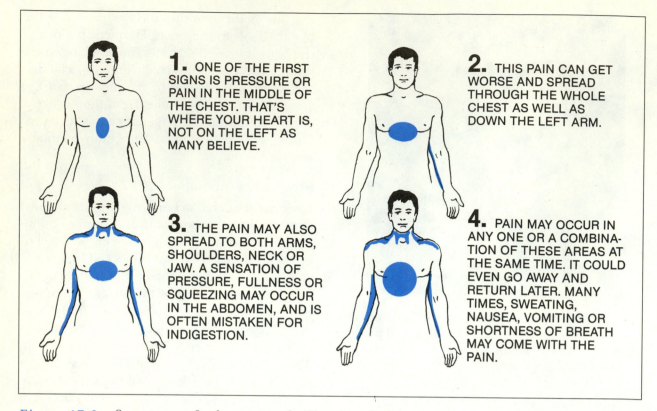

1. ONE OF THE FIRST SIGNS IS PRESSURE OR PAIN IN THE MIDDLE OF THE CHEST. THAT'S WHERE YOUR HEART IS, NOT ON THE LEFT AS MANY BELIEVE.

2. THIS PAIN CAN GET WORSE AND SPREAD THROUGH THE WHOLE CHEST AS WELL AS DOWN THE LEFT ARM.

3. THE PAIN MAY ALSO SPREAD TO BOTH ARMS, SHOULDERS, NECK OR JAW. A SENSATION OF PRESSURE, FULLNESS OR SQUEEZING MAY OCCUR IN THE ABDOMEN, AND IS OFTEN MISTAKEN FOR INDIGESTION.

4. PAIN MAY OCCUR IN ANY ONE OR A COMBINATION OF THESE AREAS AT THE SAME TIME. IT COULD EVEN GO AWAY AND RETURN LATER. MANY TIMES, SWEATING, NAUSEA, VOMITING OR SHORTNESS OF BREATH MAY COME WITH THE PAIN.

Figure 17-2 Symptoms of a heart attack (Reprinted with permission of the American Heart Association/New York City Affiliate, copyright 1987)

bruising of the skin. Use of an electrical razor instead of a blade razor is recommended for clients receiving anticoagulants. The home health aide *never* massages the legs. This could loosen a blood clot and send it directly to the lungs, causing pain and severe breathing problems or cardiac arrest. If a person's heart does stop beating, it is called **cardiac arrest.**

Congestive Heart Failure

Congestive heart failure is a condition in which the heart becomes inefficient. This condition can affect the right or left side of the heart, or even both sides at the same time. This is most often caused by heart muscle damage. Thus, the heart's pumping action is weakened. A client with congestive heart failure may have one acute attack and then develop a chronic condition. The symptoms include a cough, dyspnea, cyanosis, and retention of fluid (**edema**). Fluid (frothy pink sputum) may accumulate in the lungs causing pneumonia. Congestive heart failure can lead to chronic disability and death.

Treatment for congestive heart failure usually includes two types of drugs. One is digitalis, which slows and strengthens the heartbeat. The other is a diuretic, which reduces fluid accumulation in the body. A diuretic medication causes the client to urinate frequently to help rid the body of excess fluids. The aide should help the client remember to take medications that have been prescribed.

Diet control is an important part of the treatment for congestive heart failure. Diets usually are low in sodium and fat. A diet high in bulk helps the client avoid constipation. A person who is constipated must strain to have a bowel movement; this strain can be dangerous for any person with a heart condition. People who are overweight should restrict their calorie intake as well. The dietitian provides exact orders for diet preparation. Exercise and rest must be balanced. The correct amount of each is determined by the doctor.

Clients with congestive heart failure must stay in an upright or semiupright position

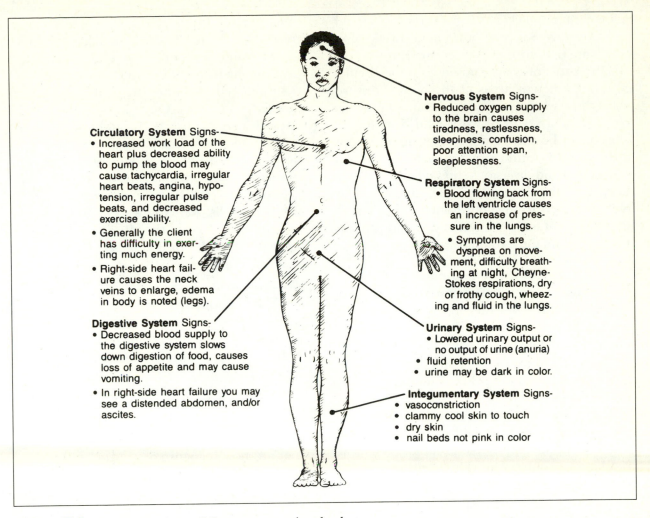

Circulatory System Signs-
• Increased work load of the heart plus decreased ability to pump the blood may cause tachycardia, irregular heart beats, angina, hypotension, irregular pulse beats, and decreased exercise ability.
• Generally the client has difficulty in exerting much energy.
• Right-side heart failure causes the neck veins to enlarge, edema in body is noted (legs).

Digestive System Signs-
• Decreased blood supply to the digestive system slows down digestion of food, causes loss of appetite and may cause vomiting.
• In right-side heart failure you may see a distended abdomen, and/or ascites.

Nervous System Signs-
• Reduced oxygen supply to the brain causes tiredness, restlessness, sleepiness, confusion, poor attention span, sleeplessness.

Respiratory System Signs-
• Blood flowing back from the left ventricle causes an increase of pressure in the lungs.
• Symptoms are dyspnea on movement, difficulty breathing at night, Cheyne-Stokes respirations, dry or frothy cough, wheezing and fluid in the lungs.

Urinary System Signs-
• Lowered urinary output or no output of urine (anuria)
• fluid retention
• urine may be dark in color.

Integumentary System Signs-
• vasoconstriction
• clammy cool skin to touch
• dry skin
• nail beds not pink in color

Figure 17-3   Congestive heart failure—systems involved

(head higher than feet). They will need frequent position changes, TED hose or Ace bandages on their legs, bedside commode or bedpan, and a bed bath. The clients will need to have their activities spaced throughout the day to prevent becoming overly fatigued. When sitting in a chair, they will need to have their legs slightly elevated.

The aide must help clients limit their activities. Clients with congestive heart failure usually cannot go up and down stairs. They must lead very quiet lives because they tire easily. Such clients get depressed because they must be dependent on others. To help reduce this feeling of dependence, the aide should give the client as much control over personal care and selection of activities as possible. Refer to Figure 17-3 for a summary of the effects of congestive heart failure.

Arteriosclerosis

Arteriosclerosis is a condition in which the arteries become hard and lose their soft, rubberlike stretchiness. It is caused by a buildup of fatty deposits on the inside walls of the blood vessels.

An important aspect of client care is to increase the client's circulation. A bath not only cleans the skin but also helps to increase circulation. Even if a client does not need a complete bath daily, the aide must wash the client's feet and massage them with lotion each day. After the feet are cleaned, a pair of cotton or wool socks may be needed. Arteriosclerosis clients often complain of cold feet. **Caution:** the home health aide must NEVER apply a hot water bottle or heating pad even if requested by the client. To warm the client's feet, the aide should give the client a second pair of socks or put a blanket over the client's legs. The socks should not fit tightly. Socks or other items of clothing which are tight further restrict circulation.

Pressure sores are caused by poor circulation in particular areas of the body. Pressure sores cause worry because the healing process is so slow. As a result of worry and discomfort, clients can be short-tempered. A home health aide should communicate with the client. Recreation and diversions should be planned to keep the client's mind off the condition. An aide will need to find out hobbies or activities that the client may be interested in and plan activities around these interests.

Contractures.   If unable to move about, the client must be protected from developing deformities. Weight from the bedcovers can press against the feet. Bedcovers should be kept loose around the feet. Bed cradles may be used in holding bedcovers off the feet. Footboards may be placed against the soles of the feet so that the foot will not drop into an unnatural position. A contracture is a condition in which muscles become shortened and stiff. The muscles freeze in an uncomfortable position. Foot drop is a kind of contracture. The client who is unable to move in bed should be repositioned regularly every two hours. This increases circulation, bringing more oxygen to the cells. Prescribed exercise and repositioning helps prevent pressure sores from forming.

Cerebral Vascular Accidents (CVA or Stroke)

What Is a Stroke?   The word "stroke" was originally used to indicate any sudden catastrophic illness. Now the term is almost exclusively used to name a sudden paralysis caused by brain damage.

Stroke is caused by a lack of oxygen and nutrients to the brain cells. This interruption of blood to the brain may be due to one of the following three reasons: an **aneurysm** (a ballooning out of the wall of an artery) that breaks open and causes a hemorrhage; an **embolus** (a moving blood clot) that causes complete blockage of an artery; or a **thrombus** (a blood clot that forms inside an artery) that can cause a blockage of blood flow to the brain cells. Brain cells deprived of circulation for even a few sec-

onds stop functioning. If the circulation stops for a few minutes, brain cells die. This causes loss of voluntary motion and results in paralysis, often in one half of the body.

Brain cells die when they are without oxygen for 4 minutes. Once brain cells are destroyed, they cannot be brought back to life. Unlike other cells in the body, new brain cells do not form to replace damaged ones. The most common cause of a CVA is high blood pressure. A CVA does not necessarily destroy all the brain cells. Remaining cells can compensate by taking over the duties of those destroyed by a CVA. For that reason rehabilitation is of vital importance.

The following material is adapted from and used with permission from a booklet prepared for in-service training. Courtesy of The Burke Rehabilitation Center, White Plains, NY, the Auxiliary and Fletcher H. McDowell, MD, Executive Medical Director:

Risk Factors in Stroke.   Often, long before a stroke occurs, there are conditions or symptoms that are now recognized as associated with an increased risk of stroke. These are:

Hypertension—sustained elevated blood pressure
Atherosclerosis (often called hardening of the arteries)—a disease in which fatty materials containing cholesterol platelets and calcium accumulate on the interior walls of the arteries. These accumulations can build up to the point where the vessel becomes obstructed.
Heart disease—(coronary artery disease, damaged heart valves)
Diabetes
Family history of heart disease and/or stroke

In addition, several conditions also may be controllable risk factors. Among these are high blood fat and cholesterol levels, obesity, physical activity, cigarette smoking, and excessive alcohol intake.

An individual who has one or more of these conditions or habits has a greater risk of developing a stroke than those without them. The risk increases with an increase in the number of factors found in a particular individual.

Statistics indicate that although stroke can happen at any age, strokes are more common in people who are 60 years or older. Men have more strokes than women. African Americans have more strokes than members of the white race.

First Signs of a Stroke.   A stroke can begin in several ways: with transient ischemic attacks; gradual onset; or sudden onset of symptoms.

Transient ischemic attack, (TIA), consists of a brief period of weakness, loss of speech, or loss of feeling that lasts from minutes to hours and then goes completely away. These attacks are due to a sudden but temporary decrease or stoppage of blood flow to a part of the brain. These attacks are important because they are a reliable warning of possible permanent stroke.

Usually a person with TIA reports one or more of the following: the sudden onset of numbness, tingling, or weakness on one side of the body, or in the hand and face on one side; temporary blindness in one or both eyes; difficulty understanding words and using them correctly; dizziness; nausea; vomiting; staggering; fuzzy speech; or a combination of these symptoms. During an attack, people do not lose consciousness, and recover with no aftereffect.

Whenever the symptoms described above occur, it is very important that a physician be notified, even if the episode seems to pass as quickly as it came. Knowing and heeding these symptoms can help to avoid a completed stroke since treatment of the underlying conditions that caused the attack often is possible, either with medications or with surgery.

When TIAs have occurred, an individual should receive a careful neurologic examination to determine if the condition causing the TIA can be corrected. Most TIAs are caused by atherosclerosis, which may block an artery, or may break up and release bits of debris, which travel through larger arteries and may block small arteries in the brain, stopping blood flow transiently to a part of the brain. Most commonly, the site of arterial disease is in the carotid artery where it divides into two large vessels—one going to the brain, the other to the face, jaw, and eye. This site is im-

portant because it is accessible to surgery and often the obstruction or plaque can be removed. Also, medications that reduce blood clotting or prevent blood platelets from clumping together can help stop TIA and reduce the chance of stroke.

Clinical evaluation of TIA usually includes an examination by a neurologist, examination of blood vessels in the arms, legs, and neck; ultrasound examination of the arteries in the neck; and often an arteriogram. The **arteriogram** is a series of x-ray pictures that show the flow of blood in the arteries, neck, and head taken after the injection of dye or contrast substance into the artery. The dye causes the arteries to stand out clearly in the x-ray picture, allowing the physician to identify sites of vessel disease and obstructions. This allows the physician to determine whether surgical correction of an obstruction is possible.

Cerebral infarction is the term used to describe the condition in which a portion of the brain dies when an artery becomes blocked and blood is prevented from reaching that part of the brain. The blockage can be the result of hardening and eventual blockage of the artery (atherosclerosis), or be caused by a blood clot in the vessel, or other substances plugging a vessel (emboli). The portions of the brain thus starved of blood, die and cannot function. The effects of the stroke, weakness, paralysis and loss of feeling, become evident in those parts of the body controlled by the affected part of the brain. When a person has a completed stroke, which means that the paralysis or loss of sensation does not go away rapidly, that person should be hospitalized to be given needed care and to be sure that there is no further progression of the stroke. Treatment of a patient after a completed stroke is difficult as there are no known remedies that can reverse the brain damage or cause nervous system tissue to regenerate. If improvement occurs in nerve function, it happens naturally. Function in a person with stroke can be adapted and improved by rehabilitation.

Risk factors which, singly or in combination, increase the chances of stroke caused by the interruption of blood flow to the brain, resulting in cerebral infarction, are the same as for TIA. Frequently, a person may have a stroke with no recognized underlying cause. Cerebral infarction is the most common form of stroke and is responsible for the majority of partially or completely disabling strokes. The most desirable form of management of this condition is prevention.

Cerebral hemorrhage means there is bleeding into the brain, which destroys or disrupts brain tissue. Normally, blood flows to the brain through arteries under high pressure. In vessels with weakened walls, the pressure may cause a rupture and blood will escape into the brain. Under high pressure, blood can spread rapidly in all directions from the point of rupture and may disrupt or damage a large area of the brain causing weakness, paralysis, loss of sensation, and frequently loss of consciousness. Cerebral hemorrhage has a high risk of being fatal.

High blood pressure is the main risk factor for hemorrhage into the brain, as almost all cerebral hemorrhages occur in clients with high blood pressure. Treatment of high blood pressure is the only satisfactory means to deal with cerebral hemorrhage. Survivors usually have severe physical disability.

Possible Aftereffects of Stroke.   Stroke can affect an individual in many different ways, depending on which part of the brain has been damaged. Among the possible consequences are:

Physical Deficits
    Paralysis or complete loss of strength or mobility in a part of the body, usually the arm, leg, and face on one side
    Weakness in a part of the body. Usually weakness is more marked in the hand than in the arm, and the arm is more affected than the leg
    Spasticity (stiffness)—a loss of muscular control with automatic muscle contraction
    Loss of sensation (feeling) in parts of the body, usually on one side
    Loss of bladder and bowel control
    Speech and language disability. Difficulty thinking of and saying words or difficulty using or understanding words
    Difficulty in swallowing
    Loss of coordination, such as unsteady gait

Perceptual/Cognitive (thinking) Problems
    Loss of awareness
    Denial or neglect of the right or left part of the environment
    Inability to understand time
    Difficulty performing tasks in proper sequence
    Disrupted sleep-wake cycles
    Uncontrolled laughter or crying
    Confusion, forgetfulness, memory loss, impaired judgment

Personal/Family Problems
    Loss of job
    Inadequate financial resources
    Loss of independence. Dependence on others who may or may not be willing or capable of accepting the new responsibility for continuing care.
    Loss of sexual capacity
    Loss of self-esteem

Psychological Problems (mood)
    Depression, apathy
    Anger, hostility
    Euphoria

Environmental Problems
    Architectural barriers in the home
    Lack of accessible transportation

Not all of these problems happen to each individual. When any of them do happen, there are degrees of difficulty. Most of these problems can be improved. However, after a completed stroke, there will always be limitations. Those with paralysis, those whose perceptual capacities are affected, or whose memory and orientation are diminished, have the greatest difficulties.

Signs and Symptoms.   The person who suffers a stroke usually loses consciousness and becomes incontinent of urine and feces. In addition, breathing becomes labored or difficult. If consciousness is not lost, the client may complain of a severe headache, slurred speech, and blurred vision. After a CVA there is usually a weakness or paralysis on one side of the body. This one-sided weakness or paralysis is known as hemiple-

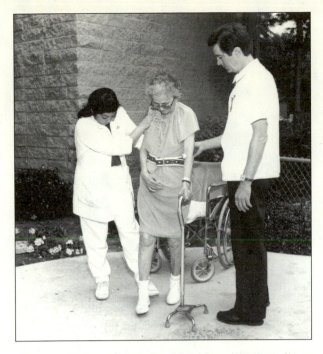

Figure 17-4 A home health aide walking a client with right side weakness. The aide is on the client's weak side. The aide is using a gait belt while walking the client.

gia, Figure 17-4. The use of muscles is temporarily or permanently lost when paralysis occurs. Thus, there may be difficulty in speaking, eating, swallowing, and even hearing. The client may take a long time to eat meals. The home health aide must be patient and permit the client to be as independent as possible. That means *assisting* with eating, not *force feeding*, in order to finish the meal.

Rehabilitation after a Stroke. A care plan will be developed by the home health team for each individual client. The plan will be implemented once the client has returned home. The goal of the plan is to have the client returned to the highest level of function as possible. The client will need to be encouraged continuously to do as much as possible with as little assistance as possible from others. At times it may be easier for an aide to dress or feed the client, but it must be remembered that the goal of care is to have the client do it, not you.

After a stroke the client will most likely have one-sided weakness. The client will need to do exercises to regain strength and function to the side of the body that is weak. If the client is unable to do the special exercises called range of motion exercises, the aide will need to do the exercises. The supervising nurse or physical therapist will train the aide to do the exercises, Figure 17-5. If the client can do the exercises without assistance from others, the exercises are called active range of motion exercises. Passive range of motion exercises are those in which the client moves with the assistance of others. Exercises will be helpful in the prevention of contractures and improve the client's self-image.

Ambulation is very important in the rehabilitation of a person after a stroke. The client may need to have a brace applied to the weak leg for support before ambulating. Check to see if the brace fits properly and does not cause skin irritation. A gait belt will need to be applied to the client's waist before standing the client. Remember to stand on the client's weak side and hold on to the gait belt when ambulating the client. Each time you ambulate the client, encourage the client to go a few steps father. This will help the client build up strength and also make the client feel like some progress is being made. Occasionally a client's sight may be affected after a stroke. Be sure when you walk a client there is a clear pathway without obstacles in the way. You, the home health aide may see these obstacles, but your client may not.

Dressing is another area where the client may need assistance. If you need to assist the client to put on a shirt, remember to put the shirt on the weak arm first and then the strong arm. If the client is unable to button the shirt, Velcro closures can be substituted in place of buttons. Elasticized waist slacks will be easier to slip on and off than pants with buttons and zippers.

Oral care is of special importance for the client with a stroke. Before meal time, it is important to do routine oral care, and if the client has dentures, encourage the client to wear them. The client may need assistance in eating or the client may need to use one of the many assistive feeding devices now available. An **occupational therapist** may work with the client in restoring the ability to eat without the assistance of others. It will be the home health aide's job to follow through with the plan designed by the

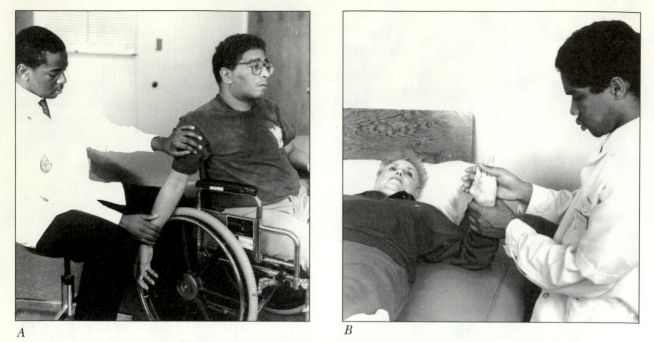

A   B

Figure 17-5   A. Physical therapist is performing range of motion exercises with a client who had a stroke. *B.* Physical therapist is doing range of motion exercises to the client's arm.

occupational therapist. The aide may need to cut the meat or open the milk carton, but once these small tasks are done, the client will be able to manage eating without assistance. Be sure to check the inside of the weak side of the mouth for food particles after the client has finished eating. The client does not have feeling on the paralyzed side and often food becomes lodged into the cheek and the client may not know it.

Bowel and bladder retaining may also be part of the rehabilitation of a stroke client. The aide should follow a schedule suggested by the nurse. The urinal, bedpan, or commode should be presented at specific times during the day and night. For example, the client who is given the bedpan after each meal and before bedtime eventually becomes adjusted to using it at that time. The body then becomes regulated. Before the client adapts to a schedule, the aide should be sure to keep the client's bed dry and clean.

Communication Problems.   The client with a stroke often has a great deal of trouble communicating. The home health aide must be patient and understanding of the speech problems. **Aphasia** is a condition in which the ability to speak is impaired. Aphasia is common after a

client has a stroke. Aphasia can affect the ability to talk, listen, read, or write. The client's speech may be slurred, distorted, and slowed. A client who has **receptive aphasia** does not understand words someone else says. In this case, it may be better to have a communication board to point to, Figure 17-6. In a few cases the client might understand all words coming into the brain, but is unable to respond appropriately. An example of this might be when an aide asks him if he is hungry and he responds with "no" and in reality he wanted to say "yes," but the answer came out just the opposite of what he wanted. This is extremely frustrating to both you and the client. This type of aphasia is called **expressive aphasia,** for the client is unable to express himself correctly. In the majority of cases in which the client just recently suffered a stroke, a speech therapist will be assisting with communication problems. The speech therapist will inform the aide of the client's type of aphasia and how to communicate more effectively. Sometimes the only words a CVA client uses are curse words or nonsense syllables. This is called automatic speech (involuntary speech). The home health aide should avoid treating the client as a child. In speaking to a stroke client, the aide should

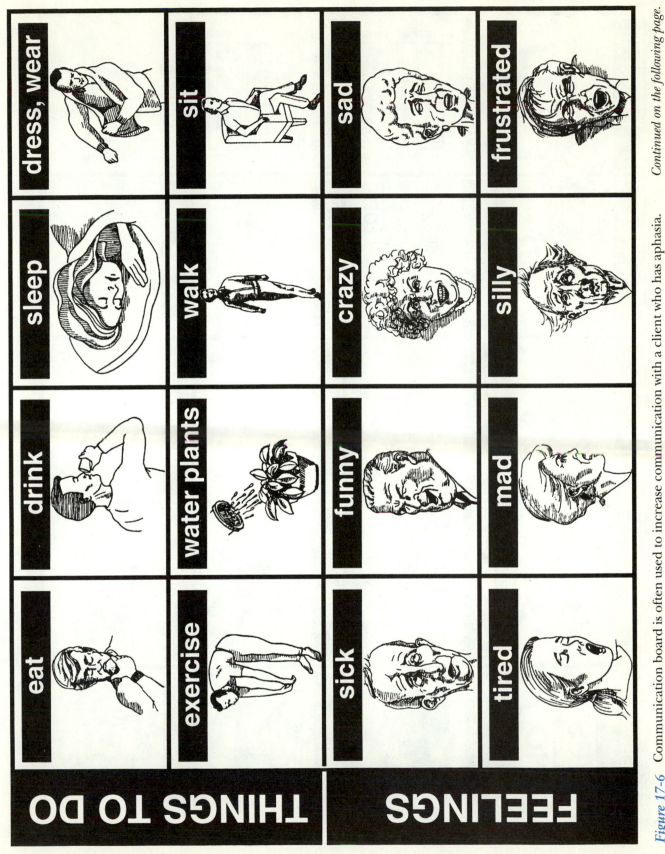

Figure 17-6 Communication board is often used to increase communication with a client who has aphasia.

Continued on the following page.

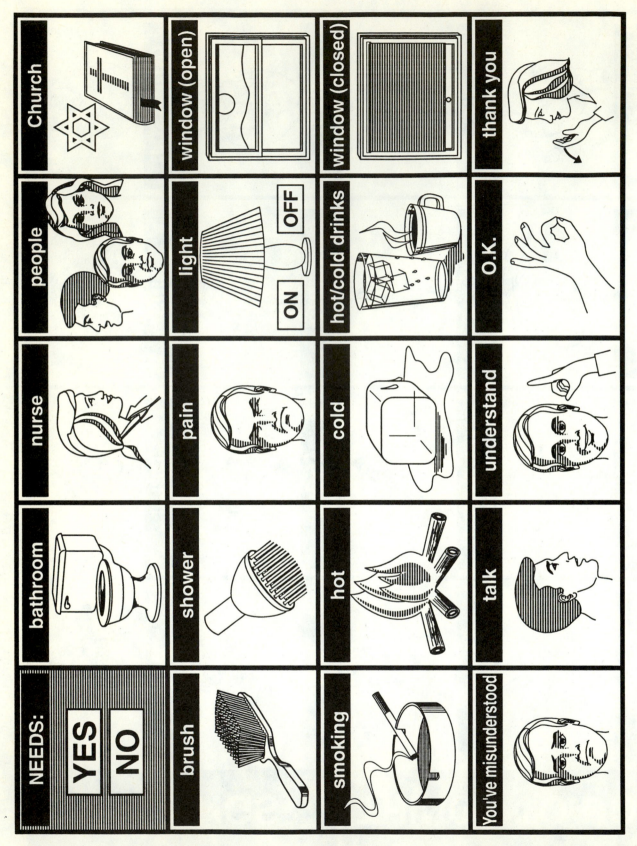

Figure 17-6 *(Continued)*

use simple sentences that require only short and simple answers from the client. Speaking clearly and simply aids the client's understanding. Stroke clients usually need a great deal of encouragement and reassurance.

Clients who normally wear glasses should continue to wear them even if their sight has been affected by the stroke. This makes the client feel less changed in outward appearance.

The same is true if the client wears dentures or a hearing aide. These courtesies show that the aide respects the client.

The home health aide should encourage clients to help themselves as much as possible. This may take more of the aide's time, but it is a form of rehabilitation. The more the clients help themselves, the more progress they will make.

SUMMARY

....

- A home health aide should have a basic knowledge of the common heart conditions. This knowledge increases the aide's awareness of the signs of distress and potential dangers to the client.
- The aide should be able to tell when the client's condition has changed and when to contact someone for help.
- The home health aide is responsible for making the client as comfortable and content as possible. The client must always be treated with concern and respect.
- The disorders of the heart and circulatory system demand special care in the following areas:

1. Diet is of utmost importance in most heart conditions. A diet prescribed by the dietitian must be followed very carefully.
2. The home health aide has an important role in assisting clients to function at the highest level of wellness possible after a stroke or heart attack.
3. Suitable exercise and rest periods are to be given as ordered by the physician.
4. Medications should be taken as prescribed.

REVIEW

1. List six risk factors that would make a client more susceptible to having a stroke or heart attack.
2. List three signs that a client may have if suffering a heart attack.
3. List four warning signs of a stroke.
4. List three causes of stroke.
5. Explain aphasia.
6. List three possible long-term physical effects of a stroke.
7. Explain the role of the home health aide in the rehabilitation of a client who had a stroke.
8. A client who has had a stroke or CVA has difficulty speaking, a sign which is called:
    a. aphasia
    b. lethargy
    c. paraplegia
    d. mutism

9. As a home health aide caring for a client with heart disease, which of the following would not be in the care plan?
   a. balance activity and rest
   b. low-salt and low-cholesterol diet
   c. observe for signs of chest pain and shortness of breath
   d. weight-bearing exercises

10. Mr. Kane has had a stroke. Which of the following signs would you expect Mr. Kane to display?
    1. aphasia   3. paralysis on one side of the body
    2. swollen joints   4. drooping lip on one side of the face
       a. 1, 2, & 3   c. all but 4
       b. all but 2   d. all are correct

11. The drug nitroglycerine may be used by clients with heart problems.
    a. true
    b. false

12. A client with a diagnosis of angina pectoris will often have mild chest pain after exercising or eating a large meal.
    a. true
    b. false

Unit *18* Caring for Clients with Arthritis

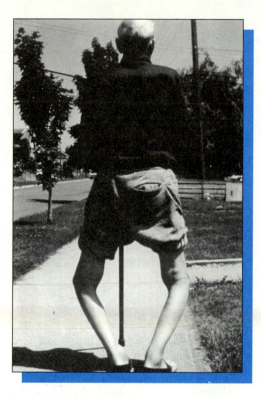

KEY TERMS
....

arthritis
degenerative
gout

joint inflammation
osteoarthritis
rheumatism

rheumatoid
steroids
tophi

LEARNING OBJECTIVES
....

After studying this unit, you should be able to:

- Describe the care given to clients with arthritis.
- Define the terms relating to arthritis.
- Discuss the exercises related to arthritis.
- Define osteoarthritis, rheumatoid arthritis, and gout.
- List two types of diets that may be prescribed for clients with arthritis.
- List three side effects of steroids.
- List two goals of an exercise program for a client with arthritis.
- Name two joints that can be replaced by surgery.

Definition of Arthritis

Arthritis means **inflammation** of a **joint.** Many people complain of **rheumatism** in relationship to their many aches and pains. The Arthritis Foundation states that arthritis is the number one crippler in the United States. It affects one in seven people. There are several types of arthritis. The two main ones are rheumatoid arthritis and osteoarthritis. A comparison of the two types is shown in Figure 18-1. Other types of arthritis are gout and ankylosing spondylitis. Arthritis affects 50% of persons over 65 years of age. Twice as many women as men are afflicted with the disease. The major warning signs of inflammatory arthritis are:

- swelling in one or more joints
- early morning stiffness
- recurring pain or tenderness in any joint
- inability to move a joint normally
- obvious redness and warmth in a joint
- unexplained weight loss, fever, or weakness
- symptoms and signs of the above persisting for 2 weeks.

Other infections such as gonorrhea, tuberculosis, syphilis, Lyme disease, and streptococcal infections can also cause arthritis. There is no cure for the disease. It can be managed with diet, medication, surgery, and exercise.

Rheumatoid Arthritis

Rheumatoid arthritis affects individuals of all ages, the very young to the very old. The cause of this condition is that the immune system that normally protects the body, works the opposite way and fights against the body. The joints of the body are generally affected the most. It is a disease that affects the whole body, not only the joints. It can occasionally cause problems with the muscles, skin, blood vessels, nerves, and eyes. Additional signs besides joint enlargement that accompany the disease are weight loss and fatigue. A client may have a very mild case, which might cause mild discomfort, or a severe case where widespread joint deformities are present. The morning is usually the worse part of the day for clients with this type of arthritis; then stiffness and fatigue are more evident. As the disease progresses, joint problems increase in severity. These deformities of the joints are usually seen in the hips, knees, wrists, fingers, and ankles, Figure 18-2.

Osteoarthritis

Another term for **osteoarthritis** is "wear and tear" arthritis. This type of arthritis affects the weight-bearing joints such as the spine, hip, and knee joints. It is most often seen in clients over 65 years of age. The cause of this type of arthritis is not clearly understood. A few of the possible causes might be attributed to the aging process, obesity, heredity, stress, trauma, unbalanced hormone levels, or overuse of the joint. The affected joint or joints become enlarged and painful. Osteoarthritis is the most common type of arthritis.

Gout is a form of arthritis that affects mainly men over the age of 40. This type of arthritis is due to the presence of too much uric acid in the client's system. The first sign of this disease is a painful "big toe." It can also affect other joints such as the foot, ankle, and wrist. These

RHEUMATOID ARTHRITIS	OSTEOARTHRITIS
affects the lubricating fluid in the joints	affects cartilage-connective tissue
inflammation	wearing down condition
system disease (total body)	health not generally affected
good and bad periods of pain	no particular good periods without pain
results in deformity	limits motion only
affects any joint	affects weight-bearing joints
affects all ages—even young people	affects older age group

Figure 18-1   Comparison of rheumatoid arthritis and osteoarthritis

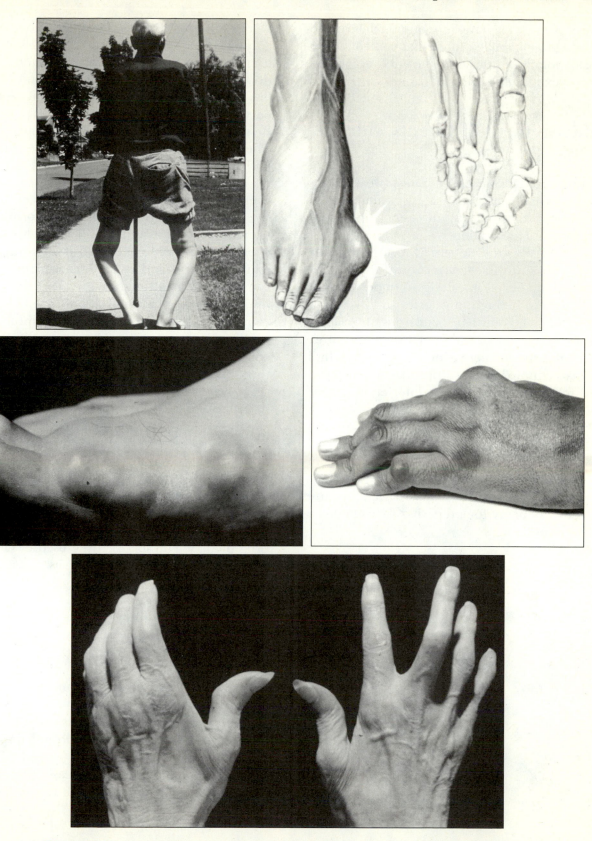

Figure 18-2   Joint deformities due to arthritis (Courtesy of the Arthritis Foundation)

areas of the body have little outpouches or protruding lesions called **tophi** that contain abnormal amounts of uric acid. The affected joint becomes extremely painful.

Management of Clients with Arthritis

Arthritis is a chronic **degenerative** (weakens and becomes abnormal) disease. It is generally managed with diet therapy, an exercise program, surgery, and medication.

The diet is individualized to meet the person's needs. If the client is overweight, the diet will need to be low in calories; if underweight, it will need to be high in calories and protein. If the client has gouty type of arthritis, the client is placed on a low purine diet (dietitian will explain this special diet to you or the client). Individuals crippled with arthritis may have a few of the following problems that interfere with their nutritional status.

- Pain may be a factor in lack of appetite.
- Decreased activity can cause weight gain, immobility, and pressure sore development.
- Impaired movement, Figure 18-3, may cause lack of energy for preparing foods and grocery shopping.

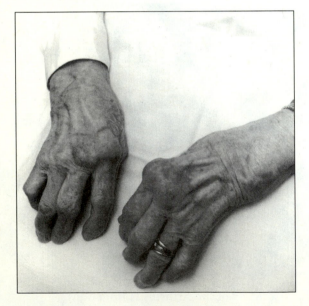

Figure 18-3 The joints of the hands are deformed because of arthritis.

You as a home health aide will be most likely employed to work in the home to assist the client with cooking, cleaning, and laundry duties. The client will be able to assist you to do a few of these tasks but will tire easily. You need to encourage the client to do as much as possible. Be sure you do not overtire or rush the client. The client will need a longer time to accomplish a task.

Another form of treatment for arthritis is exercise. Exercise can be passive (you do it for the client) or active (the client performs the exercise without assistance). The goals of the exercise program are to maintain complete joint movement and in some cases strengthen the muscles around the specific joint. The physical therapist will develop a care plan for your client. If the joints are very painful and swollen the exercises should be done gently but consistently. The exercises are usually ordered three (tid) to four times (qid) a day. It is helpful to have the client take pain medication a half-hour before the exercises are started. The client then might be more willing to cooperate and do the exercises. If the client does not exercise these joints, they will quickly become frozen or immobile. The reason for a client doing these exercises is to keep the joint mobile and maintain muscle strength.

The third method of treatment is through drug therapy. The specific drug used by clients will depend on many factors such as:

- severity of the arthritis
- tolerance to the drug (aspirin is the drug of choice, but many individuals with stomach problems cannot tolerate aspirin)
- cost
- type of arthritis (gout responds to certain drugs only)
- client's response (some clients respond positively to a drug and others do not respond at all)
- presence of other chronic diseases (if a client has a stomach ulcer, certain drugs cannot be prescribed)

There are certain side effects that a home health aide should watch for from specific drugs. If your client is taking aspirin watch for abnormal signs of bleeding such as black stools, bloody urine, ringing in the ears, and skin bruises. Other drugs used to treat arthritis are a group called **steroids.** These are powerful drugs that can cause edema, weight gain, susceptibility to infections, and elevated blood pressure.

Your nurse supervisor will inform you of the side effects to watch for in your client. More than one hundred drugs are used to treat arthritis; all have different side effects.

In the last 20 years, surgery has become successful in helping the arthritic client maintain independence. Doctors can now replace arthritic knees and hips. Surgery can also be done on the client's spine, jaw, wrist, fingers, and shoulder. An aide may be employed to care for these clients on a temporary basis after they return home from the hospital. Clients will have their own individualized plan of care designed by a team consisting of the doctor, nurse, physical therapist, occupational therapist, and case manager. You need to be fully informed of your responsibilities and what you are allowed and not allowed to do.

An aide employed in a home with a client with arthritis will need to take special care when

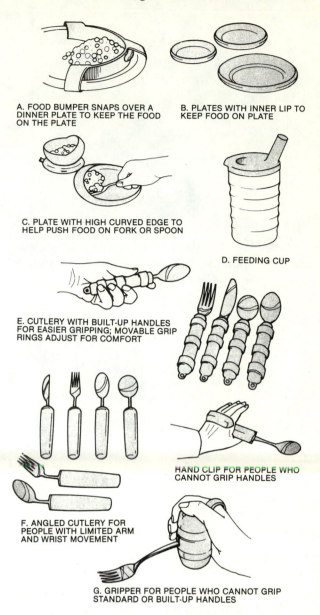

A. FOOD BUMPER SNAPS OVER A DINNER PLATE TO KEEP THE FOOD ON THE PLATE

B. PLATES WITH INNER LIP TO KEEP FOOD ON PLATE

C. PLATE WITH HIGH CURVED EDGE TO HELP PUSH FOOD ON FORK OR SPOON

D. FEEDING CUP

E. CUTLERY WITH BUILT-UP HANDLES FOR EASIER GRIPPING; MOVABLE GRIP RINGS ADJUST FOR COMFORT

HAND CLIP FOR PEOPLE WHO CANNOT GRIP HANDLES

F. ANGLED CUTLERY FOR PEOPLE WITH LIMITED ARM AND WRIST MOVEMENT

G. GRIPPER FOR PEOPLE WHO CANNOT GRIP STANDARD OR BUILT-UP HANDLES

Figure 18-5 Eating and drinking aids for the disabled (From Badash and Cheesebro, *Essentials for the Nursing Assistant in Long-Term Care*, copyright 1990 by Delmar Publishers Inc.)

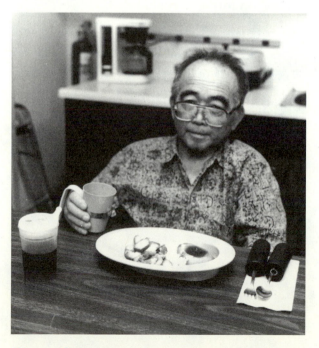

Figure 18-4 Client feeding himself using special cup, foam-handled fork, and spoon

moving or transferring a client. The aide needs to be aware that one day the client might be able to do everything but the next day very little. Encourage the client to function at the highest level of wellness possible and to be as independent as possible. Try to assist the client in making tasks as simple as possible. A suggestion might be to have Velcro closures rather than buttons on clothes. Have elastic waist slacks rather than zipper and button closures. Bars

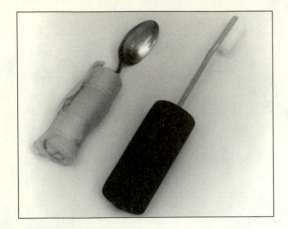

Figure 18-6   A. Assistive devices for a client with arthritis: spoon and toothbrush with large, easy-to-hold foam handles

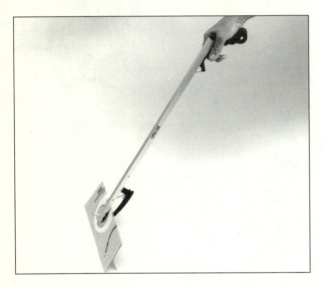

B. Assistive device is used to pick up items from the floor or to reach for items on shelves.

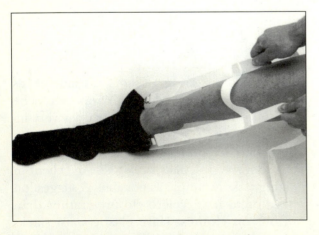

C. Using an assistive device to put on socks

may need to be placed by the bathroom and in the tub area to assist the client to get up and down. Portable whirlpool attachments can be placed in the client's tub to help soothe the client's pain. Another effective therapy is exercising or swimming in warm water pools.

Assistive devices are often used in caring for arthritis clients, Figure 18-4. Assistive devices are used mainly to maintain or increase independence, simplify tasks, reduce pain, and minimize stress on joints. Clients are more likely to use and accept simple devices over complicated devices, Figure 18-5. Your nurse supervisor will usually explain how to use these devices for your client, Figure 18-6.

In some cases the physical therapist will come directly to the home and do specialized treatments such as ultrasound or hot and cold treatments for your client, Figure 18-7. In other instances you might need to take your client (on a regular schedule) to see the physical therapist for specialized therapy.

One who suffers from arthritis can become frustrated, irritable, impatient, and depressed. If an individual has lost a job as a result of the crippling effects of the disease, he or she will worry over loss of income and cost of treatment. Sexual relationships may fail due to the pain and discomfort of the client.

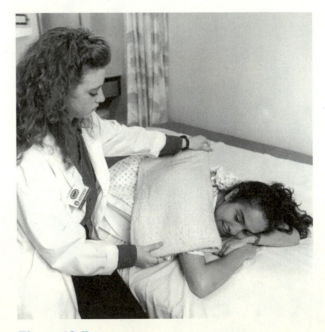

Figure 18-7   Physical therapist doing specialized treatment to client's shoulder

SUMMARY

- Arthritis is a chronic progressive disease that primarily affects the client's joints.
- Treatment of arthritis is mainly through exercise, diet, and medications.
- Osteoarthritis affects mainly the weight-bearing joints.
- Rheumatoid arthritis can affect clients in all age groups.
- Home health aides have an important role in the care of arthritic clients. The aide can assist with food preparation, personal care skills, and exercise programs.
- Arthritis cannot be cured; the degenerative process cannot be reversed, but a balanced treatment program can reduce pain and improve joint movement to allow the client to be as active as possible.

REVIEW

1. List three types of arthritis.

2. List two types of diets that can be prescribed for clients with arthritis.

3. List three side effects of steroids.

4. List two goals of an exercise program for a client with arthritis.

5. List two joints that can be replaced by surgery for a client with arthritis.

6. Describe special care that you as a home health aide would do for a client with arthritis.

7. A client has arthritis. Care will include all the following except:
   a. assistance with activities of daily living
   b. range of motion exercises
   c. use of braces or prosthesis to prevent contractures
   d. exercising painful joints gently and consistently

8. Osteoarthritis is often seen in women over 65 years of age.
   a. true   b. false

9. Rheumatoid arthritis clients experience more discomfort and pain in the evening than in the morning.
   a. true   b. false

10. Signs of inflammatory arthritis are:
    a. swelling of one or more joints
    b. inability to move a joint normally
    c. obvious redness and warmth in a joint
    d. all are correct

11. Arthritis can be treated by:
    a. drug therapy
    b. exercise program
    c. surgery
    d. all are correct

Unit *19* Caring for Clients with Cancer

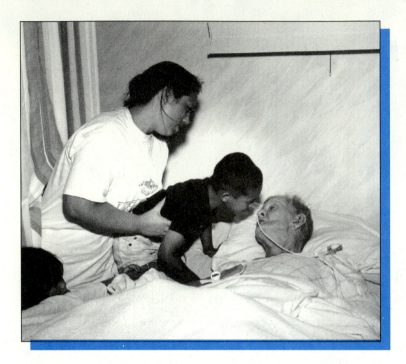

KEY TERMS
....

articulates	hysterectomy	mastectomy
benign	ileostomy	metastasis
biopsy	irrigation	metastasize
cancer	laryngectomy	pneumonectomy
carcinogen	larynx	remission
chemotherapy	lobectomy	stoma
colostomy	malignant	trachea
expectorate	mammogram	tracheostomy

LEARNING OBJECTIVES
....

After studying this unit, you should be able to:

- Identify three diagnostic tests for cancer.
- Identify six surgical procedures used in cancer treatment.
- List seven warning signs of cancer.
- Define metastasis, benign tumor, remission, and malignant.

- Name three types of treatment for cancer.
- Describe the care given to a client with cancer.
- List two precautions for an aide to take when caring for a client who is on chemotherapy.

Cancer is the uncontrolled growth of abnormal cells. In healthy tissue, body cells grow, die, and are replaced by new cells. This is a normal process that goes on day after day. Sometimes cells do not follow the rules of the body; they begin to divide quickly, steal nourishment from surrounding cells, and push normal cells out of the way. They prevent normal cells from doing their regular jobs. Finally, these cells cause changes in the body, which produce signs that indicate something is wrong. Any one of the warning signs listed in Figure 19-1 should be called to the supervisor's attention as soon as possible.

The exact cause of cancer is unknown. However, studies are beginning to show some factors that lead to the formation of cancer cells. A substance or agent that produces cancer is called a **carcinogen.** The general group of carcinogens are chemicals, environmental factors, hormones, and viruses. A chemical could be ingested with food such as red dye #2. The chemical could be inhaled as tar or asbestos. Environmental factors include such physical agents as x-rays, sunlight, or trauma. Hormones may be cancer causing because of their excess, deficiency, or imbalance. Viruses seem to upset the functions within a cell.

The way that carcinogens change normal cells into cancer cells is unclear. Therefore, a cure is not yet possible. Most physicians agree, however, that the sooner cancer is detected, the less chance it has of spreading to other parts of the body. Some tumors may interfere with body functions and require surgical removal, but they do not spread to other parts of the body. These are known as **benign** tumors. **Malignant** or cancerous tumors not only invade or destroy normal tissues, by a process known as **metasta-**

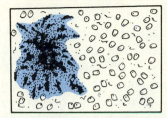

MALIGNANT CANCER GROWTH
(NO CAPSULE WITH RANDOM GROWTH)

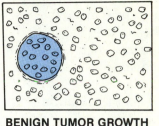

BENIGN TUMOR GROWTH
(WITH CAPSULE AROUND IT)

Figure 19-2   Growth of cancer cells

sis, the cells break away from the original tumor and move to other parts of the body, Figure 19-2. There they may form other tumors. (A cancer originating in the brain, for example, can spread or metastasize to the lungs, kidneys, or other parts of the body.) When cancer is treated early and does not reappear for 5 years, the cancer is considered to be cured or in remission. **Remission** means no longer growing or spreading.

It has been estimated that in the United States alone over fourteen hundred people a day die from some form of cancer. Since 1949 there has been a sharp rise in the number of men who develop cancer. Cancer of the lung has risen sharply in women also. Cancer of the breast, colon, and rectum occur most often among women. There are over 100 types of cancer. Cancer is second only to heart disease as the leading cause of death each year. However, statistics also show that deaths due to cancer are increasing whereas those due to heart conditions are decreasing. Research continues into the causes and possible cures for cancer.

Cancer Treatments

Several kinds of treatments may slow or stop the growth of cancer cells. Surgery is used to remove tumors and organs of the body that have

---

WARNING SIGNALS

1. Unusual bleeding or body discharge
2. A lump or thickening in an area of the body
3. A sore that does not heal
4. A change in bowel or bladder habits
5. Hoarseness or a chronic cough
6. Indigestion or difficulty in swallowing
7. A change in size, shape or appearance of a wart or mole

Figure 19-1   Warning signs of cancer

become cancerous. Sometimes surgical procedures alone are used. At other times, radiation or cobalt therapy may be used following surgery to kill any cancer cells around the surgical area. Radiation and cobalt therapy are sometimes the only treatments used. The rays are aimed deep in the body to reach cells which cannot be removed surgically. Very often, however, surrounding cells are destroyed by the rays. The site of the therapy is marked in ink on the body. The home health aide must be careful not to remove these marks when bathing the client. The marked area should not be touched by the home health aide.

Side effects of radiation therapy may include nausea, skin damage, itching of the area, and loss of hair. Some people wear wigs to cover bald heads caused by radiation.

Chemotherapy is the use of one or a combination of chemicals to attack cancer cells. Chemotherapy may be used after surgery or in combination with radiation therapy. In some cases chemotherapy works only for a short time after which it no longer kills cancer cells. New combinations of chemicals are then prescribed. This treatment, too, can cause unpleasant side effects. All of the cancer treatments cause damage to healthy cells around the cancer site. If you care for a client who is undergoing chemotherapy, you should take certain precautions to protect yourself. These precautions need to be taken the first 48 hours after the client has received chemotherapy. You need to wear gloves when handling urine or stool material. When you empty the bedpan or urinal you need to be very careful that you do not splash the contents on the toilet seat or floor or on yourself. You will need to flush the toilet twice, after emptying the contents of the bedpan or urinal or after a client uses the bathroom. After 48 hours these precautions are no longer necessary.

Common side effects of chemotherapy include nausea, vomiting, diarrhea, anemia, rash, susceptibility to infections, loss of hair, bleeding, and mouth sores. Hair loss caused by chemotherapy is usually temporary.

So-called miracle cures for cancer are sold in many forms. Most people who market these products are only interested in making a profit from the misfortune of others. Some people with cancer choose to take experimental drugs. However, a person is wiser and safer to follow the advice of a trustworthy physician. The best treatment plans are based on sound research.

Caring for Clients with Cancer

Proper nutrition and special diets are a very important part of cancer care. Clients should be given foods they like unless otherwise ordered by the doctor. Four to six small meals a day are usually preferred. If meals look attractive and are served nicely they may stimulate the client's appetite. Usually these diets are high in protein and calories. It is often necessary to supplement the diet with liquid nutritious supplements such as Ensure or similar products. The client's appetite is usually better in the morning. Be sure to give your client good oral care to stimulate the desire to eat, then follow with foods the client likes.

Clients in the later states of cancer become very thin and weak. They will need assistance in all their activities of daily living. They will need excellent skin care to prevent skin breakdown. Their bodies need to be bathed with a mild soap and lotioned frequently during the day. They need to be positioned every 2 hours. It is recommended that at least twice a day the client be allowed to sit in a comfortable chair to give the back a rest and also to increase the circulation. An air mattress, egg crate mattress, or sheepskin can be used in the bed to try to make the client as comfortable as possible.

Occasionally the room where the client's bed is may need a room deodorizer. It is not uncommon for cancer clients to have a distinguishing odor even after a bath. As a home health aide you can place a deodorizer in the room to mask this odor.

The goal of cancer therapy in the final stages is to keep the client as comfortable as possible with the least amount of pain. Your nurse supervisor will discuss with you when the client may have the pain medication. If the pain is not controlled by the medication that is ordered, you will need to inform your nurse supervisor. As the cancer spreads in the client's body, the pain may become more severe and less tolerated by the client. Occasionally just a change of position or a cold or warm snack may help ease the pain.

Cancer of the Female Reproductive System

Among women in the middle years, problems may occur in the reproductive system. All women should have an annual physical examination, including a Pap smear. A Pap smear detects early cellular change in the cervix of the uterus. In this test, a microscopic examination is made of cells scraped from the uterus. If repeated Pap smears show cellular changes, the physician takes a biopsy. A **biopsy** is a sample of tissue cut from the area where cellular change is present. The biopsy determines the seriousness of the cell changes. Sometimes a cone-shaped section is cut out for examination. If cancerous cells are found, a partial or complete hysterectomy may be performed. A **hysterectomy** is a major surgical procedure in which the uterus, and sometimes the ovaries and fallopian tubes, are removed.

Some women develop fibroid tumors in the uterus. These tumors are benign or noncancerous. They can become large or cause heavy bleeding during menstruation or cause pain. When these problems exist, a hysterectomy may also be needed. After any major surgery it may take from 9 to 12 months for full health to return. Very often women are depressed following a hysterectomy. For some women there is a feeling that they have lost the ability to enjoy sex. If the ovaries have been removed, hormones may be prescribed to replace those normally produced. The hormone pills help the body to adjust physically and help restore a sense of well-being. Although a hysterectomy prevents further childbearing, it does not physically prevent enjoyment of sex.

Cancer of the Breast

Another area in which women develop cancer is the breast. An excellent method of detecting breast cancer is self-examination, Figure 19-3. Each woman should self-examine her breasts monthly about 7 to 10 days after each period. A woman checks for changes in the shape of each breast, a swelling, dimpling of the skin, or changes in the nipple. She checks for lumps while lying on her back. Using flat fingers, she presses in a clockwise motion around the breast. If a lump is noticed, she should go to her gynecologist for further examination. All lumps are not malignant (cancerous). Many women have simple, benign breast tumors. Sometimes it is necessary to remove the benign tumors through surgery.

One diagnostic technique used in suspected breast cancer is an x-ray called a **mammogram.** Special x-ray studies can detect unhealthy or cancerous cells. In some cases, a biopsy is ordered if there is a suspicion of cancer of the breast. An incision (cut) is made in the breast and a microscopic examination of tissue is made at once. If cancer is diagnosed, some doctors remove only the growth itself. This can only be done when the diagnosis is made early. This procedure is sometimes known as a lumpectomy. Sometimes it is necessary to remove the entire breast tissue, underlying muscles and the lymph glands under the arm. This procedure is called a radical **mastectomy.** If there is any sign that the cancer cells have **metastasized** (spread), both breasts may need to be removed. A woman's self-image is often decreased after a mastectomy. She sees the altered shape of her body as a deformity. However, an increasing number of women who have had this surgery can talk about it quite openly. Because they have talked about their own surgery, other women have become more aware of the need to examine themselves. As a result, many breast cancers are discovered early enough for successful treatment.

Following a mastectomy, there is often a time of mental depression. It is very important for a mastectomy patient to have the support of her loved ones. She must understand that her life can continue as before. Part of this is accepting that she is just as much a woman as she was before surgery. Because the surgery may involve the underarm glands and muscles of the chest and underarms, rehabilitation is very important. Special exercises are prescribed by the doctor. After a mastectomy patient returns home, these exercises must be continued regularly. After the

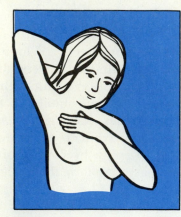
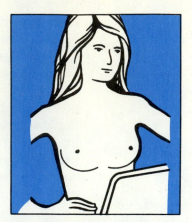
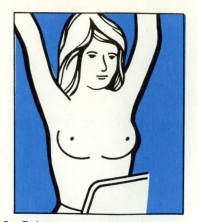

A. With the fingers flat, check for a knot, lump or thickening.

B. Flex your chest muscles and compare breast shape.

C. Raise your arms and compare breast shape.

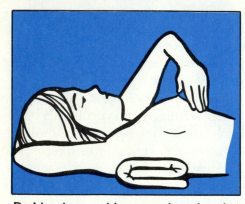
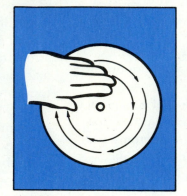
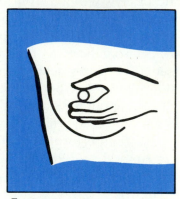

D. Lie down with a towel under the shoulder and one arm behind the head. Check again for any knot, lump or thickening.

E. Move fingers in a circular motion, inward toward the nipple.

F. Gently squeeze the nipple to check for a clear or bloody discharge.

Figure 19-3   Self-examination helps to detect breast cancer at an early stage.

incision is healed, most patients are encouraged to have a prosthesis (artificial breast) made. In some cases, the prosthesis may be surgically fitted under a flap of skin. Other prosthetic devices shaped as cups are fitted into a special bra.

Many women who have breast surgery are helped by the American Cancer Society's *Reach to Recovery Program.* This is a free service to help meet the physical, emotional, and cosmetic needs of women who had breast cancer. The Cancer Society carefully trains select volunteers, who have a previous history of breast cancer and have coped well with their own breast cancer. This volunteer and the client can talk over fears arising from this disease and their impact on a client's body and self-image and concerns for her future. The volunteer can talk about the need for exercises and how to adjust to the prosthesis that replaces her breast. This has been a very successful program and has given many women the courage to accept the loss of a breast.

Cancer of the Respiratory System

The respiratory system is on duty 24 hours a day from birth to death. Fresh air is inhaled into the body and carried to the lungs. The oxygen from the air is carried to all parts of the body by the circulatory system. As oxygen is delivered to the cells of the body, waste gases are picked up and carried back to the lungs. Carbon dioxide is exhaled and thereby expelled from the body.

Many infections and disorders can affect the respiratory system. Everyone has had a common cold. Flu, pneumonia, bronchitis, and other upper respiratory infections are some of the other illnesses affecting this system. Cancer, too, can start to grow in the lungs. Signs of lung cancer are:

• a persistent, hacking cough
• pains in the chest area
• tiredness
• a low-grade fever
• sudden weight loss
• coughing up blood
• wheezing
• recurrent bronchitis or pneumonia
• difficulty swallowing

If a biopsy (microscopic examination of tissue) shows cancer cells, surgery can sometimes be done to remove all or part of a lung. Removal of part of the lung is called a **lobectomy.** Removal of the entire lung is called a **pneumonectomy.** Lung cancer grows slowly at first. However, by the time it is diagnosed, seven out of ten cases are not helped by surgery. A person with lung cancer must be kept as comfortable as possible. Most clients with lung cancer are cared for in the home setting. The client will require oxygen therapy throughout the day. The client will most likely need to sit in the chair in order to breathe. If the client does go to bed, the bed will need many pillows because the client cannot breathe well lying down. The client will also most likely **expectorate** (spit) thick sputum. Remember to use universal precautions when handling the client's sputum.

Cancer of the Larynx

The **larynx** is the part of the trachea called the voice box. Cancer of the larynx occurs in men more often than in women. In addition, 75% of the people who develop cancer of the larynx have been heavy smokers. A common treatment for cancer of the larynx is surgical removal of the larynx, called a **laryngectomy.** To remove the larynx, a tracheostomy must be performed. A **tracheostomy** is a surgical opening made into the trachea below the larynx. The **trachea** is the airway between the nasal passages and the lungs. The tracheostomy is an artificial airway that can be used to supply oxygen to the lungs. A tracheostomy tube is placed into the artificial airway to keep it open, Figure 19-4. In some instances the tracheostomy tube is no longer being used. Instead a **stoma** is created surgically. A small dressing called a bib is placed over the stoma. This should be kept damp so that the client doesn't inhale dust or other foreign particles.

After the tracheostomy has been done, the second part of the surgery is completed and the cancerous larynx is removed. The tracheostomy tube remains in place permanently in a laryngectomy patient. After the patient has recovered from surgery, rehabilitation starts.

Speech therapy is needed to teach the patient how to talk. One of the methods is to gulp air in through the tracheostomy tube, swallow it, and then burp out words. It takes a great deal of practice to relearn speaking. Another method the laryngectomy patient may use to aid speech is an artificial larynx. A battery-powered vibrator is one type of artificial larynx. When wishing to speak, the patient places the vibrator against the side of the neck. The vibrator vibrates the air inside the patient's mouth as the patient **articulates.**

A home health aide must be tactful when caring for such clients. It may be hard to understand what the client is saying. The aide should report to the nurse supervisor immediately if the client has any difficulty breathing. Crusting

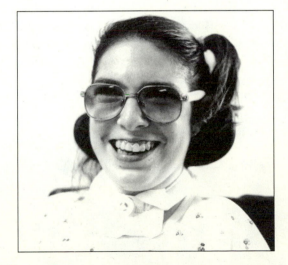

Figure 19-4   A tracheostomy tube provides an airway for this young client.

or bloody discharge from the tracheostomy also must be reported immediately.

Gastrointestinal Cancer

There is a continuous increase of new cases of gastrointestinal (stomach and colon) cancer in the United States every year. At least 93% of these individuals are over 50 years of age. Women are slightly more likely than men to develop the disease. Only lung cancer exceeds colon cancer in the number of new cases and number of deaths each year. Early detection of such cancer is an important factor in survival. One treatment for this type of cancer is to remove the diseased part of the large intestine. An opening, called a **colostomy,** is made through the wall of the abdomen. The cancerous portion of the intestine is removed. The end of the intestine remaining is pulled to the outside of the abdomen, Figure 19-5. The body wastes are expelled through this opening into a colostomy collection pouch attached to the abdomen. The area where the intestine opens to the outside is called the stoma.

After surgery, the patient is taught how to care for the stoma. Care is important since drainage from the intestine can irritate it. The patient is also taught how to irrigate the colostomy. **Irrigation** is the use of water to clean out the remaining colon. Family members are also instructed on how to help the client care for the colostomy.

In some cases, a colostomy is temporary. It may be possible to reconstruct and reconnect the intestine after several months. When this is

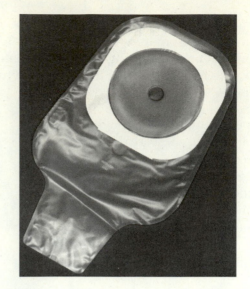

Figure 19-6 Stoma protector and drainage bag used by a client who has a colostomy

not possible, the client's rectum is surgically closed and the colostomy becomes permanent. The feces from a colostomy are fairly solid. The kind of diet prescribed for these clients helps control the type of bowel movement. Each client needs to experiment with diet and bowel habits until the best balance is found. Some people with a colostomy may be able to regulate bowel movements very well. They may only need to keep a gauze pad over the stoma. Some people are able to go swimming.

Cancer can destroy the functioning of the entire large intestine. When this occurs, the small intestine is cut and brought to the outside through the abdomen. This procedure is called an **ileostomy.** Most ileostomies are permanent. The waste discharge from an ileostomy remains liquid and drains constantly. The drainage irritates the skin.

Odors from the bag may be controlled by oral medications taken by the client or a deodorizer put into the container bag. Many different stoma appliances are on the market today, available for the client to select and use, Figure 19-6. Your nurse supervisor will instruct you on the type of appliance your client chooses to use.

Client Care

The home health aide should assist the client in cleaning around the stoma and changing the dressings and stoma bags. The aide can also

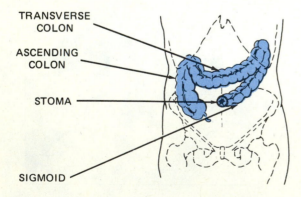

TRANSVERSE COLON

ASCENDING COLON

STOMA

SIGMOID

Figure 19-5 The cut end of the intestine is brought to the outside of the abdomen to form a stoma.

help with colostomy irrigations and sitz baths. Clients are sometimes embarrassed or ashamed of the odor and the appearance of the stoma. A home health aide must be careful not to offend the client. Aides should never show disgust at the odor or shy away from helping the client.

Skin Cancer

Skin cancer is becoming a common type of cancer, especially among the elderly. Skin cancer is most often caused by excessive exposure to ultraviolet radiation in the younger years. The lesion can be either benign or malignant. There are definite signs to watch for on the client's skin, Figure 19-7. If you notice any of these signs while bathing or working with your client, report the abnormal sign to the nurse supervisor. If detected and treated early enough, the prognosis is usually good.

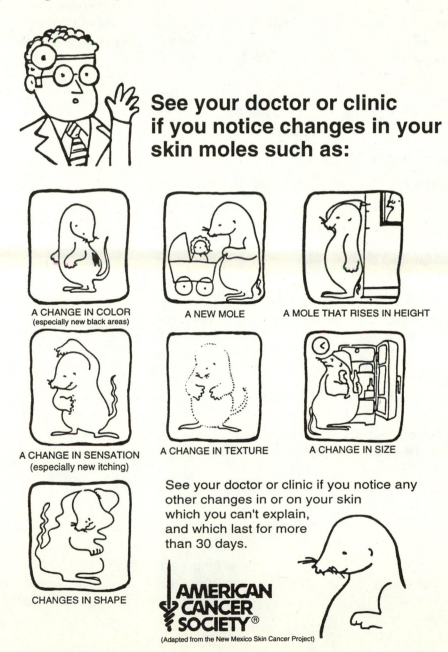

See your doctor or clinic if you notice changes in your skin moles such as:

A CHANGE IN COLOR
(especially new black areas)

A NEW MOLE

A MOLE THAT RISES IN HEIGHT

A CHANGE IN SENSATION
(especially new itching)

A CHANGE IN TEXTURE

A CHANGE IN SIZE

CHANGES IN SHAPE

See your doctor or clinic if you notice any other changes in or on your skin which you can't explain, and which last for more than 30 days.

AMERICAN CANCER SOCIETY®

(Adapted from the New Mexico Skin Cancer Project)

Figure 19-7   Seven cancer warning signs for skin moles (Courtesy of the American Cancer Society. Adapted from the New Mexico Skin Cancer Project.)

SUMMARY

* In most cases a home health aide will only be sent to care for a client with cancer after a diagnosis has been made. Usually some form of cancer treatment has been started. The client may have had surgery. In some cases the client receives chemotherapy or radiation treatments.
* When caring for a cancer client, a home health aide is given specific instructions.
* It is important that the client be kept as cheerful and comfortable as possible.
* Cancer not only causes physical pain and discomfort, but it also brings on depression and sadness.
* When caring for a client with cancer, a home health aide must be understanding and kind.
* Clients need to talk and to be listened to. Cancer clients know that they are dying. They must be helped to feel that they are still contributing members of society.
* These clients should be kept clean and comfortable. They need large doses of tender loving care.

REVIEW

1. List seven warning signs of cancer.

2. List three diagnostic tests used to diagnose cancer.

3. List six surgical procedures used in cancer therapy.

4. Define benign, carcinogen, malignant, metastasis, and remission.

5. List three types of cancer treatment.

6. Describe specialized care a cancer client may need from a home health aide.

7. List two precautions to take when caring for a client who is receiving chemotherapy.

8. Which of the following is not a warning sign of cancer?
   a. change in bowel habits
   b. chest pain radiating down arm
   c. change in mole
   d. unusual bleeding
   e. all are correct

9. Cancer of the lung is one of the leading causes of death from cancer in men.
   a. true   b. false

10. In the later stage of the cancer, the client may become very thin. The client may also suffer from constant pain. The goal of care in this phase of the disease is to keep the client as comfortable and as pain-free as possible.
    a. true   b. false

11. Match Column I with Column II.

    Column I
    ___1. remission
    ___2. benign
    ___3. carcinogen
    ___4. colostomy
    ___5. malignant
    ___6. biopsy

    Column II
    a. substance that can produce cancer
    b. no longer spreading
    c. sample of tissue cut from an area of the body
    d. an opening into the colon
    e. noncancerous
    f. cancer

12. A deodorizer is often used in a room of a cancer client to diminish the odor due to the client's cancerous condition.
    a. true   b. false

Unit 20 Caring for the Client who is Terminally Ill

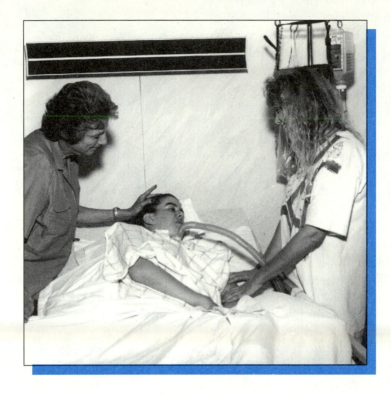

KEY TERMS
....

advanced directives	grieve	postmortem
durable power of attorney	hospice	terminally
embalming	living will	

LEARNING OBJECTIVES
....

After studying this unit, you should be able to:

- Identify some cultural influences surrounding practices related to death.
- Identify the five stages of dying as described by Dr. Kübler-Ross.
- Identify the home health aide's responsibilities when the client dies.
- Identify ways in which a person may react to the death of a family member or friend.

- Become familiar with the needs of a dying client.
- Explain the Patient Self-Determination Act.
- Define the purpose of hospice programs.
- Explain the importance of grief.

Most people in our society feel uncomfortable talking or thinking about death. This is more true today than in earlier times in history. Gathering in the room of a dying relative was a custom practiced no more than 40 years ago. Death was accepted as the natural end to life. Children openly shared the final moments of life with a dying grandparent, parent, or sibling.

This is the first time in society that three or four generations of one family are living at the same time. Death experiences in some families have been rare. In the 1980s, 80% of deaths occurred in the hospital setting and few people assisted their loved ones in their last days. Many people living today have never seen a dead body. Death to many individuals is extremely difficult to deal with. In recent years there has been a reversal of the trend of transferring a loved one to the hospital to die. The families are now allowing their loved ones to die in their own home in a familiar environment. This is due primarily to the expansion of the **hospice** program. Hospice offers a combination of physical and emotional care that involves not only the client, but also friends, family, volunteers, and home health aides. The criteria to enter a hospice program is that the client's life expectancy is less than 6 months due to a terminal illness. The client is **terminally** (final stage of the fatal illness) ill. The goal of hospice is to control uncomfortable symptoms such as nausea and make the client as comfortable and pain free as possible in the short time the client has left in this world, Figure 20-1. The primary concern of hospice is quality of life and not prolonging the client's life.

Cultural Differences

Indians and Eskimos followed customs that today may be thought of as uncivilized. The aged, ill members of Eskimo tribes were taken to an iceberg and left alone with a small amount of food. This was the accepted way to die. In certain Native American tribes, people who were ill and unable to do their share of work were taken to an isolated spot to await death. These customs were accepted as a natural and respectable way for life to end. Native Americans felt that it was good to allow life to

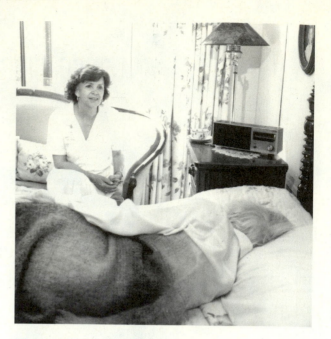

Figure 20-1 A home health aide comforting a dying client

end naturally. When human power to cure with herbs and medicines was not effective, it was time for death to come.

Medical science today has made treatments more available and more effective. In addition, advances have been made in living conditions. Clothing is warmer. Housing is better. Foods are more plentiful. Working conditions have improved. Because of these and other changes, people can expect to live for many years. Diseases once incurable have been conquered. New medicines and surgical techniques have been developed that save thousands of lives daily. Most of these medical advances improve the quality of life. However, some of the medical advances prolong life but do not always improve life. The value of life support systems is being questioned today. There are times when a client is kept alive by machines but has no awareness of being alive. These machines take over the vital functions for the client, Figure 20-2. Because of problems with the making of decisions regarding use of life support machines, a law was passed in 1991 called the **Patient Self-Determination Act.** This act requires Medicare and Medicaid home health agencies to implement procedures to increase public awareness regarding the rights of clients to make choices. The

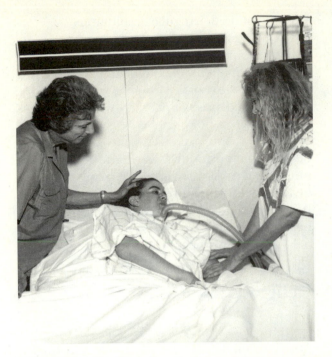

Figure 20-2   Family coping with tragedy: daughter critically injured in a car accident. The mother and grandmother remain at the daughter's side.

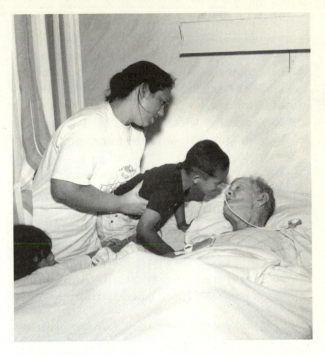

Figure 20-3   Grandson gives his grandfather a kiss. Touch is important for a terminally ill client.

law is concerned primarily with **advanced directives,** papers that specify the type of treatment the client wants or does not want under serious medical conditions in which they may be unable to communicate their wishes to the doctor or family.

Advanced directives can be done by a **living will** or by **durable power of attorney** (see samples in Appendix D). Before you start caring for a client, the decision has been made by the client what he or she wants done when seriously ill. One of these above forms has been completed already by the client. Your case manager will inform you of your client's wishes. You may have two clients with the same serious illness; one client may have mechanical life support and the other one only pain medication to keep him comfortable. The doctors are just following the client's wishes. This should ease the burden on the family and also the doctor in making the decision to use mechanical life support or not.

Changing attitudes toward death have appeared partly as a result of increased life expectancy. People seem to fear death as never before. They want to hold on to life and try not to think about death. Children are usually protected from the facts of death. When a beloved grandparent dies, children may be told that the grandparent has gone away. Since families are often separated by great distances, many children believe that their grandparents have just moved. How a family deals with death is a very personal matter, Figure 20-3. A home health aide must respect the wishes of the family in dealing with the death of a family member. The aide must be aware of the needs of the dying person and the family.

Stages of Adjustment to Dying and Death

Dr. Elisabeth Kübler-Ross has made careful studies of dying persons and their families. She has described a general pattern common to persons facing death. The pattern may apply to both the dying person and the person's family. Dr. Kübler-Ross has noted five stages of psychological adjustment to death.

1. **Denial**—This can't be happening to me; perhaps someone else, but not me.
2. **Anger**—An extension of denial; feeling that this death is unfair; bitterness and loss of faith in God; fighting against death or loss of a loved one.
3. **Bargaining**—"Dear God, I'll be good. Please, not yet—some other time, it's too soon."
4. **Depression**—Brooding, withdrawal, lack of communication; thoughts of suicide—"I'd rather kill myself than die from this disease" or, "I can't go on living if Mama dies."
5. **Acceptance**—Calmly facing what is to be or feeling a sense of peace; looking forward to release from pain and sorrow; hoping for the release of a loved one to a better world.

A home health aide who is in an environment of expected death may see these patterns develop. The aide should not offer advice to the family or client. The aide should be understanding and kind but not lose control emotionally. By knowing what to expect in the way of reactions, the home health aide is better prepared to adjust to the situation.

Sometimes a client may die suddenly and unexpectedly. Other times death is preceded by a long illness. Some people are relieved that life is ending. Some clients become unconscious just before death. Of the five senses (hearing, taste, touch, sight, smell), the last to be lost is hearing. For this reason when working with an unconscious client, the home health aide should be careful what is said in the client's presence. It would be cruel if the last words a client heard were, "Well, she's almost gone; she'll be dead by morning." The home health aide's first duty is to keep the client clean and as comfortable as possible. The client should be treated with kindness and dignity at all times. In addition, the aide should provide emotional support to the client and the family. Good communication skills are needed when dealing with the dying client and the family.

Signs of Approaching Death

Certain signs indicate that death is approaching. These signs are:

- noisy, labored, irregular respirations
- irregular and weak pulse
- cool, moist, and clammy skin
- incontinence (bowel and bladder)
- body muscles relax, jaw opens
- diminished sense of pain

When death occurs, family members may be highly emotional. The home health aide must remain calm as there are many details to be taken care of. Figure 20-4 lists the duties of a home health aide when the client dies. A home health aide may be asked to remain on duty to help the family prepare for the funeral.

Religious and Cultural Influences

Among some Jewish families, burial takes place within 24 hours after death. Religious practice forbids **embalming** the body and requires the casket remain closed. After the funeral the family may have a period of formal mourning. During this time, friends and relatives come to the home to comfort each other.

In other Jewish families and in Catholic or Protestant families, the body is usually taken to a funeral home. Friends and family meet at the funeral home during the two or three days before the body is buried. Religious practices differ from one group to another and even from family to family. Most people do recognize the need of sharing grief. This is part of the final acceptance of death. Some people weep, others

---

POSTMORTEM CARE

1. Call the case manager at once. A death certificate must be filed. Write down the time of death.
2. Do not touch the client until the case manager tells you to.
3. Call a family member after the doctor has been called.
4. Follow the case manager's instructions and clean the client's body. At death, all body functions stop.

Figure 20-4 What to do when a client dies

are angry. Some are very quiet. As people work through their emotions, they come to accept the loss. Many see that the death of an older person is less tragic than the death of a younger person. A death that is sudden is more difficult to accept than one following a long painful illness. Mixed emotions are felt by families of an AIDS client when he or she dies. Years ago people were allowed to grieve (the feeling of separation or loss) for a longer period of time; many wore black clothes for a period of time, which symbolized their "black" feelings inside. Today there are special support groups for individuals to assist them in the grieving process.

Death is usually a cause of crisis within a family. Some people may need special help to face the crisis of death. It usually takes several months to readjust to the loss of a loved one. The most difficult adjustment period is the first 2 or 3 months.

SUMMARY

- Dying is not accepted by everyone in the same manner. Many cultural influences affect the client's and family's concept of death. Besides the cultural differences, personal differences exist.
- Dr. Elisabeth Kübler-Ross has done research that shows five stages of adjustment to death: denial, anger, bargaining, depression and ac-

ceptance. People commonly pass through some or all of these five stages.
- The aide must be calm and perform the necessary duties when a client dies.
- Hospice is an organization that assists individuals who are terminally ill to be as comfortable and pain free as possible.

REVIEW

1. List the five stages of psychological adjustment to death.

2. What should the home health aide do if the client dies while the aide is on duty?

3. List three cultural influences surrounding death and dying.

4. List three ways in which a person may react to the death of a family member or friend.

5. List two goals of the hospice organization.

6. Explain what the grieving process is.

7. Describe two ways a home health aide can comfort a dying client.

8. List four signs of approaching death.

9. Two examples of advanced directives are durable power of attorney and living will.
   a. true   b. false

10. During which of the five stages of dying would a client most likely say, "If only I could live to see my oldest daughter get married"?
    a. denial   c. bargaining
    b. anger   d. acceptance

11. When a client is dying and a family member is always present, one important thing that the home health aide can do is to:
    a. tell the family member all the details about the client's illness
    b. ask the family member questions on how the illness started in the client
    c. try to cheer the family member up by talking about current events in your life
    d. provide emotional support for the family and not offer any advice

12. Signs that death is approaching include:
    a. eyes may stare blankly in space
    b. respirations slow down and are moist
    c. arms and legs become cold as circulation slows down
    d. all are correct

13. The last sense to leave the dying client is
    a. taste   c. hearing
    b. sight   d. touch

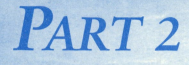 PART 2

Practical Applications

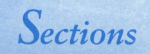 *Sections*

6   Homemaking Services

7   Health Care Services

8   Employment

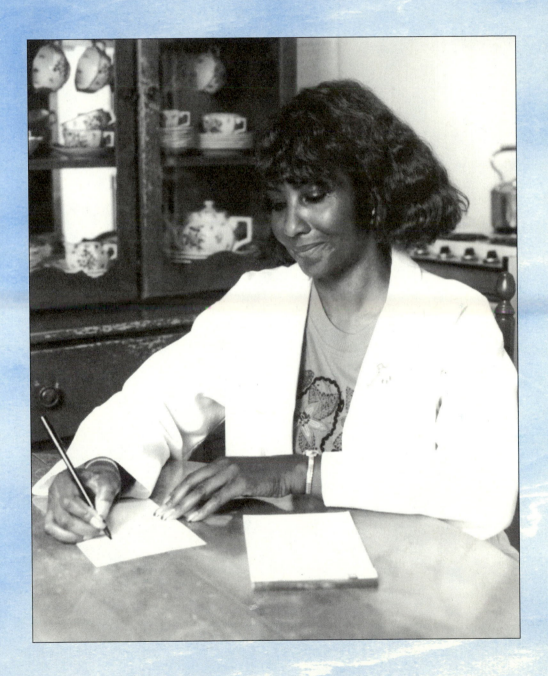

Section 6

Homemaking Services

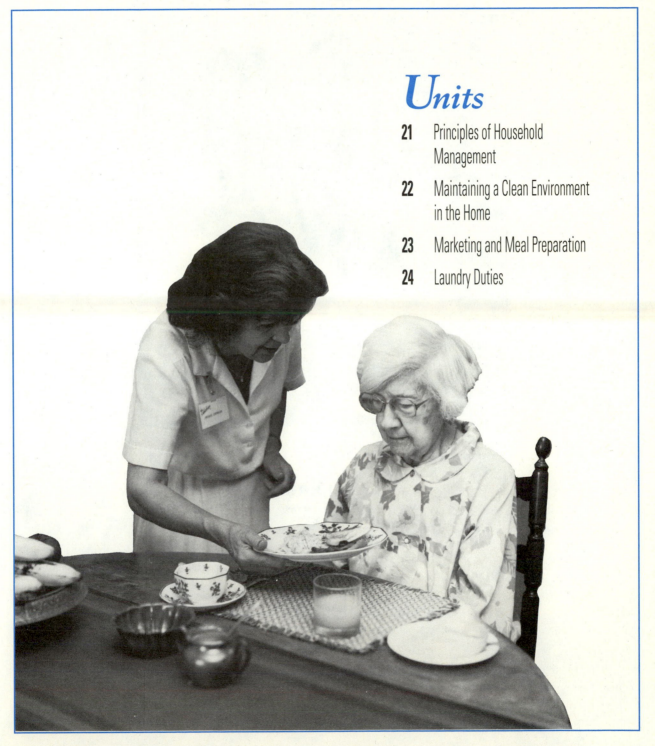

Units

21 Principles of Household Management

22 Maintaining a Clean Environment in the Home

23 Marketing and Meal Preparation

24 Laundry Duties

261

Unit 21 Principles of Household Management

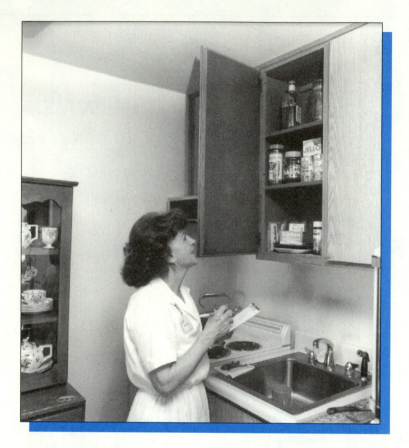

KEY TERMS

. . . .

instinct   myth

LEARNING OBJECTIVES

. . . .

After studying this unit, you should be able to:

- List at least four tips used to plan and organize tasks.
- Explain how to care for major home appliances.
- State some ways to combine client care and household tasks.

Managing a household is considered by many to be a mindless routine that requires no special ability. It has often been assumed that a person (especially females in the traditional role of wife, mother, and homemaker) was born with the talent and **instinct** (inborn knowledge) to care for a home. In fact, one of the most foolish **myths** is the belief that anyone can run a home.

Actually, managing a household is like operating a daily 24-hour business. Homemakers raise children, manage a budget, provide a clean and livable house, prepare and serve meals, and handle home accidents. It requires intelligence, understanding, and physical labor.

Home health aides not only run their own homes but take on a second job of assisting others to run their homes, Figures 21-1 and 21-2. Many home health aides have a basic knowledge of keeping up a house. However, the habits developed in their own homes may not be suitable to all working situations.

The units covering homemaking skills are presented to introduce homemaking techniques to the beginner. However, even the experienced homemaker may learn some helpful new tips.

The aide should realize that each home situation may offer different challenges. A professional home health aide must adapt to the phys-

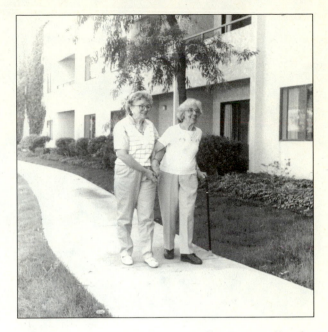

Figure 21-2   A few of your clients may live in apartment complexes.

ical surroundings of each job. This adjustment requires the aide to use whatever appliances and supplies the client has available. The aide must remember to show as much care for the property of others as is shown for personal property. The equipment and furnishings used by the home health aide belong to the employer. Reasonable care must be used. The aide should read directions and ask questions before using unfamiliar equipment. If equipment has frayed cords or appliances do not work, they should be repaired. The aide should notify the case manager or family so that repairs can be made. When using any cleaning product or appliance, the labels and directions should be read carefully. This not only makes for proper use, but can limit the number of accidents that might happen. Using rubber gloves helps avoid skin irritation caused by soaps or household chemical products. When performing regular household duties, the aide should make a list of any items in short supply. Toilet paper, laundry products, food, or other necessities should be purchased before the house supply runs out.

Sometimes a home health aide handles the client's money. Always get a receipt for any purchases you make and place the receipts in a special place. If there is any doubt about what an

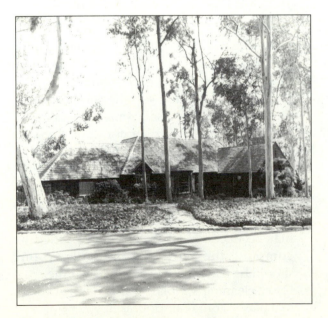

Figure 21-1   You will be working in many different home settings: a single family dwelling.

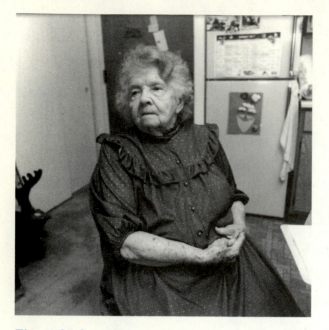

Figure 21-3   Often a client will ask you to do a task a certain way. You should follow the client's directions unless they contradict agency policy. You should know your agency-approved plan of action in these situations.

item costs, or if the client has any questions on where the money was spent, you can quickly verify your expenditures. Honesty in money matters is an absolute necessity.

When you are in a client's home and the client requests a cleaning job done a certain way even though you know a better way, you should follow the client's directions, Figure 21-3. The client is indirectly paying your salary and can have things done the way he or she likes to have them done. A few of the homes you will be going to might be very dirty and unkept for years; if you are assigned to work at this home for 3 hours, you will not be able to clean it in that short time and get everything spotless. Your client might think differently. If this situation exists, you need to discuss this with your case manager.

Planning and Organization

No house takes care of itself. In a home where everything seems neat, the homemaker has probably used a set of well-organized plans. An important duty of the aide is to plan, organize, and carry out the tasks completely. The home-

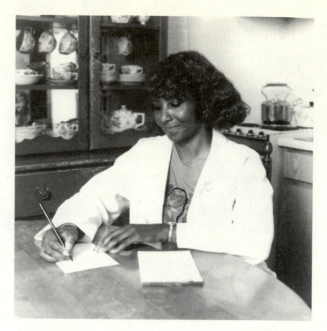

Figure 21-4   An aide is planning her work assignment and listing the supplies she will need.

maker who plans the work, organizes the tasks, and starts doing them will find the work load lightened. A home health aide will be given instructions for each assignment. The care of the client is of primary importance, but the household tasks cannot be ignored. The aide should take a few minutes each morning to plan the tasks that should be completed by the day's end, Figure 21-4. This can save time and energy.

- Carry a pad and pencil in the pocket of your uniform. Make a note of household supplies that may be needed in each room.
- Post a list of needed supplies on a kitchen bulletin board, or use a small magnet and put the list on the refrigerator door. Remind family members that if they use the last bar of soap or roll of bathroom tissue they should add the item to the list.
- Before starting to clean a room, the aide should stop to think which cleaning supplies may be needed. All the supplies needed to complete the work in a particular room should be taken to the room at one time.
- Carry cleaning supplies from room to room in a plastic container or basket.
- Prevent buildup of dirt by tidying rooms, dusting, wiping surfaces, and sponging up spots as soon as possible.

- Keep a sponge in the kitchen and bathroom for quick wipe-ups.
- Use a tray to carry dishes to and from the table.
- Schedule major jobs for a certain day of the week. For example, vacuum and wash floors on Friday so the house will be ready for weekend use; launder and iron one day; plan weekly marketing on Monday or Wednesday; defrost refrigerator, clean oven, or straighten drawers or cabinets on a day when nothing big is planned.
- Arrange to do two or three tasks at one time. A load of laundry can be put in the machine just before lunchtime. While the machine is running, lunch can be prepared and served to the client. If the laundry has to be done in the laundromat, it can be planned for the

APPLIANCE	PURPOSE AND USE	CARE AND CLEANING
Refrigerator	To retard spoilage of perishable foods. Door should be kept closed when not in use. Temperature control should be set so as to keep foods fresh but not to freeze them. Most refrigerators have zoned cooling. Store foods in a specific area. Meats to be used within 2 or 3 days belong in the meat storage compartment. Fruits and vegetables are kept in the bottom area, milk and dairy products on top shelves. Store leftovers in small airtight containers and use as soon as possible.	Discard leftovers if unused in 3 days. Wipe interior with warm water and baking soda to remove stale odors. At least every 3 or 4 weeks remove shelves and drawers. Wash them in water and detergent. Rinse thoroughly. Place a box of baking soda in refrigerator if odor still present.
Freezer compartment of refrigerator	Store frozen foods and weekly meat supply. Mark date of storage and use older products first. Frost-free refrigerators have a tray at the bottom. This tray should be pulled out and cleaned every 2 or 3 months. Persons with lung disorders may be sensitive to the dust and vapors from this area.	To defrost, put pan of hot water in emptied compartment. Turn control knob to defrost. Empty pan under freezer so water does not flood rest of refrigerator or floor. DO NOT USE SHARP KNIFE TO PRY ICE LOOSE. THIS COULD DAMAGE FREEZER COILS. When defrosting is completed, wipe inside with warm water and baking soda. Turn control on and replace foods. If any food has thawed completely, use it at once—do not refreeze foods.
Freezer	Offers large, cold storage area and maintains a constant temperature. Foods may be stored for long periods of time. Some foods cannot be stored longer than 6 months. Instructions on care and wrapping foods for the freezer appear later in the text.	Defrost twice a year. If frost-free model, remove foods and wipe inner surfaces with damp cloth and baking soda.

Figure 21-5   Proper use and care of household appliances reduces the need for repairs and the risk of personal injury.

Continued on the following page.

APPLIANCE	PURPOSE AND USE	CARE AND CLEANING
Stove	Heats food for boiling, broiling, or baking. Uses gas or electricity as a fuel source. Keep pot holders and dish towels away from flame or heat unit. Never use the oven when it is greasy—FIRE HAZARD. Turn off stove when finished cooking. When using gas stoves, be sure the pilot light is burning before turning on gas jet of the burner. When lighting the oven, first light match, then turn on gas jet and put flame to it. Keep body turned away from open oven door for safety. If oven does not light, turn off jet and try again in a few minutes. Make sure gas jet is turned OFF when through using oven.	Wipe up spilled foods at once. Wipe off stove surface once a day. Scour burners and burner pans once a week. When cleaning the oven, follow instructions on cleaner can. Clean as often as needed. When daily spills and grease are cleaned up, a full oven cleaning is not needed as often. Self-cleaning ovens—follow manufacturer's instructions.
Microwave oven	Read instructions before using. Used for rapid food defrosting, quick heating of leftovers, baking, and cooking. Use only the recommended dishes or supplies (paper, plastic) in the microwave. Never use metal containers.	Wipe clean with damp cloth, following instructions in operator's manual. Soap may be used; rinse well and dry interior. If you are unsure about care and cleaning, ask a family member for a demonstration.
Dishwasher	Washes dishes at a high water temperature; most dishwashers sterilize dishes. Rinse plates and utensils before placing in dishwasher—or turn on prewash cycle immediately after loading. Use *only* the dishwashing detergent. Wait until there is a full load before putting on wash cycle. (Saves water and electricity.) Do not put plastic, cast iron, or wooden items in dishwasher.	Clean filter once a week and wash interior with water and mild soap, rinse with damp cloth. **Caution:** Do not touch coils in dishwasher.
Garbage disposal	Appliance in sink which cuts up discarded food and disposes of it. Follow instructions in manufacturer's guide. Be careful to dispose only the food items listed, not bones or paper. **Caution:** Keep hands away from unit while in operation.	**Caution:** Do not try to repair; call for plumber if it breaks down. After using, rinse drain with hot water.
Garbage compacter	Crushes garbage to save storage space. Follow instructions in manufacturer's guide. Use it only for those items recommended by manufacturer.	Call professional repairman.

Figure 21-5   *(Continued)*

APPLIANCE	PURPOSE AND USE	CARE AND CLEANING
Washing machine	Soaks and agitates clothing. Load as instructed—use correct water temperature for type of clothing. Use soap and bleach as needed according to instructions. Do not overload.	Clean out lint trap. About once a week wipe out inside with soap and water to get rid of grit. Take off agitator and clean carefully. Wipe outer surface after use.
Dryer	Tumbles and heats clothing to dry them. Load according to instructions, using temperature recommended for type of clothes.	Clean lint trap after each use. Wipe outer surface after use. Call repairman if machine works poorly.
Small appliances Automatic blender Mixer Electric fry pan Slicing machine Electric knife Percolator Automatic coffee maker	Follow operating instructions. If you are unsure how to use it, do not use it. Pay special attention to all safety precautions provided by the manufacturer with the appliance.	Wash surface and store conveniently and carefully. Make sure the electric unit does not come in contact with water. Wash coffee maker with soap and water after using. Rinse thoroughly. Once in a while run a cycle of water and baking soda through pot to clean coffee oils away.

Figure 21-5   *(Continued)*

same day as the weekly marketing. While hand laundry is soaking, the ironing could be started.
• Learn how to use and care for the equipment in the home, Figure 21-5. Most appliances have an instruction manual. Read it before using the equipment. After using equipment, clean it so it will be ready for the next use. Store small appliances close to where they are used.

Preventing Injuries in the Home

Outside the House

• Use special caution when walking outdoors on wet or icy pavement.
• Clear all pathways and outdoor steps of litter and obstructions, Figure 21-6.

Inside the House

• Wipe up spills immediately.
• Avoid wearing socks and smooth slippers on uncarpeted floors or stairways.

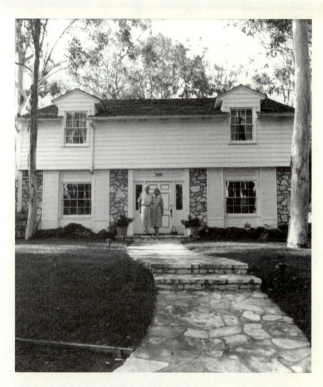

Figure 21-6   A clear pathway to a client's home will prevent injuries, especially in the client with vision and balance problems.

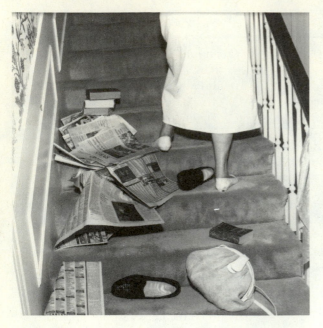

Figure 21-7   An unlighted and cluttered stairway is a good place for accidents to happen.

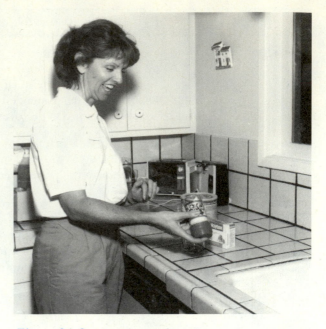

Figure 21-8   A clean and uncluttered countertop makes cooking easy.

- Use nightlights in bathrooms and keep bedside lamps and phone within easy reach.
- Keep a flashlight within easy reach at bedside.
- Arrange the kitchen so heavy cookware and frequently used items are within easy reach.
- Invest in a sturdy step stool with handles.
- Make sure all hallways and stairways are well-lighted and free of clutter, Figure 21-7.
- Consider using a shower chair in shower if client is unsteady when standing.
- Install smoke alarms and be sure batteries work.
- Remove all clutter and debris in traffic areas.
- Store medications in safe area that is cool, dry, and out of reach of children.

Combining Client Care and Household Tasks

The order in which tasks are done is not always important. If one knows just what should be completed by the end of the day the work can be arranged around the client's needs. After the client's bath and after the bed linens are changed, the aide may decide to clean the client's room. The kitchen could be cleaned after the breakfast meal, Figure 21-8. The client's bathroom cleaning could be done after the bedpan has been used and emptied into the toilet bowl. These examples show how to pair client care procedures with homemaking duties. This technique saves time and energy by avoiding many extra steps a day.

SUMMARY

- Caring for the client's home is an important part of a home health aide's job. This requires learning how to use and care for equipment and organizing time effectively.

- Although the physical care of the client is of primary importance, providing a clean and safe environment is also necessary.

REVIEW

1. List four tips to use in planning and organizing your work.
2. Explain routine cleaning tasks for major appliances.
3. List two ways to combine client care and household chores.

Unit 22 Maintaining a Clean Environment in the Home

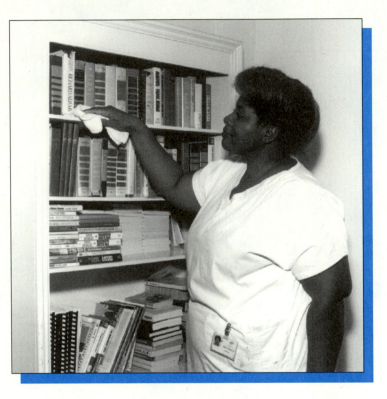

KEY TERMS

mildew   pathogens   sanitary

LEARNING OBJECTIVES

After studying this unit, you should be able to:

- Name three factors that determine the aide's cleaning plan.
- List five cleaning tasks done daily.
- List five cleaning tasks done weekly.
- List five cleaning tasks done only periodically.
- Describe the correct method for separating and disposing of garbage.

- Identify at least four steps used in cleaning a kitchen.
- Identify daily bathroom care that family members should perform.
- Identify two bathroom cleaning tasks the aide does daily.

The aide is normally expected to do general cleaning in the living room, dining room, family room, and bedrooms. Home health aides set up their own routines for completing daily household tasks. There is no one pattern to be followed. The factors to be considered include:

- the needs of the client
- the size of the home
- the ages of people living in the home
- the number of people living in the home

When you take on the responsibilities for home care, it is good to have a master plan. Some tasks must be done several times a day. Some should be done daily or weekly. Others need only be done occasionally.

Home furnishings represent a costly expenditure for most families. Furniture and carpets should last for many years. The life of furniture and upholstery can be increased by proper care and attention. The home health aide should remember that the furnishings were expensive to buy, but would be even more expensive to replace. Cleaning has been made easier with modern electrical equipment and new cleaning products. These factors make it possible to clean quickly on a day-to-day basis, Figure 22-1. Big jobs done weekly or several times a year are also done much easier than in the past.

Daily Cleaning Tasks

Certain tasks should be done every day to keep the house neat and clean. Some daily duties need to be done whether or not they have been assigned. The aide is expected to tidy rooms and clean up spills when they occur. Daily cleaning should not require longer than an hour or an hour and a half. The following duties should be done every day.

- Pick up toys, magazines, newspapers, and clothing. **Caution:** Do not discard any of these items without the permission of the client.
- Fluff cushions and pillows, make the beds or change linens when necessary.
- Dry dust furniture, lamps, and knickknacks, Figure 22-2.
- Wipe off windowsills and radiators.
- Empty ashtrays and wastebaskets.
- Remove spots and stains using a suitable cleaning product. Test the product first by

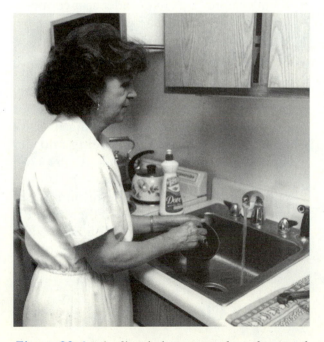

Figure 22-1   A client's home needs to be cared for properly. It is a continuous process to keep it clean and orderly.

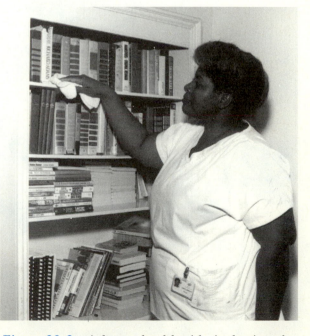

Figure 22-2   A home health aide is dusting the bookshelves. Dusting is a task that needs to be done daily.

trying it on a hidden spot. See whether the carpet bleeds or fades. After cleaning a difficult spot, cover it with a clean white cloth until the area dries. Never use soap on carpet stains. Dried soap attracts dirt and can cause permanent damage. To avoid spreading the stain, work from the outside of the stain toward the center (clean to dirty).

Weekly Cleaning Tasks

Weekly care can be done in more than one way. The aide may want to change the bed linens in every bedroom on the same day. On the other hand, the aide may prefer to completely clean and arrange one bedroom at a time. The aide's decision can vary with each assignment. The aide should always consider the needs of the client before making out a schedule.

- Change bed linens throughout the house, Figures 22-3 and 22-4. The client's bed may need to be changed more often.
- Vacuum floors and carpets, Figure 22-5, getting under furniture where dirt may lodge.

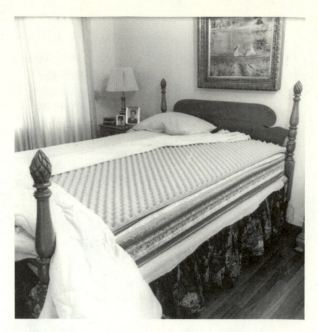

Figure 22-4   Clean linens are being applied to the client's bed. Note the neat and tidy appearance of the bedroom.

Change or empty the vacuum cleaner bag as required; discard the dirt in a large paper bag. Avoid bumping the furniture and woodwork with the vacuum cleaner.
- Wipe windowsills and frames.
- Vacuum upholstery and under seat cushions; vacuum lamp shades and wipe away cobwebs.
- Damp or wet mop floors. Oiled dust mops are preferred by some people.
- Polish the furniture. Handle knickknacks carefully when dusting. Use a flannel cloth, old diaper, or cheesecloth. Use one cloth for dry dusting, another for polishing. Do not dust and polish until vacuuming and dry mopping have been completed. Pour polish onto the polishing cloth. **Caution:** Do not pour polish directly onto the furniture. Use long strokes along the grain of the wood. Refold cloth and add more polish as needed. Be careful not to spill polish on upholstery or carpets.

Periodic Cleaning Tasks

Certain areas in the home do not require frequent cleaning. However, the aide should check these areas to be sure that dust and dirt do not

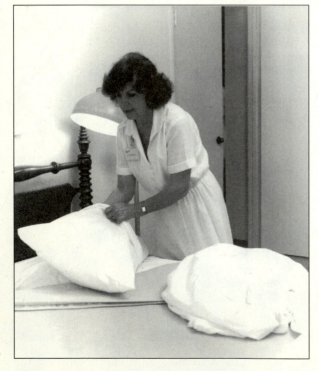

Figure 22-3   An aide strips the dirty linens from the client's bed.

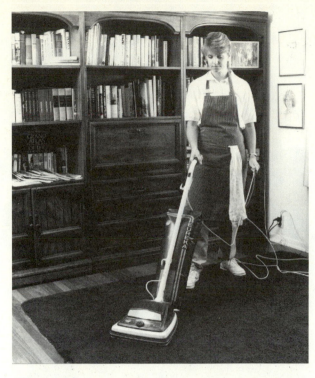

Figure 22-5   An aide is vacuuming the living room, a weekly task.

collect. The following tasks can be done on an occasional basis.

- Remove cobwebs from the ceilings, walls, curtains, and shades. Use a long-handled dust mop covered with a clean cloth.
- Remove small pictures from the wall and dust behind them. Dust the frames and glass.
- Wipe mirrors or use glass cleaner on them as needed.
- Remove books from shelves and dust both books and shelves.
- Clean lamp bases. Replace burned out bulbs as needed.
- Damp wipe lighting fixtures on walls or ceilings, Figure 22-6.
- Hand wash decorative plates and table ornaments in mild soapsuds.
- Vacuum draperies and window blinds, Figure 22-7.
- Launder small area or throw rugs.

Kitchen Maintenance and Cleaning

In many homes, the kitchen is the center of family life. For this reason, keeping the kitchen in order probably requires more organization

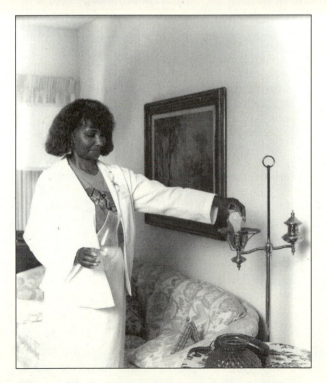

Figure 22-6   Minor tasks, such as changing a light bulb, are often part of the home health aide's duties.

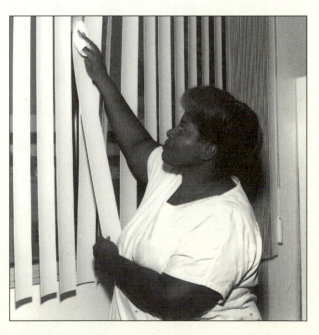

Figure 22-7   Cleaning the window blinds is a task that needs to be done on a regular basis.

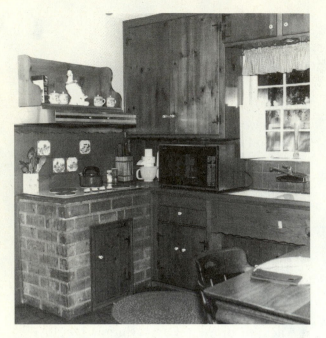

Figure 22-8   An example of a neat and orderly kitchen

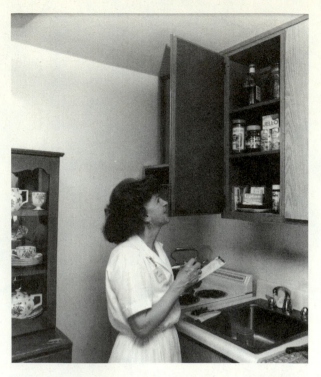

Figure 22-9   An aide is checking the cupboards for needed supplies.

than any other room in the home, Figure 22-8. Not only must the aide prepare and clean up after each meal, but products must be replaced as they are used, Figure 22-9. Wastes must be discarded, leftovers stored for future use, and special menus and snacks prepared for the client. Kitchen work may seem to be an endless cycle. With the right attitude it can be challenging and satisfying when it is done well. With a little effort, attractive and nutritious meals can be made. These meals can improve the client's physical condition; however, they must be made in a clean and healthful environment.

Following are some reasons for keeping a kitchen clean and neat:

• Germs are less likely to grow in a clean kitchen.
• It is easier to prepare meals in a neat area.
• It is quicker to find equipment and supplies that have been properly stored.
• Clean dishes, utensils, and pots are ready for use.
• Accidents are less likely to happen when floors are free of spills.
• Insects (flies, roaches, ants) and rodents (mice or rats) are less likely to appear when food and garbage are properly put away.

Maintaining order is an easier task when the kitchen area is clean. The aide who keeps up with small cleanup jobs will find that this practice makes work easier, Figure 22-10. When these tasks are left undone, kitchen work becomes overwhelming, Figure 22-11. Routine cleanup procedures usually take no more than 15 to 20 minutes after each meal. Major tasks such as cleaning drawers and cabinets require more time. The aide should schedule these duties to be done at times when routine tasks are light and the client is resting or has visitors.

Disposing of Garbage

Place a heavy plastic bag in a waste container or garbage can. It is required in some areas to separate the glass containers and cans from the recyclable materials, Figure 22-12. You will need to separate the garbage according to your local guidelines. In some areas of our country, you will need to place the garbage in specially marked plastic bags. In other states, you may need to save all aluminum cans to be returned to the store for reimbursement. Empty garbage and trash often to prevent

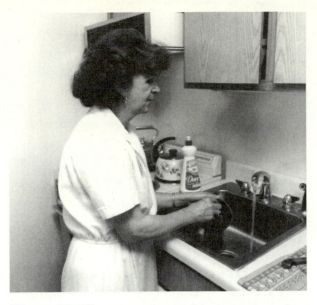

Figure 22-10   Keeping the kitchen clean is a continuous daily task.

odors from forming and help in preventing ants, mice, and roaches from being attracted to the area. You might need to spray the garbage container with a disinfectant.

Dishwashing

If the client has an infectious disease, wash the client's dishes and utensils separately from the other family dishes. Rinse these dishes and utensils in boiling water. This is an aseptic technique used to prevent the spread of germs (**pathogens**) to other members of the family. When washing the family's dishes by hand, use hot water and liquid detergent. Wash the dishes in the following order: cups and glassware, utensils, plates and bowls, pots and pans. If the water becomes greasy, drain the sink and add fresh water and detergent. After washing them with detergent, rinse the dishes completely with hot water. Place the dishes in a drainer. Air drying is more **sanitary** than drying with a dish towel. Lay a clean dish towel over the dishes as the rest of the kitchen is cleaned. After the dishes are dry, put them away in cabinets.

Some homes are equipped with automatic dishwashers. Before placing dishes in the dishwasher, scrape and rinse them well. Some machines have a rinse cycle prior to the wash cycle. When using these machines, hand rinsing the dishes may not be necessary before loading. Pour dishwasher detergent into the correct area labeled on the machine. **Caution:** Do not use soap powder or liquid detergent. Run the dishwasher only when it is fully loaded. Water and electricity are wasted when the dishwasher is

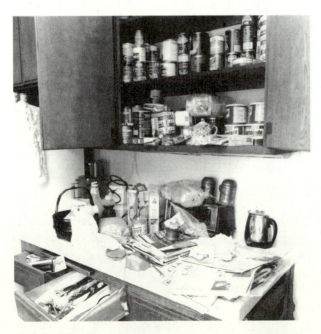

Figure 22-11   An example of an untidy kitchen

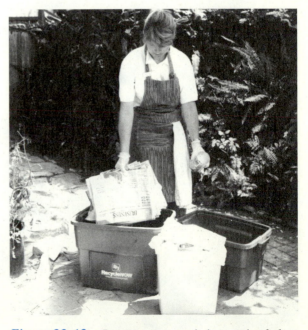

Figure 22-12   In many areas, it is required that garbage be separated into recyclable and nonrecyclable items.

half empty. Pots and pans should be hand washed, rinsed, and stored when dry.

Wiping Surfaces

Use a cloth or sponge, warm water and detergent to wipe the table, countertops, wall behind the stove, stove top, and outside surfaces of the refrigerator and microwave oven. Be sure to remove grease or splashes caused from cooking foods.

Use a cloth or sponge and vinegar to wipe out the inside of the refrigerator. The inside of the microwave oven should be wiped with warm water and carefully dried.

Wipe the sink; use scouring powder if necessary. Scouring powder helps remove stains and marks left by pans or food wastes. After scouring, be sure to rinse the sink completely. **Caution:** Always check with your client before using scouring powder on the sink as many new sinks can be damaged by scouring powder.

Cleaning the Floors

Wipe up any spills with a cloth, sponge, or paper towel as soon as they occur. Do not wipe with a sponge or cloth that is used for other surfaces; keep a separate cloth or sponge for floors only. For general sweeping, use a dust mop or broom. Gather crumbs and dirt on a dustpan and empty the dustpan into a garbage container. Damp mop floors at least once a week. If blood or other body fluids are spilled on a tile floor, you are required to wear gloves and wipe it up with a solution of 10 parts water to 1 part bleach, Figure 22-13.

Cleaning Cabinets and Drawers

Dishes, glassware, and utensils should be stored in clean cabinets and drawers. Water vapor, smoke, and grease from cooking cause a buildup of oily film on kitchen surfaces. The film collects on both the inside and the outside of closed cabinets. The outside of cabinets should be cleaned at least once a week. The inside should be cleaned several times a year. The cleaning product used will depend on the type of cabinet being cleaned. Metal, formica, and wood require different types of cleaning products. Drawers will remain neat if kitchen items are put away in order. Drawers should also be cleaned out several times a year.

Storing Cleaning Supplies

Cleaning products should be stored in a place that children and confused adults cannot reach. **Caution:** Many cleaning products are poisonous. Swallowing even a small amount of a poison can be fatal. In a home where children are living, do not store products under the sink. A high cabinet with a door is the best place to store cleaning products. Brooms, mops, and rags should be put away after use.

Bathroom Maintenance and Cleaning

Bathrooms must be given special care in homes where there is illness. The natural dampness in a bathroom causes the growth of molds and **mildew,** which are unsightly and cause odors. Moisture provides an environment ideally suited for the growth of microorganisms, which may be present in the home. For this reason, the home health aide must be particularly concerned with cleaning techniques, Figure 22-14.

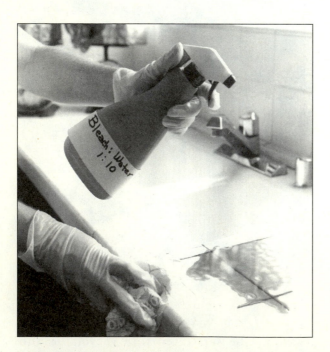

Figure 22-13 To clean up blood and body fluid spills, use a solution of bleach and water.

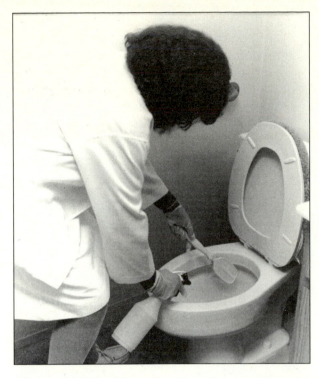

Figure 22-14   The client's toilet needs to be cleaned routinely.

Daily Care by Family Members

If more than one family member uses the same bathroom, each must assume certain responsibilities as a matter of courtesy to the rest of the family. After shaving, brushing the teeth, and washing, the sink should be rinsed out. After bathing or showering, the tub or shower should be wiped out with cleanser. Instruct family members to remove loose hair from the tub or shower floor. This practice helps avoid drain clogs. The toilet must be flushed after each use. Combing or brushing hair while standing over the wash basin should be avoided. Loose hairs are unpleasant to look at and can clog the drain. Towels should be hung neatly or put into the laundry hamper after use.

Daily Care by the Home Health Aide

Bathrooms are used frequently throughout the day and can easily become dirty. The aide should encourage family members to help in keeping the bathroom neat. In addition, a thorough cleaning reduces the risk of spreading disease. The following duties should be done on a daily basis.

- Wash and rinse all surfaces in the bathroom. The outside of the toilet as well as both sides of the toilet seat should be cleaned daily. The shower floor and walls, wall tiles, shower curtain, towel racks, windowsills, and radiator should also be cleaned daily. Use hot water, detergent, and disinfectant.
- Use a damp cloth to remove water spots from the walls around the sink. Clean the bathroom mirror with a glass cleaner, rinse off the soap dish, and wipe off the toothbrush holder.
- Damp mop bathroom floor.
- Using bathroom cleanser and sponge or cloth, clean and rinse sink and tub.
- Using brush and bowl cleaner, clean the inside of the toilet bowl. Be sure to scrub the area under the top rim of the bowl.
- Bleach in water can be used to remove mildew and mold.
- Empty wastebasket contents into a plastic bag. Line the clean wastebasket with a plastic liner.
- If needed, place a new roll of toilet paper on the roller. If the existing roll is running low, place a fresh roll nearby for easy replacement.
- A laundry hamper kept in the bathroom should be wiped out regularly using hot water and detergent. It is best to wash the client's linens daily. When emptying the family laundry hamper, transfer clothing directly to a laundry basket. Never put soiled clothing on the floor. Germs from the clothing can be transferred to the floors or germs on the floor can be transferred to the clothing. People walking across the floors can transfer these germs to all areas of the home. Hold dirty laundry away from the body as it is transferred from place to place.
- If possible, open the bathroom window and ventilate the room for a few minutes. Spray around the tub and sink drain with a disinfectant or air freshener.
- Add fresh towels and face cloths to the towel racks. Make a note of any bathroom supplies that need to be purchased such as shaving cream, toothpaste, soap, tissues, toilet paper, etc.
- Do not use the same container for both dirty and clean laundry.

Weekly Care by the Home Health Aide

Some tasks do not need to be done daily. The duties with each home assignment vary. The aide makes the judgment as to how often duties should be done. The following tasks can be done weekly or whenever necessary.

- Clean shower stall to remove lime buildup.
- Launder bath mats, small rugs, and throw rugs as needed. **Caution:** Do not put rubber-backed mats into the dryer.

- Tidy the linen closet to make it neat.
- Clean the medicine chest. With permission of the family, throw out old medications. Prescription medicines are normally dated and are marked as to length of time they may be safely used. All medicines should be labeled. It is unsafe to use medicines from unlabeled bottles.

SUMMARY

- Certain household tasks must be done daily, others once or twice a week, and still others on a weekly or bimonthly basis.
- The home health aide should develop a cleaning schedule that works well. The aide should try to keep to that schedule so the working day is evenly paced and the chores don't become overwhelming.

REVIEW

1. Name three factors you should think of before developing a cleaning plan.
2. List five household tasks that need to be done daily.
3. List five household tasks that need to be done weekly.
4. List five cleaning tasks done only periodically.
5. Describe the correct procedure for disposing and separating trash in your area.
6. Identify four steps necessary to clean a kitchen.
7. Identify daily bathroom care that family members or you need to do.
8. Identify two bathroom cleaning tasks the aide does daily.

Unit 23 Marketing and Meal Preparation

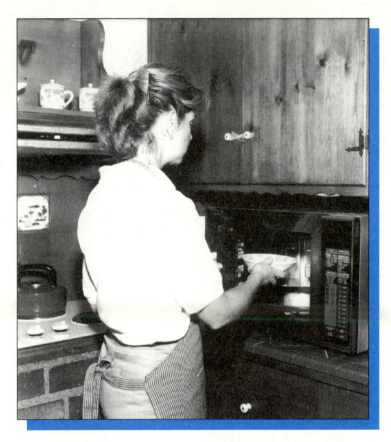

KEY TERMS
....

bulk

convenience foods

delicatessen

fermented

perishable

produce

staple items

LEARNING OBJECTIVES
....

After studying this unit, you should be able to:

- List four guidelines for planning menus.
- State eight guidelines for buying foods.
- List four guidelines for storing food.
- Name five guidelines for preparing meals.

Marketing and meal preparation require time and use of special skills. Planning nutritious meals and buying foods the family can afford require knowledge and use of judgment. Storing foods properly is also important. The aide, like the homemaker, develops these skills with study and practice.

Menus and Shopping Lists

Most meal planning is done for an entire week. Weekly planning saves the aide from making frequent trips to the market. The following steps are helpful planning guides.

- Sit down with the client and/or client's family and ask what foods and menus they want. This could be an important activity for the client as it may foster the client's feelings of being useful and in charge of the care.
- Plan menus for a full week. Make sure that the menu follows any specific guidelines provided by the client's physician.
- Be sure all **staple items,** such as spices and seasonings that are needed for each planned meal, are on hand.
- Make a shopping list and include all items needed in the household, Figure 23-1. Shopping time can be reduced by organizing the shopping list so that all items of one type are under one heading.
- Look in the newspaper and check the prices of products advertised. Cut out any coupons of items on the shopping list.
- Plan to use only the amount of money budgeted for food and supplies.

Purchasing Food

Purchasing food is simplified when planning is well thought out. Planning which is done in the home saves the aide time in the store. Marketing should be done at a time when the client can be safely left alone. The aide can sometimes shop while the client has a visitor. Shopping at home is an excellent activity for the housebound client and this is especially true of food shopping. It has several advantages. The client can become involved and interested in choos-

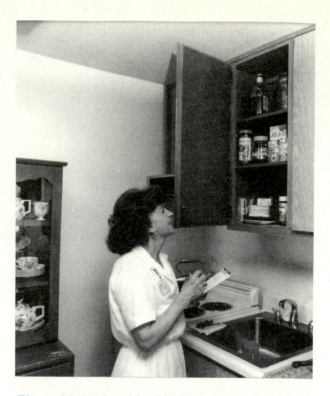

Figure 23-1   An aide checking the cupboard for needed groceries

ing foods, planning meals, and, even more importantly, saving money. This activity helps the client remain aware of the "life beyond illness" and can actually make the client feel better and more hopeful about the future. How do you shop at home for food? By reading newspaper and magazine ads and clipping coupons and company offers. One can actually see how prices differ from store to store within a single geographic area. If the client is able to read and has the energy to look through papers and magazines, this might be a challenging and economical way to pass the time.

Check with the client's local grocery store to see if it has special days that the disabled or elderly can shop and receive extra discounts or assistance. Many large grocery stores have special individual motorized carts to ride while shopping at their stores. Volunteers might be available in your community or through the client's church to assist the client to shop or actually do the shopping for the client. If at all possible, it is very beneficial to get your client out of the house and involved in the actual grocery shopping. This gives the client a chance to see other people and also make choices in the grocery shopping. Another benefit is for the client to actually see the "real" cost of food and how expensive certain items are.

A smart shopper plans ahead. Sometimes the supermarkets are inconvenient to reach. If it is necessary to expend extra time, bus or taxi fares, or gas and wear and tear on the car to get there, then it is unwise to use that store. If, however, several markets are located within the same general area, it pays to take advantage of money-saving brand or store coupons and buy items at the store where the price is lowest. When prices are particularly low on staple items such as paper and household cleaning supplies or canned goods, then, if money and storage space are available, extra amounts may be purchased. Practical guidelines for shopping are presented in the following list.

- Avoid going to the grocery store when you are hungry. Sweets and foods not on the shopping list are more likely to be bought when the shopper is hungry.
- If there is time, walk through the store with the shopping list in hand. Compare prices and decide on the best buys for the budget. If the allowed money won't cover all the items, make substitutions. For example, if beef prices are very high, buy ground beef instead of cube steak. If the quality of fresh **produce** is poor, buy frozen or canned vegetables.
- Select the needed foods by starting at one side of the store and moving from aisle to aisle. Compare the prices of brand names and store brands. Read labels. Do not be swayed by advertising slang such as jumbo, king size, giant, or economy. Buy the size best suited to the needs of the client or family. Large quantities are not practical if they cannot be stored.
- Do not buy sale items unless the client normally uses them and has storage space for them. A bargain the client cannot use is no bargain at all.
- If the client needs to prepare food when you are not there, you may need to purchase nutritious **convenience foods** that the client can prepare with little assistance.

- Be aware of how much area is available for storage of food. Use this space wisely and purchase items that are going to be needed within the month only.
- If a client just wants a small amount of a dish, it may be wise to purchase a small serving of this in the **delicatessen** rather than preparing a large dish and throwing it away in a few days.
- If only one person is living in the home, it may be wise to put the bread in the freezer and remove when needed.
- Powdered or dried milk can be a money saver. Dry milk mixed with water can be added to a quart of skim or whole milk. The flavor may be the same or better and it costs less. The nutritional value is the same as in whole milk.
- Fresh fruits and vegetables are less expensive during their growing season. Compare fresh vegetable prices with canned and frozen vegetable prices while vegetables are in season. Out of season produce is quite costly.
- Eggs have the same food value whether they are jumbo, extra large, large, or small. Brown or white shelled eggs are equally tasty and nutritious. Large eggs look better when served fried, boiled, or poached. However, for cooking or scrambling, small eggs are the best buy.
- When buying meat, consider how the meat will be prepared. Most meat cuts have the same food value. Cheaper cuts can be just as tasty when prepared with imagination and care. When comparing the price per pound, consider the waste due to bones and fat. Figure the number of servings needed and the cost per serving.
- When selecting poultry, buying the whole bird is the best choice. Buying separate parts such as the breast, legs, or thighs is more expensive.
- If there is enough freezer space in the home, meats can be purchased in **bulk;** there is a considerable saving in the cost per pound. At home, meat can be rewrapped for the freezer in smaller meal-size portions. However, do not buy more than can be used. Waste occurs from overstocking the freezer. Most meats can be safely frozen for up to 6 months.

Some meats lose flavor and food value when stored longer. Foods not properly wrapped can be ruined by freezer burn.

- Make sure meats purchased are fresh. If they do not smell, look, or feel right, do not buy them. Fresh meat will regain its shape when poked with a finger. If the meat feels slimy, slick, or soft, don't buy it. If the color is off, the meat may be spoiled already.
- Don't buy damaged cans, no matter how low the price. Cans with bulging tops, dents, or rust may contain spoiled food.
- Purchase **perishable** foods last. These include foods which spoil easily such as milk, meats, and frozen foods.

Storing Food

After returning from the market, the aide should store the purchased foods properly. Putting foods and supplies away should be done before any other major task is begun.

- Always refrigerate perishable foods immediately. Lettuce can wilt and milk will spoil if they are not refrigerated.
- Frozen fruits and vegetables should be placed in the freezer as soon as possible. Do not overstock on frozen foods.
- Wash and clean poultry before refrigerating. If poultry is not planned for a meal within 2 days, wrap and freeze it.
- Dried and packaged foods should be stored in airtight containers. Examples of airtight containers are canisters, glass jars with lids, or plastic bags. Many containers of food can be refrigerated if there is room. Otherwise they should be stored so that roaches, ants, or rodents cannot get to them. If safe storage space is limited, buy only small amounts of these foods.
- Canned goods store easily and keep very well. They should not be stored near hot water pipes or near any other source of heat.
- Paper goods and other supplies should be stored nearest the place where they will be used. Toilet paper should be stored near the bathroom and laundry supplies near the

washing machine. Cleaning products should always be stored in a closet or cabinet out of the reach of children.

Meal Preparation

To prepare nutritious meals, the aide must use foods from the food guide pyramid groups. In addition, the aide should check to see if the client has a special diet ordered or if the client has allergies to any foods. Occasionally the client may be taking medications that cannot be taken with certain types of foods. The aide should use the following guidelines when preparing meals (refer to Chapter 11):

- Follow the food pyramid daily guidelines
  6–11 Bread, cereal, rice, pasta products
  3–5 Vegetables
  2–4 Fruits
  2–3 Milk, yogurt, cheese
  2–4 Meat, poultry, fish, dry beans, eggs, nuts
  Use sparingly—salad oils, cream, butter, sugar, soft drinks, sweet desserts
- Prepare any special diet the dietitian has ordered for the client.
- Limit the use of salt in cooking and also in seasoning foods. Have salt substitute available.
- Serve skim or 2% milk to limit fat intake.
- Cook vegetables in microwave if available. This will preserve nutritional value of the vegetables.
- Prepare amounts that will be eaten in one or two meals only. Serving the same foods can decrease client's appetite.
- Have low-calorie nutritious snacks available so client does not eat high-calorie snacks.
- Be sure the meal being prepared has adequate fiber foods. Clients who are inactive may develop constipation, which can be prevented with a diet high in fiber.
- Encourage intake of water or other fluids throughout the day.
- If the client is taking a diuretic, the diet will need to be high in foods that contain potassium, such as bananas, dates, raisins, and orange juice.

- If the client is on a low-calorie diet, sugar substitutes should be used as often as possible.
- Store food in pantry at a height convenient for the client to reach.
- Avoid fried foods as much as possible. Fried foods add more fat to the diet than is necessary.
- People should limit the number of eggs per week (*not* including eggs used in preparing a dish such as custard).
- Do not overcook frozen or fresh vegetables.
- When opening cans, wash the top of the can before piercing with a can opener. This will keep dirt and germs from entering the food. If the contents spew out or are foamy or appear to have bubbles they may have spoiled and must be discarded. After a can has been opened, unused portions should be transferred to a refrigerator container and covered tightly before refrigerating.
- Check food for spoiling: sour milk, rancid butter, moldy bread, **fermented** fruits, spoiled meats.
- Plan for variety. Throughout the week serve different vegetables, meat, poultry, fish, and meat substitutes. Different spices and herbs may also be used to add variety to meals, Figures 23-2 and 23-3.
- Consider how each meal will look on the plate. For example, mashed potatoes, cauliflower, fish, and a pear (for dessert) would not look appetizing because each is white or colorless.
- Most fresh fruit and vegetables should be served raw if possible because of greater nutritional value. They should be cooked unpeeled to give the most food value. Steaming instead of boiling preserves both flavor and food value. The water from fresh vegetables is high in vitamins. This water may be added to meat stock and used for making tasty soups.
- Save whole milk for drinking. Use dry milk in preparing sauces and gravies. The food value and flavor of dry milk is equal to whole milk.
- Use leftover meats in a creative way. Add fresh mushrooms to leftover beef and make a brown sauce. Turkey hash, creamed turkey, chicken salad, or sandwiches can all be made with leftovers.

- Foods not in season may not be the best buy. However, if the client likes a certain food it is well worth the extra cost and may make a pleasant change in the diet. Fresh vegetables should be purchased in the exact amount needed to prevent spoilage.
- Practice cooking and serving meals. A good cook uses clean, unspoiled raw meats and vegetables and follows recipes. Food should be attractive and served on an attractive table or tray, Figure 23-4.

Cooking in a Microwave

Microwave ovens have been in general use for a few years, but they are not a standard appliance in all homes. If one has not had occasion to use a microwave oven here are a few simple rules.

NEVER place anything metal (including twist ties or labels with metal content) in the microwave. It will ruin the oven and probably the metal also. There are special microwave utensils, plates, and dishes that can be used as well as glass, china, and paperware. Most microwave owners will have a simple manual with instructions for proper use. Here are a few examples of ways to make use of a microwave, Figure 23-5.

- Baked potato: Wash and dry thoroughly, then prick the skin with a fork so the steam can escape. Place the potato on a paper towel or paper plate and put in the oven following instructions for timing. It can take 3 to 5 minutes to have a perfect baked potato.
- Leftovers: Place in microwave plate or dish, cover with paper towel or wax paper as recommended, and heat at the recommended setting and time. It can take as little as 2 or 3 minutes to heat up leftovers.
- Frozen vegetables: Follow instructions on package. This is an excellent way to prepare frozen vegetables as they remain crisp and taste fresh. Seasoning is done after the food is cooked so that vegetables prepared in the microwave can be appropriately seasoned to fit the needs of any diet.
- Defrost: The microwave may also be used to defrost frozen foods quickly so that they can

SEASONINGS AND SPICES*	USES
Allspice	Particularly good with pot roast, in puddings and cereals. (Tastes like cinnamon, clove, and nutmeg.)
Anise	In tossed green salad and other vegetable salads. It can be used with pot cheese.
Caraway Seeds	Give flavor to bread, pot cheese, cabbage, cauliflower, cereals, and cookies.
Cardamom Seeds	Good with curries, soups, and meats.
Cayenne	Few grains will be enough to season vegetables, meats, fish, poultry, soups; vegetable, meat, fish, poultry, or egg salads.
Chili Peppers	Seasoning soups, rice, dried peas or beans, meat, fish, pot cheese.
Cinnamon	Flavors cereals, bread, pot cheese, vegetables such as beans, cabbage, cauliflower, carrots, cucumbers, eggplant, lentils, onions, and peas.
Cloves	Can be used in much the same way as cinnamon; particularly nice for flavoring tea.
Coriander Seeds	For seasoning stews, curries, soups, and fish.
Curry Powder	To season soups, stews, rice, chicken, eggs, meat, fish, and vegetables.
Garlic	Flavors soups, sauces, salads and salad dressings, meat, fish, poultry, pot cheese, dried peas or beans.
Ginger	Used in much the same way as cinnamon.
Mace	Flavors meats, fish, poultry, soup, sauces, stews, potatoes, carrots, snap beans, peas, cabbage, and cauliflower.
Dry Mustard	Seasons meats, fish, salad dressings, vegetables, eggs, pot cheese, fish, poultry, and all salads.
Nutmeg	Used the same way as mace.
Paprika	Gives a bright garnish to vegetables, meats, eggs, pot cheese, fish, poultry, and all salads.
Pepper	Adds flavor to meats, fish, poultry, eggs, and vegetables.
Poppy Seeds	Used as toppings for bread, rolls, cookies, and cakes. Good with pot cheese and in salad dressings.
Sesame Seeds	Used on rolls, buns, and bread.
Turmeric	Seasons meats, fish, and poultry.

*Spices and many seasonings are highly perishable unless kept in tightly closed containers. They should be bought in small quantities and renewed at least once a year.

Figure 23-2   Seasonings and spices add variety and taste to meals.

be chosen and prepared at the last minute. Meats seem to taste better when cooked by traditional methods on top of the stove or in oven or broiler. However, there are recipes in the microwave manual for cooking all sorts of food.

- Reheat: If for some reason, a client's food has become cold (a telephone call interrupting the meal or an emergency of some sort), a microwave-proof dinnerplate can be placed directly in the microwave and in just a minute, the meal will be heated thoroughly without loss of flavor or appetite appeal.

Herb and Part Used	Uses in Cooking
Basil — leaves	Italian tomato dishes, soups, ragouts, salads, meats, sauces, fruit drinks.
Bay — leaves	For flavoring soups, stews, sauces.
Chervil — leaves and sometimes fleshy roots	In place of parsley, in fine herbs, salads, sauces, soups. In omelettes.
Chives — leaves	In fine herbs, salads, omelettes, or anything for which a delicate onion flavor is desired.
Dill — seed and young tips	Added to melted sweet butter or salt-free margarine, it makes a fine sauce for fish. In mashed potato, in tossed green, potato, fish, or vegetable salads. Sprinkled on broiled chops.
Sweet Marjoram — leaves	Sprinkled over beef, lamb or pork. Used in veal stew, chopped meat, meat balls. In fine herbs, salads, and fish dishes. Cooked with zucchini.
Mint — leaves	Flavors sauces, vegetables, jellies, fruit drinks, vegetable and fruit salads, custards, puddings.
Oregano	Can be rubbed over meat before roasting or broiling or it can be put in the water during the cooking of meat and fish. Used with veal, pork, soups, potatoes, vegetables and fresh salads. (Closely related to marjoram and has a similar flavor.)
Parsley — leaves	In fine herbs, for soups, sauces. Popular with boiled potato and many other vegetables. With meat, fish, eggs and with vegetable, meat, or fish salads.
Rosemary — leaves	To flavor roast lamb and veal, meat stews, poultry sauces, stuffings.
Sage — leaves	In stuffing for meat, poultry, fish. In fish chowder.
Savory — leaves	Excellent with snap beans, dried peas, lentils. Also good in chopped beef, gravy, meat stew, and croquettes. Can be sprinkled over fish before baking or broiling.
Tarragon — leaves	Flavoring for vinegar, sauces, and salad dressings, chicken and other meats. For egg and tomato dishes, sandwiches. In fine herbs.
Thyme — leaves	In fine herbs, in stews, soups, sauces, salad. With meat, poultry, fish, tomato dishes. Can be combined with melted butter and served over carrots, onions and peas.

Figure 23-3   Herbs may also be used to enhance the taste and appeal of many foods.

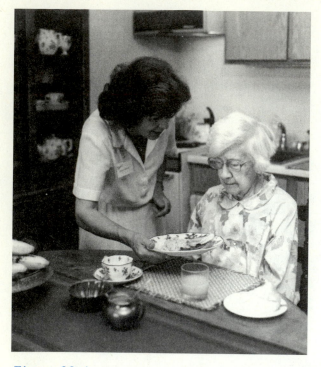

Figure 23-4   An aide is serving the client an attractive meal. Notice the neat and attractive table.

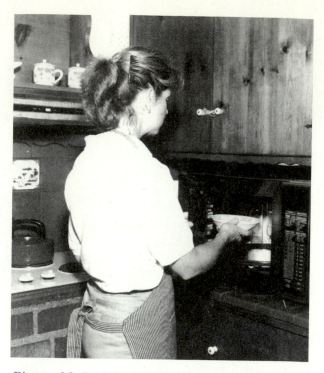

Figure 23-5   Microwave cooking is a fast and convenient method of cooking for a client.

SUMMARY

- Meal preparation and marketing are an important part of the home health aide's responsibilities.
- The aide must follow any specific guidelines provided by the client's dietitian when preparing meals.
- When purchasing food, the aide must keep within budget limits.
- Food should be properly stored.

- Contrasting the color and texture and attractively arranging the food will do more to increase the client's appetite than just throwing it on the plate.
- An aide needs to try to balance two things when preparing meals for the client: modern nutritional thinking and the preferences and choices of the client.

REVIEW

1. List four guidelines for planning menus.
2. List eight guidelines to remember when grocery shopping.
3. List four guidelines for storing foods.
4. Name five guidelines to remember when preparing meals.

Unit 24 Laundry Duties

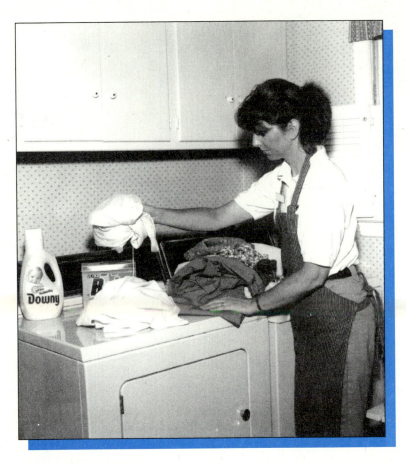

KEY TERMS

agitator   permanent press   polyester fabrics

LEARNING OBJECTIVES

After studying this unit, you should be able to:

- Identify two ways to sort clothes for washing.
- Identify the best time to perform mending.
- Identify several methods for removing stains.
- Explain how to wash clothing and bed linens from a client with an infectious disease.

Clothes and household linens are a major expense for most families. The home health aide must be responsible for giving suitable care to these items. Correctly sorting, washing, and ironing clothes requires careful attention.

Sorting Clothes and Linens

Most clothing can be machine washed. However, some articles of clothing must be dry cleaned; others must be hand washed. Most of today's clothes have labels with instructions for proper care. If an item is not labeled, the aide must be able to judge from its appearance. If there is any doubt, the aide should ask a family member which washing method is best.

In general, cotton fabrics can be washed in hot water. Blends of cotton and polyester and cottons of light color should be washed in warm water. Chlorine bleaches are only used for white cottons. There are special bleaches for nylon and **polyester fabrics.** Be careful to follow instructions when using bleaches. Dark fabrics are washed separately from light fabrics, Figure 24-1. Many homemakers wash dark clothes in cold water with cold water detergent. When sorting clothes for the laundry, use the following tips:

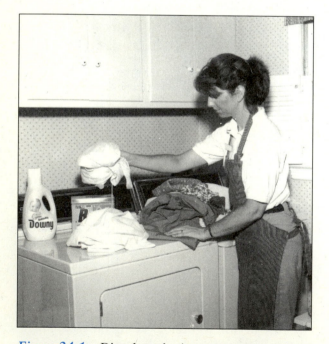

Figure 24-1   Dirty laundry is separated according to white and dark colors before the clothes are placed in the washing machine.

- Sort the clothes according to color. Do not wash white clothes with dark items. If possible wash towels separately. You may use a separate load for lingerie and other fabrics needing a gentle cycle.
- Make a separate pile of clothes that must be hand washed or dry cleaned.
- As each item is sorted, check it for spots that might require special care. Collars of shirts and dresses and spots from food or other stains may need special care, Figure 24-2.
- Turn pockets inside out. Be sure to remove pens, pencils, paper, coins, or other items in the pockets.
- Shake dirt, sand, or grass out of clothing before placing it with the other clothes.
- Remove belt buckles or ornaments that might be ruined in the washer.
- Hand wash separately those fabrics in which the colors run or bleed.
- Make sure dark socks do not get mixed with the light or white loads.

Loading the Washing Machine

Loading differs depending on whether the family has a top or front loading machine. Before operating the washing machine, the aide should read the directions. If the aide is still in doubt, a family member should be asked to assist. Improper use of a machine could cause personal injury or damage to the clothing or the machine.

- Most top loading machines will allow you to add the clothes first and then fill the machine with water. Pour in correct amount of detergent, Figure 24-3. Add bleach if necessary. Make sure the bleach mixes well with the water before adding the white clothes. Add softener if necessary. Close the machine and set dial at correct setting. Modern detergents recommend washing clothes for no longer than 12 minutes in the wash cycle.
- For front loading machines, add detergent and softener as indicated. Put in the clothing and close the door tightly. Set dial for correct setting.
- Unload clean wet laundry into clean container or basket. Hang outside if allowed or

STAIN	HOW TO REMOVE
Blood	Presoak in cold water; if stain is stubborn rub in detergent, then launder using safe bleach.
Butter, oils	Rub cornstarch on spot or use powdered cleaning product or cleaning fluid according to instructions.
Chocolate	Soak in cold water, and rub detergent directly on stain. Launder in water as warm as the fabric allows.
Coffee, tea	Pour hot water directly on spot, then wash as usual. Use water as hot as the fabric allows.
Cosmetics	Presoak in detergent and water, then launder.
Crayon and candle wax	Scrape off as much as possible. (Crayons have a wax base.) Place blotting paper under spot and on top of spot. Rub hot iron over blotter. The wax should melt into the blotter. Launder, using safe bleach and detergent.
Deodorants	Presoak area with white vinegar, rinse, and launder.
Fruits	Rinse in cold water. If stain is stubborn, put 1 tablespoon of baking soda in a quart of water to neutralize the acid. Rinse and launder.
Grass	Rub detergent into the spot. Launder with safe bleach and detergent.
Ink, magic marker, felt tip pens	Remove washable ink by rubbing cold water and detergent into the spot. Ballpoint pens make a stain that can be removed with dry cleaning fluid. Permanent or unwashable inks must be removed by a professional dry cleaner.
Lipstick	Remove with cleaning fluid. Make sure the fluid will not ruin fabric by testing on an inside seam area.
Meat juice, eggs	Scrape off, then sponge area with cold water. Rub in detergent and launder.
Rust	Use dry cleaning fluid, then wash as usual.
Scorch (mark from hot iron)	Dampen a white cotton cloth in cold water to which a small amount of bleach has been added. Quickly rub over the scorched spot. Turn the iron to a cooler setting—wait until the spot has dried, then proceed with ironing. Deeply scorched items may need to be patched.

Figure 24-2   Guidelines for removing stains

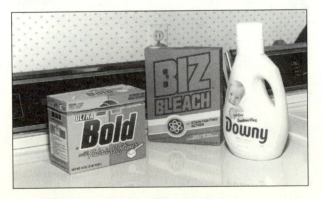

Figure 24-3   Common household products used in doing the client's laundry

place in dryer. Figure 24-4 shows a typical laundry room.

• Be sure you do not overload the washing machine.

Pathogens such as HIV, which causes AIDS, are not airborne. However, when handling bed linens and clothing of an infected client, wear gloves and separate the items from other laundry. Bed linens of clients with infectious or contagious diseases should be washed with detergent in the hottest water possible (at least 160°F), using the longest washing cycle. If water

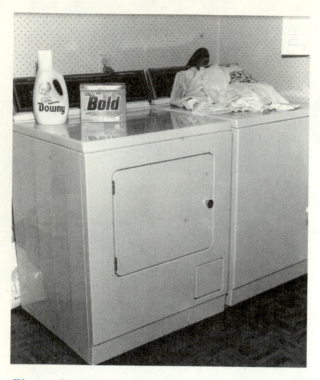

Figure 24-4   Laundry rooms with washer and dryer are quite popular today.

temperature is less than 160°F, bleach germicide should be added to the water. Ask the case manager to provide clear instructions so that laundry can be done correctly and safely.

Some clients will not have washing machines and dryers. In that case, you may have to take the dirty linens and clothing to a laundromat. Some apartments do have laundry rooms that are used by the tenants. If it is necessary to use laundromats or laundry rooms, the home health aide should schedule laundry time when it is safe and convenient to be away from the client and, when using an apartment laundry room, at a time when the machines are available. It might be a good idea to talk to the apartment superintendent and arrange for a regular time for you to use the machines.

When using laundromats and laundry rooms, the aide will need quarters or other small change and should make certain that there is plenty of change on hand. Usually, it is best to take the soap, bleach, and other necessary supplies from the client's home. If you purchase them from vending machines, the cost is much more. A good idea when using "community" machines (ones that are

used by many people), is to wipe them on the inside with a damp cloth before starting to do the wash.

Drying, Ironing, and Mending

Not all clothing requires high heat or long drying cycles. Towels, heavy pants, and sweat shirts usually take the longest time to dry. Nylon, polyester, or any **permanent press** fabrics can be dried quickly. Permanent press clothing should be removed from the dryer as soon as the tumbler has stopped. If clothes are hung or folded at once, few wrinkles will form in them.

Large items such as sheets and blankets should be placed in the dryer separately or no more than two at a time. Folding sheets and blankets as soon as the drying process is finished helps to prevent wrinkling. Some clothing items may need to be drip-dried or laid flat to dry, blocking to shape (such as sweaters). These items usually are not to be wrung out because this twists the fabric fibers.

Cotton clothing that needs to be ironed should be folded neatly. Folding clothing before ironing keeps out unwanted creases and makes ironing easier, Figure 24-5.

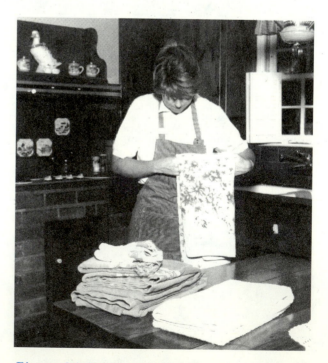

Figure 24-5   An aide folding clean laundry before putting it away

- Set up the ironing board and set heat to correct temperature for steam or dry ironing.
- Gather hangers to be used for those items that will need to be hung.
- Prepare needles and thread of various colors. Stick the needles at the broad end of the ironing board ready to be used to replace buttons or mend small tears or split seams. Just a few extra minutes spent while handling the ironing to make these small repairs will save time and trouble later. The clothes will be ready for use or storage at once.
- While the ironing is being done, other loads can be put through the wash and dry cycles. Clean the lint traps in the washer and dryer after use. Wipe the inside and outside of machines so they will be ready to use the next time.
- Take the clean and ironed items and store them properly.

SUMMARY

- Follow instructions on the washing machine, sort clothing before placing in the machine, and use the proper detergent and the correct water temperature.
- When using a commercial machine (in a laundromat or in an apartment laundry room), take a damp cloth and wipe out the machine before using it. Some people are careless and leave the machines dirty. Wiping the machines before use will help to ensure clean laundry.
- When doing a client's laundry and ironing, the aide should take care to do it properly; this is taking suitable responsibility.
- Unload clean clothes into a clean container.
- Be sure to wear gloves when handling linen soiled with body fluids.

REVIEW

1. Describe two ways of sorting clothes to be washed.
2. Explain the best time to perform mending.
3. Identify several methods of removing stains.
4. Explain how to wash infected client's laundry.
5. When working in the home you are to use your time wisely. It is also important to do good quality work. Why are these two traits important?
   a.
   b.
6. You are assigned to do the following tasks in the home for Mr. Tan, a 95-year-old man who is paralyzed on his right side. You are allowed 4 hours to do the tasks. How would you plan your work?
   a. shower
   b. oral care—dentures
   c. shave
   d. apply topical ointment to both legs
   e. change his bedding
   f. walk outside for at least two blocks
   g. cook two balanced meals
   h. do his laundry for the week

Section 7

Health Care Services

Units

25 Introduction to Client Care Procedures

26 Infection Control and Universal Precautions

27 Restorative Care

28 Bathing

29 Daily Care

30 Feeding and Toileting

31 Collecting Specimens and Catheter Care

32 Vital Signs and Measurements

33 Hot and Cold Applications

34 Rectal Care

35 Special Treatments

36 Infant Care

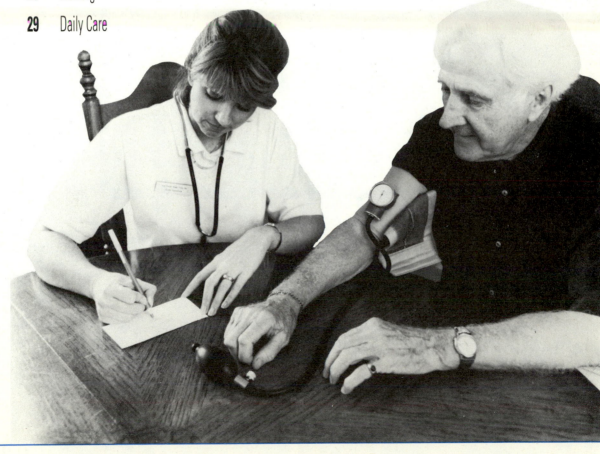

Unit 25 Introduction to Client Care Procedures

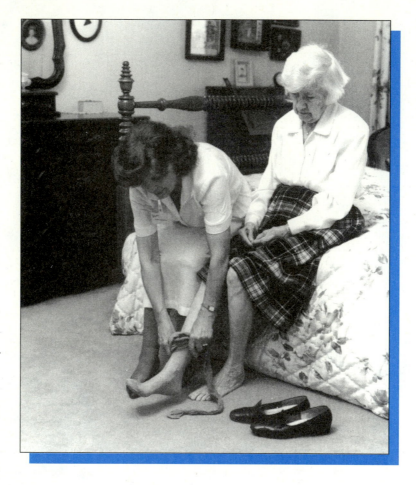

LEARNING OBJECTIVES

After studying this unit, you should be able to:

- List the rules for carrying out client care procedures.
- Describe how to provide privacy for the client during procedures.
- State when the aide's hands should be washed.

- Explain why it is necessary to give an explanation to the client before doing any procedure.
- Recognize those procedures which you, as a home health aide, are not permitted to do because of state mandated guidelines or agency's policies.

Almost all clients would prefer not to have someone besides themselves do basic tasks for them. Most people prefer to be independent rather than dependent on others for care. The skills you will be using on your clients have special ways for them to be done. The particular method is called a **procedure.** The procedures you will be doing are in most instances basic tasks, but they have been developed to save you effort, help you organize your work, prevent injury to the client, and be sure you do all the necessary steps. Procedures also show clients that they can expect consistency of care from all aides. Your case manager will inform you of the skills you are permitted to perform for the client and also what procedures are allowed to be done by the home health aide in your state.

In some cases, a client may be receiving special and specialized treatments at home, which require special machines. These pieces of equipment are known as durable equipment. Often rental of such equipment is expensive. Decisions to use such items are made by the doctor and the client or client's family. For instance, home dialysis machines are used by those who have little or no kidney function. Dialysis requires several hours on the machine to remove the impurities from the blood. An aide may be expected to check the client's progress and make sure that the machine is functioning. Other durable equipment sometimes used in home care includes respirators, tube feeding or intravenous feeding equipment, and oxygen tanks. Unless aides are specially trained, qualified, certified, and permitted by law to operate such equipment, they must not attempt to do so. However, an aide will probably be shown by the case manager what to look for, what to observe, and what to report when such equipment is in use.

As a home health aide goes from case to case, the client care procedures vary. Each client has special needs and will require different procedures. As experience is gained, the home health aide develops a pattern of providing safe and proper care. However, no amount of experience excuses taking shortcuts in giving client care.

Table 25-1 provides a list of the client care procedures covered in this text. When performing any of these procedures, the aide should always keep in mind the following basic guidelines.

1. Involve the client as an active participant in each procedure. If possible, allow the client to decide when care such as bathing or shaving is to be done. This allows clients to feel more in control of their lives and is good therapy.
2. The aide's hands should always be washed before carrying out any procedure.
3. The aide should plan ahead and know what equipment and supplies will be needed.
4. Equipment and supplies should be placed as close as possible to save time and energy while giving the client care.
5. Explain to the client what is going to be done and the reason for doing it, Figure 25-1. The aide should keep in mind that being cared for may make clients feel they do not have control of their lives. Clients may feel they are being forced to do things they do not want to do. It is extremely important for the aide to get the client's cooperation and consent before doing any procedure. If the aide communicates in an easy and natural way, clients feel more important and are usually more cooperative. For example, in the morning ask whether the client needs the bedpan or urinal or needs help getting to the bathroom. Help the client to wash and brush teeth before breakfast. You might say, "Good morning. Did you sleep well? It's about time for breakfast." Let the client talk and LISTEN to what the client is saying. At bathtime and bed changing time say, "After your bath and back rub I will get your bed ready for the day." Try to get the client interested in what is being done. Participation makes the client more cooperative and understanding of treatments.
6. Provide privacy for the client during a procedure. The client should have privacy when using the bedpan, having a bed bath, or while having the bed linens changed. Talk to the client before these procedures. Plan what to do in case the phone or doorbell rings while in the middle of such procedures. Perhaps a "Do Not Disturb" sign

UNIT 16 CARING FOR CLIENTS WITH DIABETES
1. Testing Blood

UNIT 26 INFECTION CONTROL AND UNIVERSAL PRECAUTIONS
2. Handwashing
3. Gloving
4. Putting On and Removing Personal Protective Equipment
5. Collecting Specimen in Isolation

UNIT 27 RESTORATIVE CARE
6. Maintaining Body Alignment
7. Turning the Client Toward You
8. Moving the Client Up in Bed Using the Drawsheet
9. Log Rolling the Client
10. Positioning the Client in Supine Position
11. Positioning the Client in Lateral/Side-lying Position
12. Positioning the Client in Prone Position
13. Positioning the Client in Fowler's Position
14. Assisting the Client from Bed to Chair
15. Assisting the Client from Chair to Bed
16. Transferring the Client from Wheelchair to Toilet/Commode
17. Performing Passive Range of Motion Exercises
18. Assisting the Client to Walk with Crutches, Walker, or Cane
19. Lifting the Client Using a Mechanical Lift

UNIT 28 BATHING
20. Assisting with Tub Bath or Shower
21. Giving a Bed Bath
22. Giving a Partial Bath
23. Giving a Back Rub
24. Giving Female Perineal Care
25. Giving Male Perineal Care
26. Special Skin Care and Pressure Sores

UNIT 29 DAILY CARE
27. Assisting with Routine Oral Hygiene
28. Caring for Dentures
29. Shaving the Male Client
30. Dressing and Undressing Client
31. Applying Elasticized Stockings
32. Making an Unoccupied Bed
33. Making an Occupied Bed
34. Giving Nail Care
35. Shampooing the Client's Hair in Bed
36. Assisting the Client with Self-administered Medications

37. Inserting a Hearing Aid
38. Caring for an Artificial Eye

UNIT 30 FEEDING AND TOILETING
39. Feeding the Client
40. Measuring and Recording Fluid Intake and Output
41. Giving and Emptying the Bedpan
42. Giving and Emptying the Urinal

UNIT 31 COLLECTING SPECIMENS AND CATHETER CARE
43. Collecting a Clean-catch Urine Specimen
44. Caring for Urinary Catheter
45. Connecting the Leg Bag
46. Emptying a Drainage Unit
47. Retraining the Bladder
48. Collecting a Sputum Specimen

UNIT 32 VITAL SIGNS AND MEASUREMENT
49. Taking an Oral Temperature
50. Taking a Rectal Temperature
51. Taking an Axillary Temperature
52. Taking the Radial and Apical Pulse
53. Counting Respirations
54. Taking a Blood Pressure
55. Measuring Weight and Height

UNIT 33 COLD AND HEAT APPLICATIONS
56. Applying an Ice Bag, Cap, or Collar
57. Applying a K-Pad—Dry or Moist
58. Performing a Warm Foot Soak

UNIT 34 RECTAL CARE
59. Giving a Commercial Enema
60. Giving a Rectal Suppository
61. Training and Retraining Bowels
62. Applying Adult Briefs
63. Collecting a Stool Specimen

UNIT 35 SPECIAL TREATMENTS
64. Applying Unsterile Dressing and Ointment to Unbroken Skin
65. Caring for Casts
66. Changing an Ostomy Bag
67. Assisting the Client with Oxygen Therapy
68. Assisting with Cough and Deep Breathing Exercises

UNIT 36 INFANT CARE
69. Assisting with Breast-feeding and Breast Care
70. Giving the Infant a Sponge Bath
71. Bottle-feeding the Infant

Table 25-1   Client Care Procedures

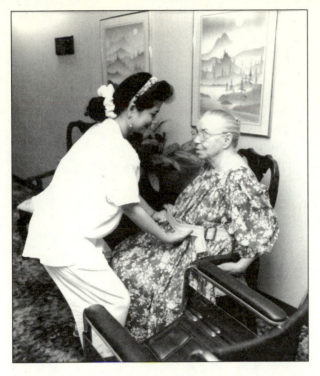

Figure 25-1   Always tell the client what you plan to do.

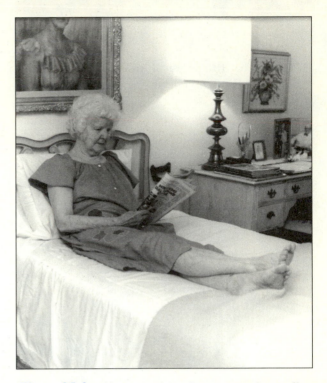

Figure 25-2   Always put equipment and supplies away after use and leave the client's room neat and tidy.

can be put on the door and the phone taken off the hook. (Remember to tell other family members if this is done.) The client will be able to relax without worry of interruptions.

7. Complete client care procedures as quickly and carefully as possible. Procedures cannot be timed. However, if the client is on the bedpan and there are no results, remove the bedpan. Do not wait until the client becomes uncomfortable. Tell the client to call when the bedpan is again needed.

8. Do not embarrass the client in any way. Aides should treat clients as they themselves would wish to be treated.

9. After a client care procedure is completed, remove all equipment and supplies. Clean and store the equipment and supplies at once so that the client's room is neat and orderly, Figure 25-2.

10. The aide should keep a pad and pencil handy to make notes of signs and symptoms that need to be reported (temperature, pulse, respiration, weight, blood pressure, etc.).

11. Using a form provided by the agency, check off each procedure as completed. Write up any incident that is unusual and if in doubt or uncertain about any incident, behavior of client, or unusual circumstance, call your case manager.

12. Follow all safety precautions when working with the client; report unsafe conditions to the agency and work carefully so as not to endanger yourself.

13. Above all, treat your client with dignity and do not cause any harm to the client.

SUMMARY

....

- Caring for the physical, emotional, and medical needs of the client involves both the aide and the client.
- Aides must recognize procedures they are not permitted to perform because of state mandated guidelines and agency policies.
- If a task or procedure is not charted, it is assumed not done by your case manager.
- It is vital to gain the cooperation and participation of the client.

- If the client is helpless, the aide must do all the work as efficiently and safely as possible.
- For the client who is able, the aide should let the client actively assist in the procedures.
- The aide must always provide safety, privacy and an explanation of what is being done and the reason for the procedure.

Unit *26* Infection Control and Universal Precautions

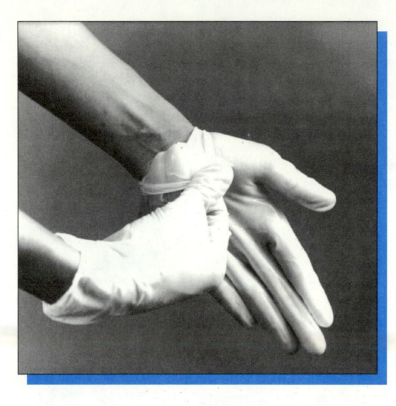

CLIENT CARE PROCEDURES

. . . .

2. Handwashing
3. Gloving
4. Putting on and Removing Personal Protective Equipment
5. Collecting Specimen in Isolation

NOTE: All procedures are not allowed in all states. Make sure you are aware of limits as outlined by state guidelines.

LEARNING OBJECTIVES

. . . .

After studying this unit, you should be able to:

- Demonstrate clear ability to perform all the procedures.
- Explain the purpose of each procedure.
- State when the procedures should and should not be done.
- Identify precautions to be taken for each procedure.

Client Care Procedure **2:** Handwashing

Purpose

- To prevent the transfer of disease-producing organisms from person to person or place to place.

NOTE: The hands of the home health aide must be washed before and after each client contact; before preparing food; before and after each meal; after blowing the nose or sneezing, combing hair, using the bathroom; and after handling soiled items such as linens, clothing, or garbage.

Procedure

1. Collect the items needed for handwashing and bring them to the bathroom or kitchen sink.

   soap
   soap dish
   towel (paper towels preferred)
   washbasin (if needed)
   orange stick (optional)

2. Using a clean paper towel turn on water and adjust temperature. Wet hands with fingertips pointing down, Figure 26-1.

3. Apply soap—either liquid or bar.
4. With fingertips pointing down, lather well. Rub your hands together in a circular motion to generate friction, Figure 26-2. Wash carefully between your fingers and rub fingernails against the palm of the other hand to force soap under the nails. Keep washing for 10 to 15 seconds. Be sure to clean under fingernails, Figure 26-3.

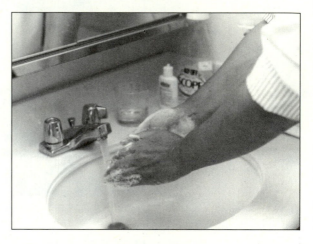

Figure 26-2 Lather hands well; be sure to use friction between the hands.

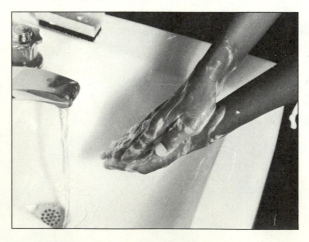

Figure 26-1 Wet hands, apply soap, and point fingertips down in the sink.

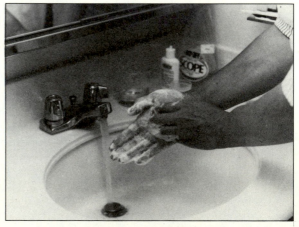

Figure 26-3 Always clean your fingernails.

5. With fingertips still pointing down, rinse all the soap off. Be careful not to lean against the side of the sink or touch the inside of the sink because germs are there.

6. With clean paper towel or cloth hand towel, dry hands. Take clean paper towel and turn off faucet, Figure 26-4. Do not turn off faucet with clean hands because the faucet handles are contaminated.

7. Discard the paper towel in the wastebasket. Hand towels can be placed in a laundry hamper.

8. Apply hand lotion if hands are dry or chapped.

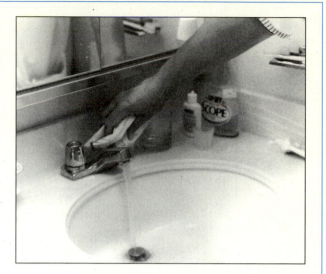

Figure 26-4 Turn off faucet with dry paper towel.

Client Care Procedure 3: Gloving

Purpose

• To prevent the spread of infections

NOTE: Gloves should be worn for most personal care procedures. Always wear gloves when doing procedures in which you have contact with body fluids. Wear gloves when you are giving mouth care, perineal care, handling excretions and body fluids, for example, emptying a bedpan, changing soiled linens, bathing a client with an open skin lesion, and collecting specimens.

Procedure

1. Wash your hands.
2. With your dominant hand, usually the right, pull out one glove and slide it on to your other hand.
3. With the gloved hand, pull out another glove and slide your dominant hand into it.
4. Interlace your fingers to make the gloves comfortable and adjust the top of the gloves to stay flat.

Removal of Contaminated Gloves

1. Use your dominant hand to grasp the opposite glove on the palm side, about 1 inch below the wrist, Figure 26-5.

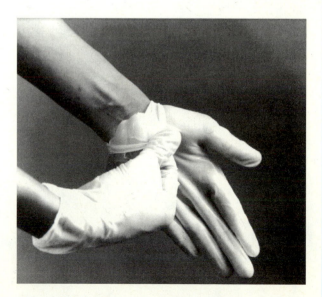

Figure 26-5 To remove gloves, grasp glove on the palm side.

Continued on the following page.

2. Pull the glove down and off so that it is removed inside out and keep hold of that glove with the fingertips of the gloved hands, Figure 26-6.

3. Using your ungloved hand, insert the fingers into the inside of the remaining glove down and off, inside out, so that the glove you are holding with your fingertips is now inside the glove that you are taking off, Figure 26-7.

4. Drop both soiled gloves together into waste receptacle (which is a double bag), Figure 26-8.

5. Wash your hands.

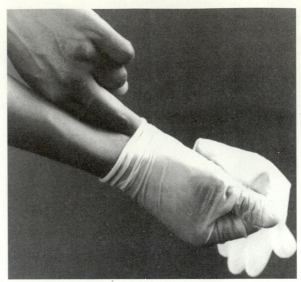

Figure 26-7   Use your ungloved hand, insert fingers into inside of remaining glove, turn inside out so glove you are holding is inside glove you're removing.

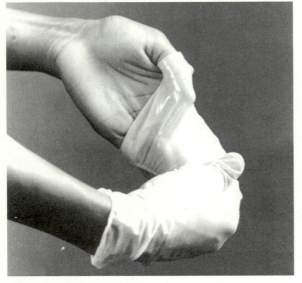

Figure 26-6   Pull glove down and off, inside out.

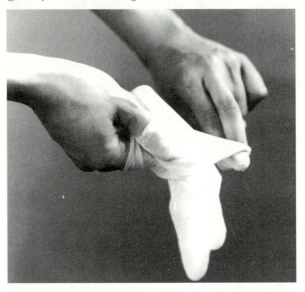

Figure 26-8   Drop gloves into proper waste container.

Client Care Procedure 4:
Putting On and Removing Personal Protective Equipment

Purpose

- To prevent contaminating the aide's clothing

- To prevent the spread of germs through the respiratory tract

Procedure

1. Assemble personal protective equipment, Figure 26-9.
2. Remove wristwatch and place on clean paper towel.
3. Wash your hands.
4. First piece of equipment to apply will be the mask.
5. Adjust the mask over your nose and mouth. Tie the top strings first and then the bottom strings. Your mask must always be dry, so that droplets are not absorbed into the paper of the mask. If the mask becomes wet, you must replace it.
6. Unfold and open the gown, so that you can slide your arms into the sleeves and your hands come right through. Slip the fingers of both hands inside the neckband of the gown and grasp the two strings at the back and tie into a bow, so that they can be undone easily after the procedure is completed, Figure 26-10. Reach behind you, overlap the two edges of the gown so that your uniform is completely covered and then secure the waist ties, Figures 26-11 and 26-12.
7. **Remember:** Your moisture-resistant gown is only worn once and is then discarded in a container for contaminated linen.

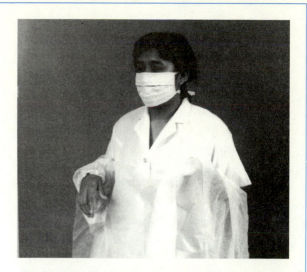

Figure 26-10   Putting on gown

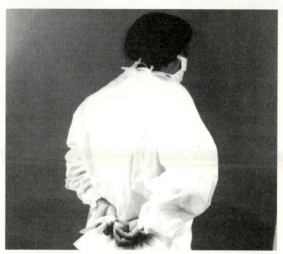

Figure 26-11   Tie waist ties in back

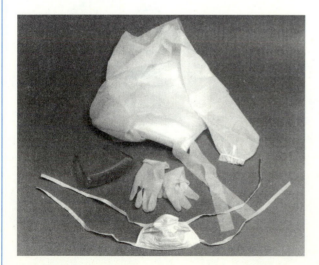

Figure 26-9   Examples of protective barriers

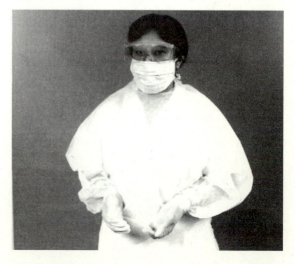

Figure 26-12   Properly masked, gloved, and gowned aide

Continued on the following page.

Removing Contaminated Gown and Mask

1. Undo the waist ties of your gown.
2. Wash hands.
3. Undo your mask, bottom ties first, then top ties. Holding top ties, drop mask in appropriate waste receptacle.
4. Undo neckties and loosen gown at shoulder.
5. Slip finger of right hand inside left cuff without touching outside of gown and pull gown over left hand. With your gown-covered left hand, pull gown down over right hand and then right arm.
6. Fold gown with contaminated side inward and dispose of it into the appropriate receptacle.
7. Wash hands.
8. Remove watch from paper towel and place back on wrist.

Client Care Procedure 5:
Collecting Specimen in Isolation

Purpose

- To obtain and send specimen to laboratory without spreading germs from the client's home

Procedure

1. Assemble equipment:

   clean specimen container, cover, label
   paper towels
   gloves
   plastic transport bag

2. Fill in label with client's name, date, time, and type of specimen.
3. Remove cover from the container and place all the equipment on the clean paper towel.
4. Wash your hands and put on gloves.
5. With gloved hands, pick up the specimen and place it in the container so that you do not contaminate any part of the container, Figure 26-13.
6. Remove gloves and wash hands.
7. Using the paper towel, pick up the container without touching it with your bare hands.

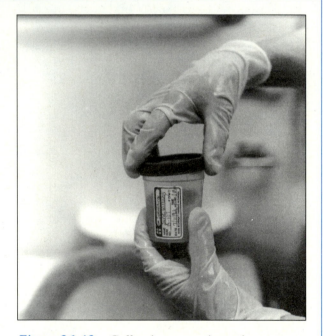

Figure 26-13   Collecting a specimen in isolation

8. Place the container in the plastic bag and seal it.
9. Send specimen to the laboratory per instruction of your nurse supervisor.

Unit 27 Restorative Care

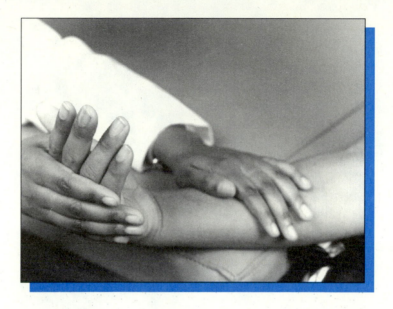

CLIENT CARE PROCEDURES

6. Maintaining Body Alignment
7. Turning the Client Toward You
8. Moving the Client Up in Bed Using the Drawsheet
9. Log Rolling the Client
10. Positioning the Client in Supine Position
11. Positioning the Client in Lateral/Side-lying Position
12. Positioning the Client in Prone Position
13. Positioning the Client in Fowler's Position

14. Assisting the Client from Bed to Chair
15. Assisting the Client from Chair to Bed
16. Transferring the Client from Wheelchair to Toilet/Commode
17. Performing Passive Range of Motion Exercises
18. Assisting the Client to Walk with Crutches, Walker, or Cane
19. Lifting the Client Using a Mechanical Lift

NOTE: All procedures are not allowed in all states. Make sure you are aware of limits as outlined by state guidelines.

LEARNING OBJECTIVES

After studying this unit, you should be able to:

- Demonstrate clear ability to perform all procedures.
- Explain the purpose of each procedure.
- Identify precautions to be taken for each procedure.
- Use proper body mechanics for both client and aide doing each procedure.

- Move the client without injury to either client or aide.
- Identify altered body alignment.
- Increase client independence and aid rehabilitation.

Client Care Procedure **6:**
Maintaining Body Alignment

Purpose

- Position client to prevent injury and promote client's comfort

Procedure

1. Observe alignment of client in sitting or lying position.
2. If sitting up—is head erect and spine in straight alignment, Figure 27-1?
3. If sitting up—is body weight evenly distributed on buttocks and thighs?
4. If sitting up—are feet supported on floor and are ankles comfortably flexed?
5. If sitting up—are forearms supported on armrest, or on lap, or on table in front of chair?

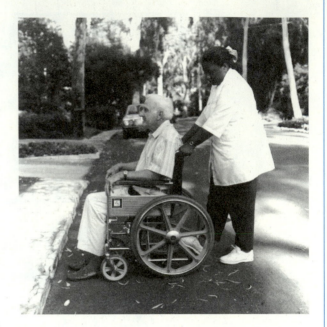

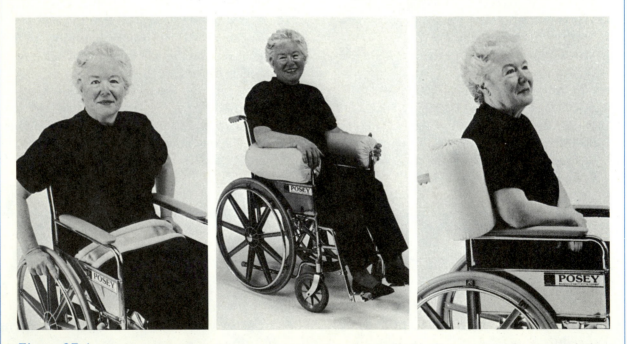

Figure 27-1   Supports help position patients and maintain body alignment without restricting movement. Clients are supported and protected without being restrained. (Photo courtesy of J.T. Posey Co., Inc. From Hegner and Caldwell, *Nursing Assistant, A Nursing Process Approach,* 6E, copyright 1992 by Delmar Publishers Inc.)

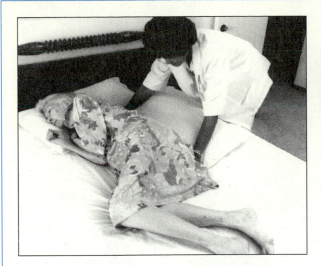

Figure 27-2 Aide checks body alignment of resting client.

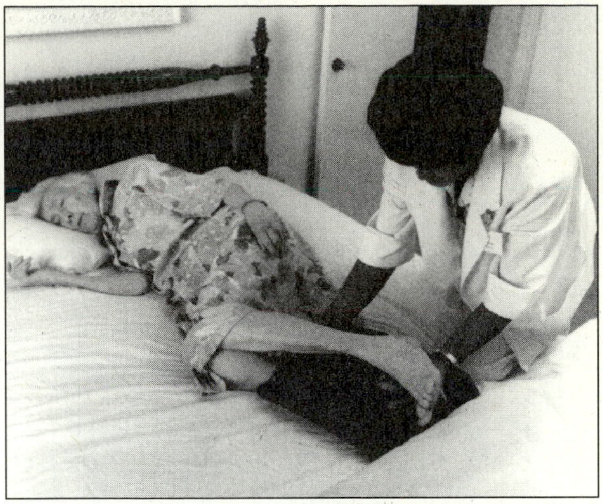

Figure 27-3 Check to see if the hips and legs are in correct alignment.

6. If lying on side—are pillows and positioning supports correctly placed, Figures 27-2 and 27-3?

7. If lying on side—is spinal column in correct alignment?
8. If lying on side—are arms positioned over the chest?

Client Care Procedure 7:
Turning the Client Toward You

Purpose

- To make the client more comfortable
- To change the client's position to improve circulation and reduce skin pressure

Procedure

1. Wash your hands.
2. Tell client what you are going to do.
3. Lift client's far leg and cross it over the leg that is nearest you.
4. Lift the far arm over the chest, bend the elbow, and bring the hand toward the client's shoulder.
5. Place the hand nearest the head of the bed on the far shoulder and place your other hand on the client's hip on the far side.
6. Brace your thighs against the side of the bed and smoothly roll client toward you. Make sure that the client's upper leg comes over and bend it at the knee to ensure that the new position is stable.
7. Go to opposite side of bed and place your hands over the client's shoulder and pull upper body to the center of the bed. Place your hands over client's hips and pull the rest of the client's body to the center of the bed and into good body alignment.
8. Place a pillow against the client's back and secure it by pushing part under the client's back.
9. Support the knee, ankle, and foot of the upper leg with a pillow, which also prevents the knees and ankles from rubbing against each other and causing skin irritation. Cover client.
10. Wash your hands.
11. Document procedure completion, time, and client's reaction.

Client Care Procedure 8:
Moving the Client Up in Bed Using the Drawsheet

Purpose

- To move client up in bed with minimum discomfort
- To relieve pressure on body parts

NOTE: Very often a client will slide down in the bed away from the headboard. This is uncomfortable for the client. The sheets become wrinkled and undue pressure may be placed on the body prominences, allowing the formation of pressure sores.

Procedure

1. Wash your hands.
2. Tell client what you plan to do. Have your partner stand on the opposite side of the bed to assist you.
3. Place pillow at the head of the bed to protect the client's head. Roll both sides of the drawsheet or flat sheet folded in fours toward the client. Place the client's feet 12 inches apart, so that they will not bump together as you move the client.
4. With the hand nearest the client's feet, firmly grasp the rolled drawsheet or folded sheet. With the other hand, both of you cradle the client's head and shoulders and firmly grasp the top of the rolled drawsheet or folded sheet.
5. Turn your body and feet toward the head of the bed. Keep your feet about 12 inches apart and bend your knees slightly to achieve good body mechanics as you lift the client.
6. Coordinate your lift—on the count of three, together lift the drawsheet and the client up toward the head of the bed without dragging the client, Figure 27-4A. Align the client's body and limbs so that the client is straight and comfortable.

7. Place the pillow back under the client's head, Figure 27-4B, and tighten the drawsheet. Replace the covers and make the client comfortable.
8. Wash your hands.
9. Document completion of the procedure, time, and client's reaction.

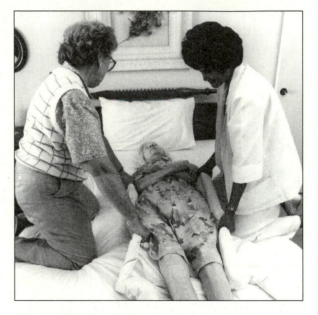

Figure 27-4A   Lifting a client up in bed using a drawsheet

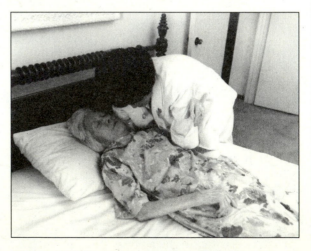

Figure 27-4B   Be sure to position client's head comfortably.

Client Care Procedure 9:
Log Rolling the Client

Purpose

- To ensure the spinal column is kept straight because of special medical conditions

NOTE: You will need help to perform this procedure.

Procedure

1. Wash your hands.
2. Tell client what you plan to do.
3. With both you and your helper on the same side of the bed, remove the top covers.
4. Place your hand and arm under the client's head and shoulder. Your helper places his arms under the client's body and legs. On the count of three, lift the client toward you as a single unit.
5. Do not allow the client to bend and use good body mechanics yourselves by bending your knees and keeping your backs straight.
6. Place a pillow lengthwise between the client's thighs and legs and fold the client's arms over the chest.
7. Go over to the other side of the bed. You are in a position to keep the shoulders and upper body straight and your helper is positioned to keep the client's lower body, hips, and legs straight. Reach over the client and roll the drawsheet firmly against the client. On the count of three, the client is rolled toward you in a single movement, keeping the client's head, spine, and legs in a straight position.

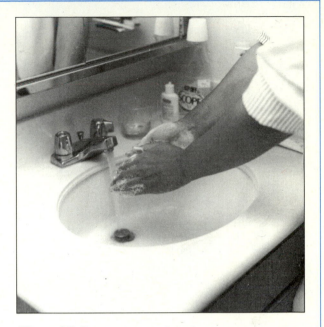

Figure 27-5 Wash your hands.

8. To maintain the client's new position and alignment, place pillows against the spine and leave the pillow between the client's legs. Other small pillows or folded towels can be placed under the client's head and neck and under the arms for support.
9. Fold the drawsheet back over the pillows supporting the spine. Make sure the client's alignment is straight and that the client is comfortable. Arrange covers for the client.
10. Wash your hands, Figure 27-5.
11. Record this repositioning, time, and any observation you made.

Client Care Procedure 10:
Positioning the Client in Supine Position

Purpose

- To make client more comfortable
- Assist the body to function more efficiently

Procedure

1. Wash your hands.
2. Tell client what you plan to do.
3. Place pillow under the client's head, so that the client's head is about 2 inches above the level of the bed. The pillow should extend slightly under the shoulders, Figure 27-6.
4. Have client's arms extended straight out with palms of the hands flat on the bed. The arms can be supported by pillows or covered foam pads placed under the forearms and extending from just above the elbows to the ends of the fingers.
5. Place a small pillow or rolled towel along the side of the client's thighs and tuck part of the support under the thigh, ensuring that the part under the thighs is smooth. This maintains alignment of the hips and thighs and helps prevent the hips from rotating outward or externally.

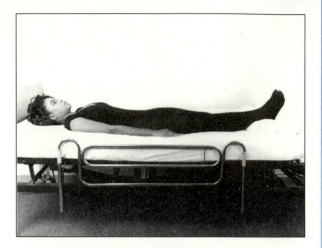

Figure 27-6   A client in supine position before placement of pillows. The head may be elevated slightly with a pillow and the arms may also be supported with pillows. Trocanter roll may be placed along the side of the client's thighs to keep legs in good alignment.

6. Place a pillow under the back of the ankle to relieve pressure on the heels.
7. Wash your hands.
8. Document the time and position change and the client's reaction.

Client Care Procedure 11:
Positioning the Client in Lateral/Side-lying Position

Purpose

- To provide for client comfort
- To relieve pressure on body parts

Procedure

1. Wash your hands.
2. Tell client what you plan to do.
3. Go to opposite side of bed from the direction you are planning to turn the client toward.
4. Cross the client's arms over the chest. Place your arm under the client's neck and shoulders. Place your other arm under the client's midback. Move the upper part of the client's body toward you.
5. Place one arm under the client's waist and the other under the thighs. Move the lower part of the client's body toward you.

6. Turn client to opposite side. Pull shoulder that is touching the bed slightly toward you. Pull buttock that is touching the bed slightly toward you. Place pillow under back and buttocks. Place bottom leg in extension and flex upper leg. Place small folded blanket or pillow between the upper and lower leg.

7. Place pillow under client's head. Rotate the upper arm to bring it up to the pillow with the palm facing up. Place the other arm on a pillow that extends from above the elbow to the fingers. Extend the fingers.

8. Check the client's position to see if the body is in good vertical alignment, Figure 27-7.

9. Wash your hands.

10. Document time, change of position, and client's reaction.

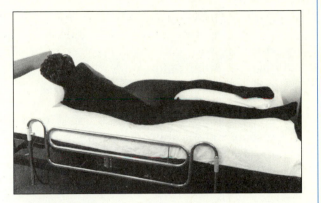

Figure 27-7A   Lateral/side-lying position

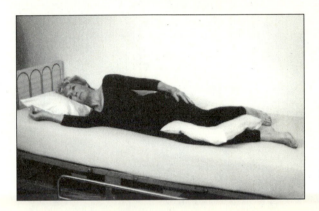

Figure 27-7B   Right lying (lateral recumbent) position. (From Hegner and Caldwell, *Nursing Assistant, A Nursing Process Approach,* 6E, copyright 1992 by Delmar Publishers Inc.)

Client Care Procedure 12:
Positioning the Client in Prone Position

Purpose

- To relieve pressure on body parts
- To provide for client comfort

NOTE: Most elderly clients are not able or do not like to be in this position. Before turning a dependent client prone, make sure client's arms are straight down at sides to avoid injury while turning. Never leave an older client in this position more than 15 to 20 minutes.

Procedure

1. Wash your hands.

2. Tell client what you plan to do.

3. Turn client on abdomen. Check to see if spine is straight and face is turned to either side.

4. Legs are extended. Arms are flexed and brought up to either side of head.

5. A small pillow can be placed under the abdomen, especially for women as this reduces pressure against their breasts.

Continued on the following page.

An alternative method is to roll a small towel and place it under shoulders to reduce pressure.

6. Place another pillow under lower legs to prevent pressure on toes, Figure 27-8.
7. Client can also be moved to foot of bed so feet extend over mattress. This is an alternative method for preventing pressure on toes.
8. Wash your hands.
9. Document time, position change, and client's reaction.

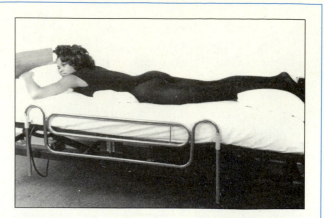

Figure 27-8   Prone position

Client Care Procedure 13:
Positioning the Client in Fowler's Position

Purpose

- To provide client comfort
- To aid in breathing
- To position client so the client can engage in activities such as eating, reading, watching television, visiting

NOTE: If the client is weak or frail, the sitting position may be hard for the client to maintain. Supporting the client with pillows may help the client maintain the sitting position.

Procedure

1. Wash your hands.
2. Tell the client what you plan to do.
3. Check to see if the client's spine and legs are straight and in the middle of the bed.
4. Support client's head and neck with one, two, or three pillows. If client has a hospital bed, raise bed to 45° angle.
5. Knees may be flexed and supported with small pillows.
6. Pillows may be placed under each arm from elbows to fingertips to support shoulders.

7. Place pillow or padded footboard against feet, Figure 27-9.
8. Wash your hands.
9. Document time, position change, and client's reaction.

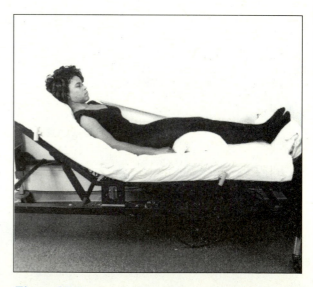

Figure 27-9   Fowler's position

Client Care Procedure 14:
Assisting the Client from Bed to Chair

Purpose

- To move client from one location to another safely and without discomfort

NOTE: There should be a specific transfer procedure for each client who is not an independent, self-transfer

Procedure

1. Wash your hands.
2. Tell the client what you plan to do.
3. Assemble needed equipment.

   wheelchair   client's shoes and socks
   transfer belt

4. Place chair so client moves toward client's strongest side. Set chair at 45° angle to bed. Lock wheels.
5. Assist client to sit at edge of bed, Figure 27-10A.
6. Wait a few seconds to allow the client to adjust to sitting position. Assist client to put on shoes and socks.
7. Apply transfer belt. Make sure the belt is not too tight or too loose.
8. Spread your feet apart and flex your hips and knees, aligning your knees with client's.
9. Grasp transfer belt from underneath. Rock the client up to standing on the count of three, Figure 27-10B, while straightening your hips and legs, keeping knees slightly flexed.
10. If client has a weak leg, press your knee against it or block client's foot with yours to prevent weaker leg from sliding out from under the client.
11. Instruct client to use armrest on chair for support and be sure to flex your hips and knees while lowering client into chair. Remove transfer belt.
12. Check alignment of client in chair and make adjustments accordingly, Figure 27-10C.
13. Wash your hands.
14. Document time, position change, and client's reactions.

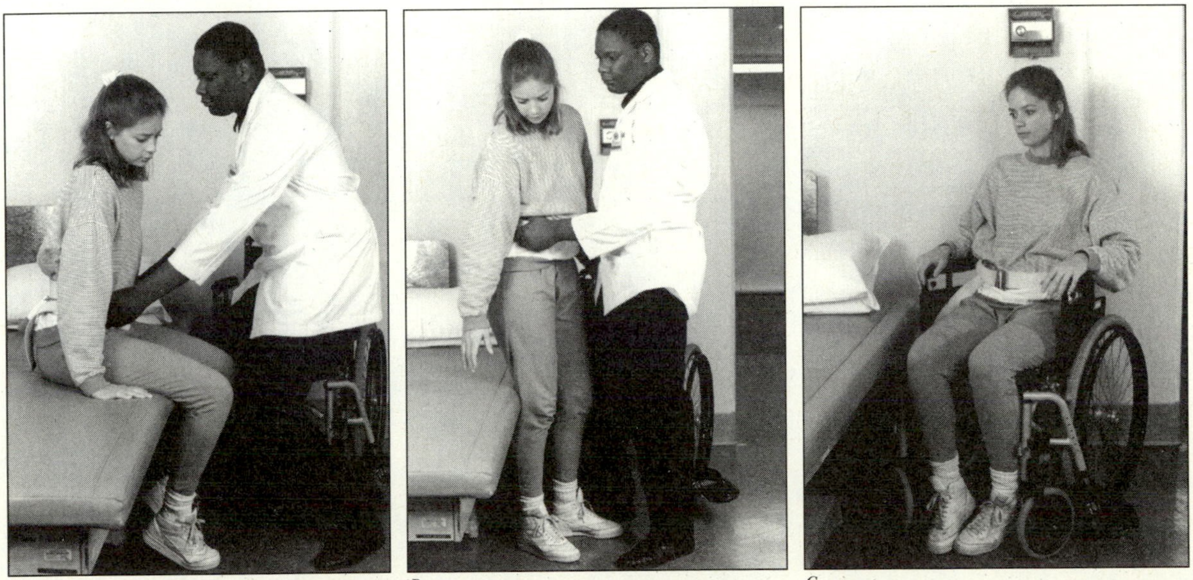

A   *B*   *C*

Figure 27-10   *A.* Lift belt is applied to client. An aide holds onto belt to assist the client to stand. *B.* Client stands and pivots on her good leg. *C.* Client is positioned comfortably in chair.

Client Care Procedure 15:
Assisting the Client from Chair to Bed

Purpose

- To change client's position
- To transfer client safely from one location to another

Procedure

1. Wash your hands.
2. Tell client what you plan to do.
3. Position client with strong side toward bed with wheelchair at 45° angle.
4. Apply transfer belt and place both hands on front of the belt. Instruct client, if able, to put feet flat on the floor and hands on the chair. On the count of three, have client push up to standing position. While standing, have the client pivot (turn) on strong leg toward the bed. Have the client lower himself/herself to the bed to a sitting position.
5. Remove shoes, socks, and transfer belt. Assist the client to lying position. Position client in comfortable position and in good alignment.
6. Wash hands.
7. Document time, change of position, and client's reaction.

Client Care Procedure 16:
Transferring the Client from Wheelchair to Toilet/Commode

Purpose

- To enable client to sit on toilet for normal excretion of body wastes

NOTE: It is essential to have grab bars, preferably secured to the wall, but they can be attached to the toilet seat.

Procedure

1. Wash hands.
2. Tell client what you plan to do.
3. Have client in wheelchair with strong side nearer to the toilet or commode.
4. Lock the wheelchair. Apply transfer belt. Lift foot pieces out of way.
5. Loosen clothing on the client, but not too loose that the slacks fall while transferring.
6. Have client lean forward in chair and place feet apart. Have client place hands on armpiece and on the count of three push up. Place your hand on the transfer belt.
7. Stand client up and have client place strong arm on grab bars, Figure 27-11. You continue to hold onto the transfer belt and slowly lower client onto the

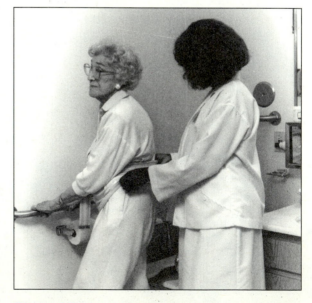

Figure 27-11   Assisting the client to the toilet with client holding onto grab bars

toilet or commode. Have client hang onto grab bar while you drop the client's pants.

8. Remove belt and move wheelchair out of way.

9. Provide privacy for client. Check often to see if client is all right. Give client toilet paper.

10. Assist the client as needed, return to wheelchair and prior activity.

11. Wash client's hands and your hands.

12. Document bowel movement or urination.

Client Care Procedure 17:
Performing Passive Range of Motion Exercises

Purpose

- To increase muscle tone and strength in the client's body
- To restore function to injured parts of body
- To prevent joint stiffness and contractures

NOTE: Do not perform the exercises until you have received instructions specific for your client's joints. When possible, support the extremity above and below the joints being exercised. If the client shows pain or discomfort, stop the exercise and document it. The head can be exercised if specifically ordered by the physical therapist. Exercises can be done in bed or in the chair. It is important to keep the client covered or clothed to prevent unnecessary exposure during the procedure.

Procedure

1. Wash your hands.

2. Read any special instructions for these exercises for your client.

3. Tell client what you plan to do. Ask client to assist as much as possible.

4. Exercise the shoulder.
   Supporting the upper and lower arms, exercise the shoulder joint. Abduct (away from the body) the entire arm out at right angles to the body, Figure 27-12A, and then adduct (bring back to the midline of the body) the arm back to

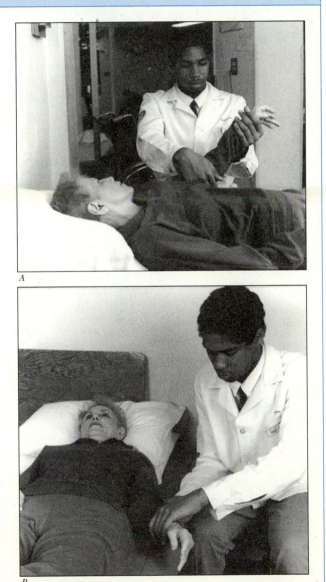

Figure 27-12   Exercising the shoulder joint

Continued on the following page.

the center of the client's body, Figure 27-12B.

5. Exercise the elbow.

   Bend elbow, keeping the arm close to the body. Bring the fingers to touch the shoulder. Lower the fingers to touch the bed, Figure 27-13.

6. Exercise the forearm.

   Bring the arm out to the side. Rest it on the bed. Take the client's hand and rotate the arm, palm up and palm down, Figure 27-14.

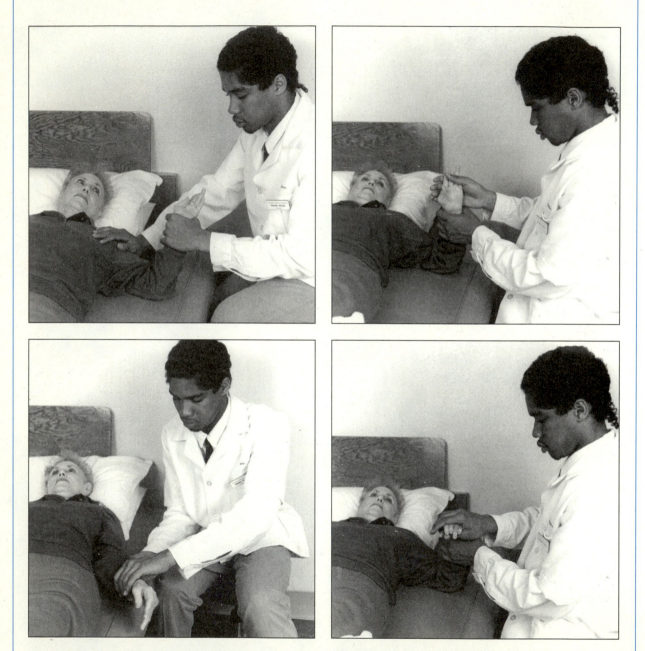

Figure 27-13   Exercising the elbow

Figure 27-14   Exercising the forearm

7. Exercise the wrist and fingers.
   Take the client's hand and move the hand forward and back, Figure 27-15A, B. Move the hand side to side. Curl the client's fingers and straighten them, Figures 27-15C, D. Spread the fingers apart and rotate the thumb. Touch all fingers to thumb, Figure 27-15E.

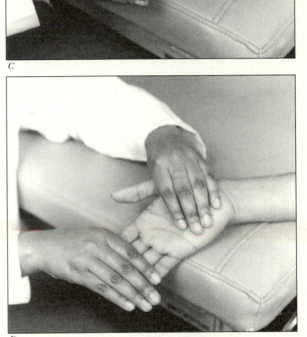

C

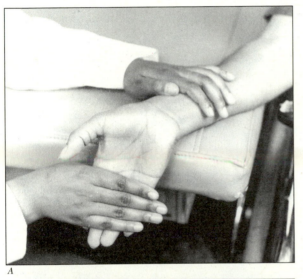

A

D

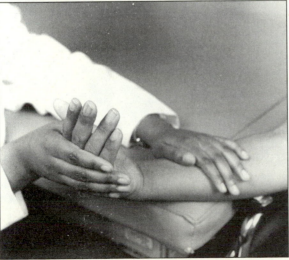

B

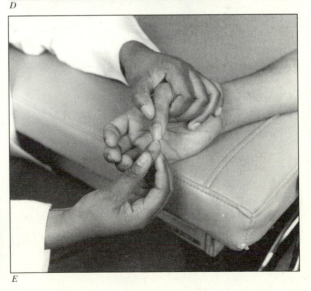

E

Figure 27-15   Exercising the wrist and fingers

Continued on the following page.

8. Exercise the knee and hip while the client is lying on the back.
Bend the knee and raise it to the chest, Figure 27-16. Bring the leg out to the side and back. Cross one leg over the other leg. Allow the leg to rest on the bed with the knee straight and the heel resting on the bed. Rotate the leg inward and outward.

9. Exercise the ankle.
Bend client's knee slightly and support lower leg with one hand. With other hand, bend client's foot downward (plantar flexion) and then bend client's foot toward client's body (dorsiflexion), Figure 27-17. With client's legs extended on bed, place both hands on client's foot and move foot inward and then outward.

10. Exercise the toes.
Bend (flexion) and straighten (extension) each toe. Do abduction and adduction with each toe as you did with the fingers.

11. Go to other side and repeat movements for each joint.
12. Wash hands.
13. Document the completion of the exercises and client's reactions.

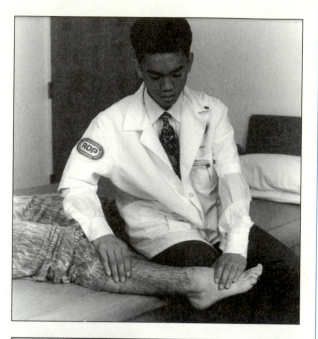

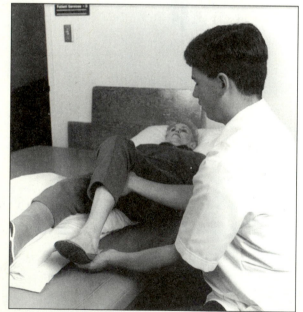

Figure 27-16   Exercising the knee and hip

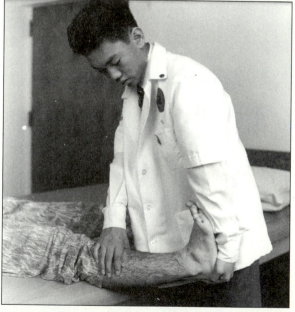

Figure 27-17   Exercising the ankle and foot

Client Care Procedure 18:
Assisting the Client to Walk with Crutches, Walker, or Cane

Purpose

- To provide support and maintain balance as client walks

NOTE: There are three basic walking patterns. With a nonweight-bearing pattern, all the weight is placed on the arms and uninvolved leg. Partial weight-bearing means that minimal weight is placed on the toes. However, most weight is still on the arms and the uninvolved leg.

To walk in a nonweight-bearing pattern, the client uses crutches, Figure 27-18. The physical therapist measures the client to select the correct length of crutches. The therapist also teaches the client how to walk with the crutches.

To walk in a partial weight-bearing pattern, the client can use crutches but often uses a walker. The walker is a curved metal frame with four legs. It is a walking aid that gives maximum stability as the client moves. The client steps forward while holding onto the walker with both hands. Some walkers have wheels so that the client does not have to lift up the walker between steps, Figure 27-19.

A cane is used when the client is strong enough to bear full weight on both legs. A standard cane should not be used as a weight-bearing aid. A special cane with four short legs, called a quad cane, is designed to bear a small amount of weight only, Figure 27-20. A cane is primarily used for balance. Check rubber tips on the canes, walkers, and crutches as they wear out quickly if used on sidewalks.

Always have client wear good supportive shoes with nonskid soles. Instruct clients to pick up feet and not to look at feet, but to look straight ahead.

Procedure

1. Wash your hands. Apply transfer belt unless instructed not to.
2. Always walk on the client's weak side.
3. Walk slightly behind the client holding onto the transfer belt from behind.

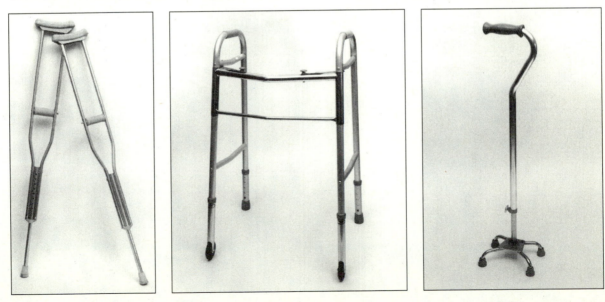

Figure 27-18   Crutches   *Figure 27-19*   Walker with small wheels   *Figure 27-20*   Four-point (quad) cane

Continued on the following page.

4. For the client using crutches, hold onto the transfer belt if the client feels uncomfortable using the crutches, Figure 27-21.

5. For the client using a walker, instruct the client to place the walker firmly before walking. If the client is strong enough, the walker and the weaker leg can be moved forward at the same time.

6. For the client using a cane, Figure 27-22, instruct the client to hold the cane in the hand opposite the weaker leg. If the right ankle has been injured, the client should hold the cane in the left hand.

7. Balance is a judgmental situation. If the client has poor balance, the aide should

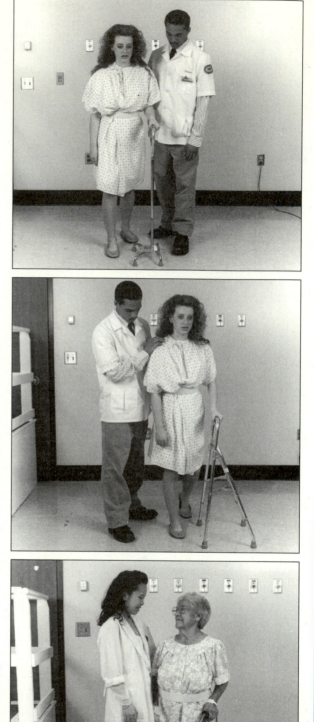

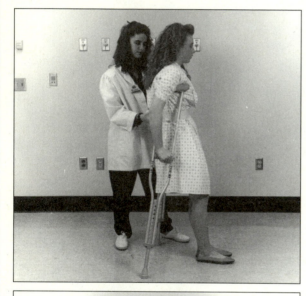

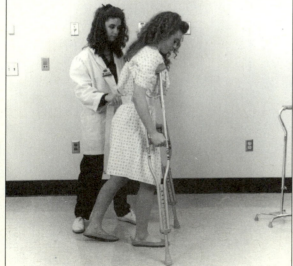

Figure 27-21   Crutch walking

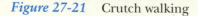

Figure 27-22   Using various types of canes

support the weak side. If the client has good balance and can walk without assistive devices, the aide should use a transfer belt for safety reasons.

8. Wash your hands at completion of the procedure.
9. Document how far the client walked and client's reaction.

Client Care Procedure 19:
Lifting the Client Using a Mechanical Lift

Purpose

- To transfer client from one place to another, usually from bed to chair
- To safely transfer a client who is heavy or has no weight-bearing ability

NOTE: Check slings, chains, and straps for frayed areas or defective hooks. Two types of slings are supplied with the Hoyer lift: hammock style and two-piece canvas strips. The hammock type can be made out of mesh or canvas. This type of sling is better for clients who are weak and need support, Figure 27-23. The canvas strips can be used for clients with normal muscle tone.

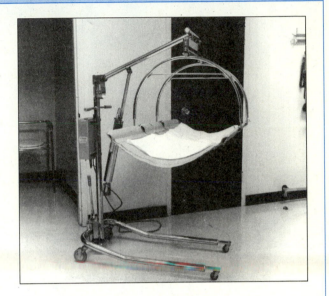

Figure 27-23   Mechanical lift

Procedure

1. Wash your hands and assemble equipment.
2. Tell client what you plan to do.
3. Position chair near bed and allow adequate room to maneuver the lift.
4. Roll client away from you.
5. Place hammock sling or canvas strips under client to form seat; with two canvas pieces, lower edge fits under client's knees (wide piece); upper edge goes under client's shoulders (narrow piece).
6. Go to opposite side of bed and pull hammock or strips through.
7. Roll client supine into canvas seat.
8. Place lift's horseshoe bar under side of bed (on side with chair). Have base of lift in maximum open position and lock.
9. Lower horizontal bar to sling level by releasing hydraulic valve. Lock valve.
10. Attach hooks on strap (chain) to holes in sling. Short chains/straps hook to top

holes of sling; longer chains to bottom of sling. Point hooks to the outside when attaching.
11. Fold client's arm over the chest.
12. Pump handle until client is raised free of bed, but no higher than necessary.
13. Using steering handle to pull lift from bed and maneuver to chair.
14. Roll base around chair. Slowly release check valve and lower client into chair.
15. Check to see if client is positioned correctly. Unhook chains or straps and remove lift.
16. If straps are used, they can be removed. If the hammock sling is used, sling will remain underneath client so it is in position for transfer back to bed.
17. Wash your hands.
18. Document transfer, time completed, and client's reactions.

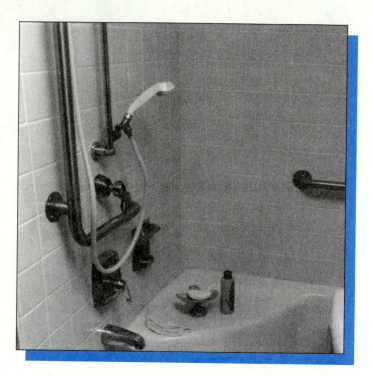

CLIENT CARE PROCEDURES

20. Assisting with Tub Bath or Shower
21. Giving a Bed Bath
22. Giving a Partial Bath
23. Giving a Back Rub

24. Giving Female Perineal Care
25. Giving Male Perineal Care
26. Special Skin Care and Pressure Sores

NOTE: All procedures are not allowed in all states. Make sure you are aware of limits as outlined by state guidelines.

LEARNING OBJECTIVES

After studying this unit, you should be able to:

- Demonstrate clear ability to perform all procedures.
- Explain the purpose of each procedure.
- State when the procedures should and should not be done.

- Be aware of precautions to take with each procedure.
- Demonstrate the use of universal precautions when doing each procedure.

Client Care Procedure 20:
Assisting with Tub Bath or Shower

Purpose

- To clean and refresh the client
- To check client's skin for signs of irritation
- To stimulate circulation in the skin

Procedure

1. If possible, plan the tub bath or shower for a time convenient for the client. A tub bath or shower should not take more than 15 minutes unless there is a special reason for a longer bath.
2. Assemble needed supplies and place in bathroom, Figure 28-1.

   clean clothing
   bath seat or stool
   2 washcloths and towels
   shampoo (if needed)
   plastic pitcher (if shampooing client's hair)
   hose attachment
   comb and brush
   skidproof bath mat
   soap

3. Wash hands.
4. Tell client what you plan to do.
5. Fill tub one-third full with warm water. **Caution:** Test the temperature with a thermometer or on inside of wrist to be sure it will not burn the client. Place a skidproof bath mat in the bottom of the tub. If client is taking a shower, regulate the flow and be sure the temperature is correct. The water should be about 115°F (46°C).
6. Assist the client to sit on a chair or on the closed toilet seat. Help the client undress. Place soiled clothing in the hamper. Close the bathroom door so the client will not be chilled.

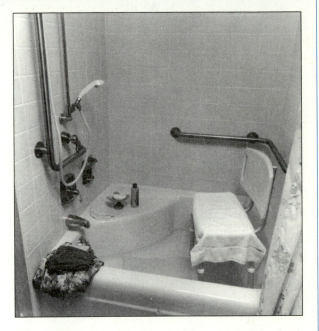

Figure 28-1   Gather equipment needed for bath.

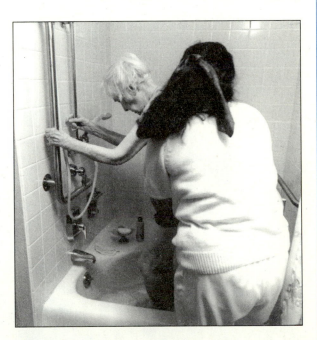

Figure 28-2   Instruct client to hold onto grab bars.

Continued on the following page.

7. For a tub bath, help client to sit on the edge of the tub. If there is a safety bar, have client hold onto it. When client has gained balance, help the client to turn and lift both legs into the tub. Give assistance by supporting the client under the arms and helping the client to slowly sit down in the tub facing the faucets. If the client cannot sit in the tub, place a bath stool in the water. Help the client to sit on the stool, Figures 28-2 and 28-3.

8. If the client needs a shampoo, wet the hair and rub in shampoo, lather, and massage head. If possible, have the client tilt head back. Pour water over the head using the pitcher or attach the hose to the faucet and use it to rinse the head. Repeat shampoo, massage, and rinse. Client may hold a washcloth over the eyes during the shampoo to prevent soap entering the eyes.

9. Give the client a washcloth and soap. Allow the client to do as much as possible. Assist as necessary, Figure 28-4. If shower is running, make sure the flow is not too heavy; check water temperature often.

10. Remain beside the tub at all times during the bath or shower. **Caution:** Be ready to help the client at any moment. If the client should feel faint, empty water from the tub, cover the client with a towel to avoid unnecessary chilling, and lower the client's head between the client's knees.

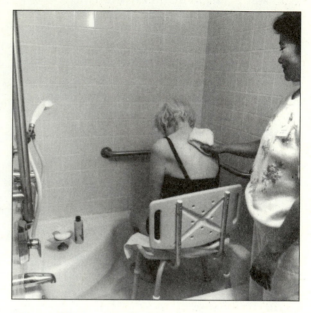

Figure 28-4   Assist the client in washing her back.

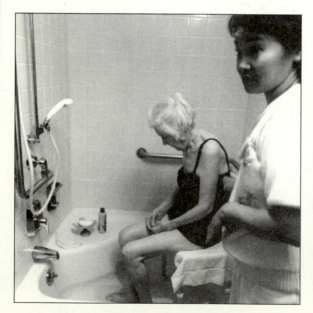

Figure 28-3   Have client sit on tub chair.

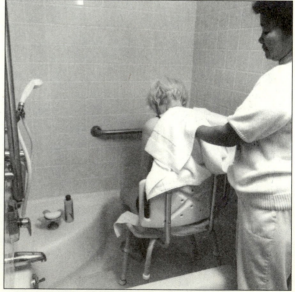

Figure 28-5   Dry client's back.

11. For a tub bath, help the client raise out of the water. Assist the client out of the water. Assist the client to sit on the edge of the tub. Bring client's legs over to outside and assist the client to stand. Allow the client to sit on the closed toilet seat or the chair.

12. Make certain that the client's body is thoroughly dry. Help dry difficult areas such as the back and shoulders, Figure 28-5. Be sure underarms and area under breasts are completely dry. Pay special attention to the feet. Dry soles of feet and between toes. Apply lotion to the client's skin as required, Figure 28-6.

13. For a shower, make sure the client is completely washed and rinsed and then turn off the shower. Towel dry and assist client out of the shower area.

14. Assist client to dress in clean clothes.

15. Help client back to bed, to a wheelchair, or to a lounge chair.

16. Return to the bathroom and drain and clean tub, Figure 28-7. Place dirty clothes and towels in the hamper. Put supplies away.

17. Wash hands.

18. Document procedure, any observations, and client's reaction.

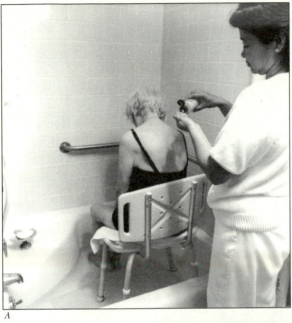

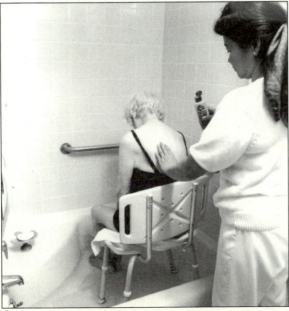

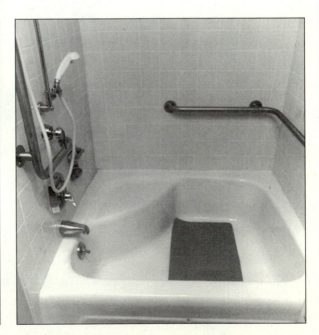

Figure 28-6   A. Place lotion in your hands to warm. B. Apply lotion to client's back.

Figure 28-7   Be sure to clean tub after the bath.

Client Care Procedure 21:
Giving a Bed Bath

Purpose

- To clean and refresh the client
- To stimulate circulation
- To observe the body for signs of irritation

NOTE: The bed bath is usually given in the morning. This procedure is one of a series of procedures performed in the same time period. This will require the home health aide to organize and plan ahead. All materials and supplies needed can be gathered and placed conveniently so that each separate procedure can be completed easily.

- If client needs to use the bedpan, offer it before the bath.
- Gather supplies needed for making the bed and put them near at hand.

- Organize materials needed for oral hygiene, denture care, and nail care to move easily into the procedures if needed.

Procedure

1. Gather supplies for the complete series of procedures including:

   soap and gloves
   washcloths and towels
   fresh clothes
   body lotion
   orange stick
   change of bed linens
   bath basin, two-thirds filled with water
   adult brief if needed

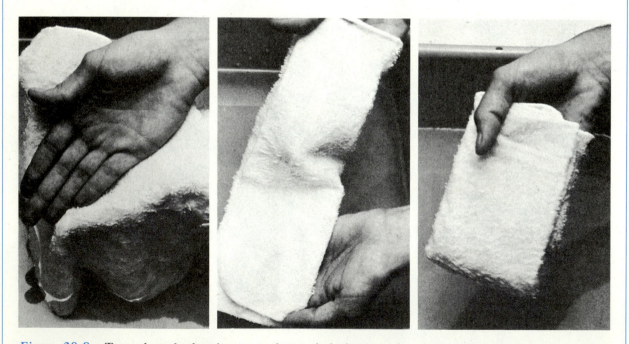

Figure 28-8   To make a bath mitt, wrap the washcloth around one hand, bringing free end over palm, and bringing the free-hanging end up over palm and tucking in the end. (From Hegner and Caldwell, *Nursing Assistant, A Nursing Process Approach,* 6E, copyright 1992 by Delmar Publishers Inc.)

2. Close windows to prevent a draft from blowing on the client. Place a "Do Not Disturb" sign on the door to avoid interruptions.
3. Wash your hands.
4. Tell client what you plan to do.
5. Remove blankets, leaving the top sheet covering the client. Place one pillow under client's head.
6. Pull out bottom part of top sheet so it covers client loosely. Remove client's clothing.

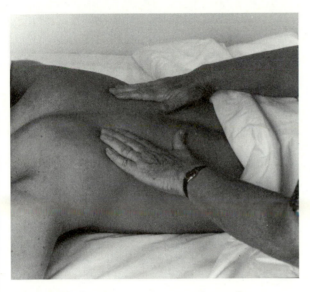

Figure 28-9 Use long, smooth strokes as you apply the lotion.

7. Place a basin of water on the chair or dresser at the bedside.
8. Assist client in moving to side of bed nearest you.
9. Moisten washcloth, squeeze out excess water. Form a mitt by folding a washcloth around one hand, Figure 28-8.
10. Wash the client's eyes first. Wipe from the inner corner to the outer corner of the eye. Keep soap out of eyes. Wash the face, ears, and neck. Pat dry with the face towel.
11. Lift client's farthest arm and lay a bath towel under the area to keep bed dry. Wash with soap, rinse, and pat dry, making sure the arm, underarm, and hand are cleaned and thoroughly dry. Repeat for other arm. Apply underarm deodorant or bath powder if client desires.
12. Give nail care using an orange stick to clean nails. Trim nails *if allowed*.
13. Place towel over client's chest, then pull sheet down to waist. Working under the towel, wash with soap, rinse, and dry chest. Rinse, dry, and powder area under a woman's breasts carefully to prevent skin irritation and redness. Replace sheet over chest.
14. Have client bend one knee. Fold sheet up from the foot of the bed. Expose the thigh, leg, and foot. Place a towel under

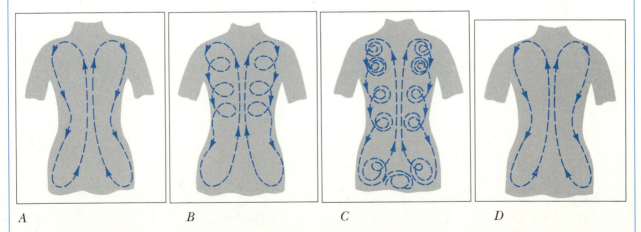

A   *B*   *C*   *D*

Figure 28-10   Strokes to be used during the back rub. *A.* Soothing strokes. *B.* Circular movement. *C.* Passive movement. *D.* Soothing strokes. (From Hegner and Caldwell, *Nursing Assistant, A Nursing Process Approach*, 6E, copyright 1992 by Delmar Publishers Inc.)

Continued on the following page.

the area, and put the basin on the towel, placing client's foot in basin. Wash and rinse foot. Remove the foot from the basin and dry it well.

15. Remove the basin from the bed. Follow the same procedure for the other leg and foot.

16. Lightly apply lotion on legs and feet if skin is dry (never massage legs).

17. Change the water in the basin before proceeding with the bath. If at any time during the bath, the water becomes dirty or cool, change it.

18. Assist the client to move toward your side of the bed. Place bath towel lengthwise by the client's back and buttocks. Starting at the hairline use long, firm strokes while washing the back.

19. Give the client a back rub starting at the base of the spine, Figures 28-9 and 28-10.

20. Prepare washcloth with soap and have client wash the genital area, if able. Rinse the cloth and have client wipe and dry the genitals, if capable.

21. Spread the towel under client's head and comb or brush hair.

22. Assist the client into clean clothes.

23. Remove the basin, dirty linens, and the other equipment away from the bed.

24. Change the bed linens using the procedure for making an occupied bed.

25. Leave the client in a comfortable position. After all the activities, the client may require a rest period.

26. Wash your hands.

27. Document procedure and time, observations, and client's reaction.

Client Care Procedure 22:
Giving a Partial Bath

Purpose

- To clean and refresh body

NOTE: To give a partial bath, the same procedure is followed as a bed bath, but the legs and feet are not washed. This type of bath is given on the days a complete bed bath is not given. If the client is able, this type of bath can be given by the bathroom sink.

Client Care Procedure 23:
Giving a Back Rub

Purpose

- To increase the blood circulation to the back area
- To give comfort to the client and provide relaxation
- To observe the skin for signs of skin breakdown

Procedure

1. Wash hands
2. Assemble supplies.

small towel
lotion

3. Provide privacy for the client.
4. Position client on back or side.
5. Place small amount of lotion on your hands. Rub together to warm the lotion.
6. Begin by starting at the base of the spine; rub toward the neck in the center of the back. Use both hands in one long stroke.
7. When reaching the neck, continue back down the sides of the back. When reaching the base of the spine, rub up the center again. Repeat several times.
8. If necessary, add more lotion and use a spiral motion for several minutes.
9. Remove excess lotion with small towel. Reposition client.
10. Wash hands and return supplies to proper place.
11. Record and report any sign of skin irritation.

Client Care Procedure 24:
Giving Female Perineal Care

Purpose

- To prevent infections
- To clean the genital and anal area well and prevent skin breakdown and odors

Procedure

1. Assemble supplies.

   soap
   basin
   gloves
   water
   washcloths and towel

2. Wash your hands and apply gloves.
3. Tell client what you plan to do.
4. Position client on back and place sheet or thin cotton blanket over client.
5. Position towel under client's buttocks.
6. Wet washcloth with soap and water. Help the client flex her knees and spread her legs if able.
7. Separate the vulva. Clean downward from front to back with one stroke first the inner labia and then rinse. Repeat with outer labia. Repeat on other side. Dry with the towel.
8. Help the client lower her legs and turn onto her side away from you.
9. Apply soap to washcloth.
10. Clean the rectal area by cleaning from the vagina to the anus with one stroke. Rinse washcloth and repeat until area is clean.
11. Pat the area dry with towel.
12. Cover client with sheet or blanket and make her comfortable.
13. Remove basin and supplies from bedside.
14. Remove your gloves and wash your hands.
15. Document procedure completed, observations, time, and client's reactions.

Client Care Procedure 25:
Giving Male Perineal Care

Purpose

- To prevent spread of infection
- To promote comfort and decrease odor

Procedure

1. Repeat steps 1 through 6 as for female perineal care.
2. Grasp penis gently with gloved hand. Clean the tip of the penis using gentle circular motion. You will need to pull back the foreskin if the man is uncircumcised. Start at the urinary meatus and work outward. Rinse the area well and dry. Return the foreskin to its original position.
3. Clean the remaining portion of the penis with firm downward strokes. Rinse well.
4. Wash the scrotum and pat dry.
5. Turn client to side and clean rectal area in the same way as for the female.
6. Follow steps 11 through 15 as for female perineal care.

Client Care Procedure 26:
Special Skin Care and Pressure Sores

Purpose

- To prevent skin breakdown resulting from pressure and skin irritations
- To use preventive devices
- To prevent friction resulting when skin is in contact with skin or linen

NOTE: Certain clients are at risk for the development of pressure areas leading to sores. Clients at risk are bedridden, obese, very thin, diabetic, paralyzed, and malnourished. A home health aide's role is mainly in the prevention of pressure sore development. Once a pressure sore has developed, the nurse will need to come to the client's home to treat the open area.

Assistive Devices to Prevent
Pressure Sores

1. Air mattress—This is a mattress filled with air. This works by continuously changing the pressure areas on the client's back. One can improvise an air mattress designed for camping instead of buying a medical air mattress.
2. Egg crate mattress—This is a mattress made of foam rubber that is molded like an egg crate. They are inexpensive, but effective in reducing pressure on the skin. You can also purchase one the size of a seat for the client to sit on during the day when up in a chair.
3. Water mattress—This is similar to a regular water mattress used in homes. This mattress is effective in reducing pressure on the skin, but causes problems when transferring clients in and out of bed.
4. Gel foam cushion—This is a special cushion filled with a special solution or gel. This style of cushion is effective in the prevention of pressure sores for a client who sits in a wheelchair for long periods of time.
5. Sheepskin or lamb's wool pads or elbow or heel pads—Lamb's wool pads prevent pressure sores by acting as a barrier between the client's skin and the sheets.

6. Bed cradle—This is a device to keep linens off the client's legs and feet. In the home a client may substitute a box or other device to keep linens off the legs and feet.

Special Care to Prevent Pressure Sores

1. Change client's position at least every 2 hours to reduce pressure on any one area.
2. As quickly as possible, remove feces, urine, or moisture of any kind that might be irritating the skin.
3. Encourage clients who sit in chairs or wheelchairs to raise themselves or change position every 15 minutes to relieve pressure.
4. Encourage client to eat a high protein diet if allowed and drink adequate fluids.
5. Keep bed linens clean, dry, and wrinkle free.
6. When bathing clients use soap sparingly because soap drys skin. Keep skin well lubricated.
7. Watch for skin irritation when applying braces and splints.
8. At the first sign of a reddened area, gently massage area around the reddened area. Report your observations to the nurse supervisor.

Unit *29* Daily Care

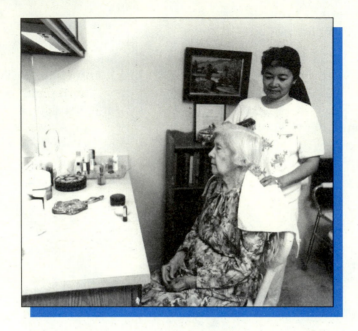

CLIENT CARE PROCEDURES

27. Assisting with Routine Oral Hygiene
28. Caring for Dentures
29. Shaving the Male Client
30. Dressing and Undressing the Client
31. Applying Elasticized Stockings
32. Making an Unoccupied Bed
33. Making an Occupied Bed

34. Giving Nail Care
35. Shampooing the Client's Hair in Bed
36. Assisting the Client with Self-administered Medications
37. Inserting a Hearing Aid
38. Caring for an Artificial Eye

NOTE: All procedures are not allowed in all states. Make sure you are aware of limits as outlined by state guidelines.

LEARNING OBJECTIVES

After studying this unit, you should be able to:

- Demonstrate clear ability to perform all procedures.
- Explain the purpose of each procedure.
- State when the procedures should and should not be done.

- Be aware of precautions to take with each procedure.
- Demonstrate the use of universal precautions when handling body substances.

332

Client Care Procedure 27:
Assisting with Routine Oral Hygiene

Purpose

- To keep client's teeth and gums healthy
- To refresh client's mouth and improve appetite

NOTE: Clients who are helpless are unable to give themselves oral care. In these cases the aide must give special mouth care:

- Wash hands and apply gloves.
- Place small towel under client's head and turn head to one side.
- Dip padded tongue blade into mouthwash solution or other special solution.
- Clean teeth, tongue, and inside surfaces of the mouth. Hold an emesis basin under the client's chin to collect secretions.
- Apply pleasant tasting lubricant to lips. Repeat procedure as ordered.
- Clean and replace equipment. Remove gloves. Wash hands.
- Document procedure and time, observations, and client's reaction.

Procedure

1. Assemble needed equipment and supplies, Figure 29-1A.

   toothbrush
   toothpaste
   gloves
   glass of water
   towel
   small bowl or basin or emesis basin
   mouthwash if available
   tissues or damp washcloth

2. Wash your hands and apply gloves.
3. Tell client what you plan to do and position the client in a sitting position (if allowed).
4. Place a towel over the client's chest and

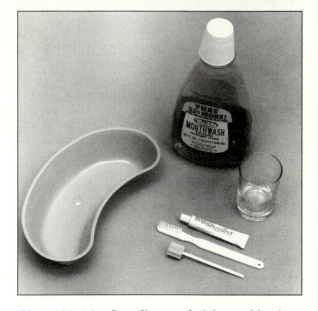

Figure 29-1A Supplies needed for oral hygiene

under the chin.
5. Moisten toothbrush and apply toothpaste.
6. Let client brush teeth, if able. If not, carefully brush the client's teeth, Figures 29-1B through 29-1E.

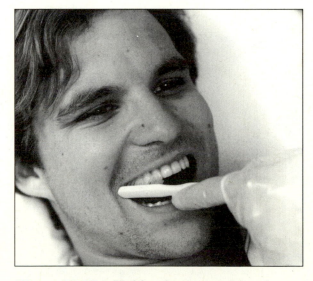

Figure 29-1B Hold soft, wet toothbrush at a 45° angle and brush back teeth.

Continued on the following page.

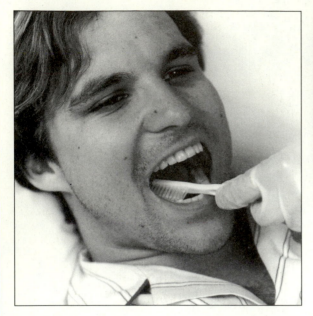

Figure 29-1C   Brush top and bottom teeth thoroughly.

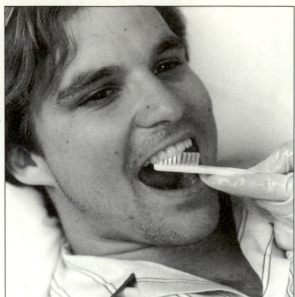

Figure 29-1D   Be sure to brush behind the front teeth.

7. Give the client a glass of water; be sure client rinses mouth well. Hold the basin underneath the client's chin and have client return the fluid. If mouthwash is available, have client rinse mouth with the mouthwash.
8. Give the client a moistened washcloth to wipe mouth.
9. Reposition client.
10. Clean and replace equipment.
11. Remove gloves and wash hands.
12. Document procedure completed and time, any observations and client's reaction.

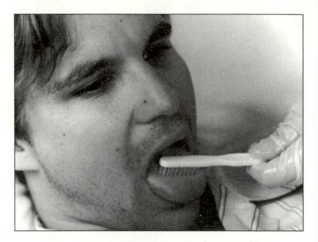

Figure 29-1E   Brush tongue.

Client Care Procedure 28:
Caring for Dentures

Purpose

- To clean dentures and refresh client's mouth
- To provide opportunity to observe client's gums for irritation or soreness
- To stimulate client's appetite

Procedure

1. Assemble the needed supplies, Figure 29-2A.

   denture cup or two small containers lined with gauze
   toothbrush and toothpaste
   mouthwash with small cup
   small towel and dampened washcloth
   gloves

2. Wash your hands and apply gloves.
3. Tell client what you plan to do.
4. Ask client to remove dentures, Figure 29-2B, helping if needed. Place dentures in padded container or denture cup, Figure 29-2C. Be very careful in handling client's dentures. They may become slippery to hold.
5. Place approximately 2 to 3 inches of water and a small paper towel in bottom of sink, Figure 29-2D. This will protect the dentures in case they are dropped. Turn on cold water and brush all surfaces of the upper and lower plate, Figure 29-2E. Rinse denture cup and place fresh gauze squares into bottom. Place dentures in cup, Figure 29-2F, and take to client's bedside.
6. Assist client to rinse mouth with mouthwash.

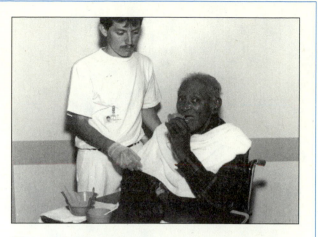

Figure 29-2B   Ask client to remove dentures.

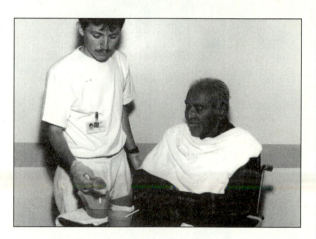

Figure 29-2C   Place dentures into container.

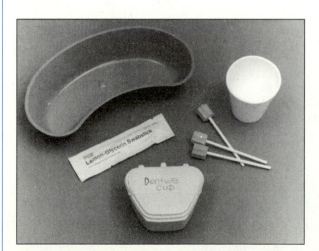

Figure 29-2A   Assemble needed supplies.

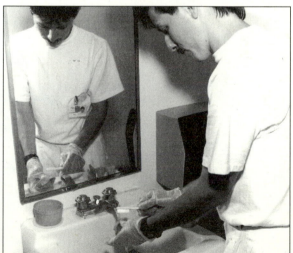

Figure 29-2D   When cleaning dentures under cool running water, protect the dentures by placing a paper towel in the bottom of the sink.

Continued on the following page.

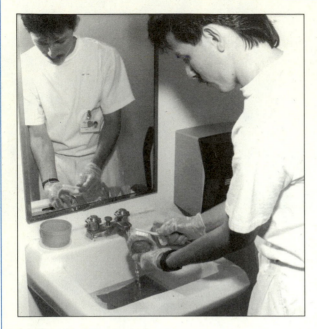

Figure 29-2E   Be sure to brush all surfaces of dentures.

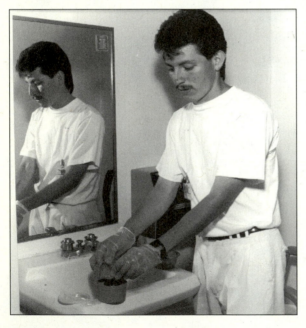

Figure 29-2F   Place clean dentures in clean denture cup.

7. A soft toothbrush or other type of applicator may be used to clean the mouth while dentures are out, Figure 29-2G. This is a good time to observe the inside of the client's mouth for signs of irritation or soreness.

8. Have client, if capable, insert clean dentures into mouth, Figure 29-2H.

9. Clean and replace equipment.

10. Remove gloves and wash hands.

11. Document procedure completed and time, observations, and client's reaction.

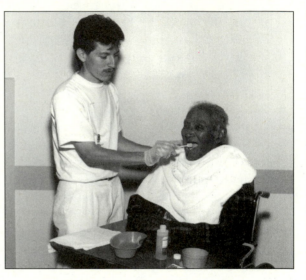

Figure 29-2G   Use toothette and clean inside of mouth. Remember to clean the tongue.

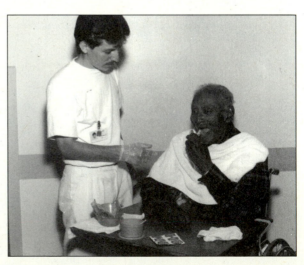

Figure 29-2H   Instruct client to place clean dentures in mouth.

Client Care Procedure 29:
Shaving the Male Client

Purpose

• To make the client comfortable and to maintain client's appearance

NOTE: Shaving can be planned for the same time as other daily hygiene tasks are done. For shaving, the electric razor is usually the easiest to use. However, it may be necessary to use a safety razor or disposable razor. In some instances, older women also may request to have facial hair shaved to improve cosmetic appearance. Remember universal precautions; wear gloves.

Procedure

1. Wash hands and apply gloves.
2. Asks client if he wants a shave.
3. Assemble needed supplies. If possible have client shave in bathroom by the mirror.

   gloves
   razor and shaving cream
   basin of hot water
   washcloth and towel
   aftershave lotion (optional)

4. Position client in sitting position and place towel under chin and across his chest.
5. Wet client's face with shaving cream, Figure 29-3A. With one hand pull the skin tight above area to be shaved. With razor in other hand, gently take short, even strokes. Shave in the direction the hair grows, Figures 29-3B through 29-3D. If client is capable, let him do as much as possible.
6. Rinse the razor frequently. After shave is completed, place used uncapped razor in "sharps" containers.
7. Change water in basin when shave is completed. Rinse the client's face in clear warm water and pat dry.

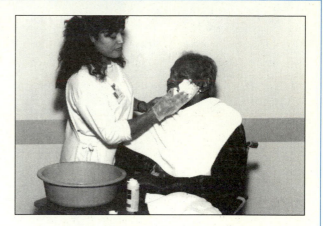

Figure 29-3A   Apply shaving cream to face.

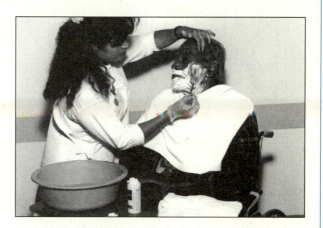

Figure 29-3B   Shave in direction of hair growth.

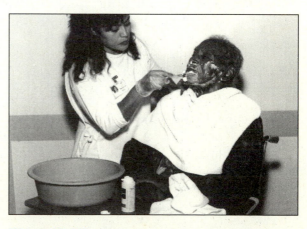

Figure 29-3C   Be sure to shave area under nose and top of chin.

Continued on the following page.

8. If desired, apply aftershave lotion. Remove gloves.
9. Return equipment and supplies, clean and rinse basin, dry and store.
10. Reposition client.
11. Wash hands.
12. Document completion of procedure and time, observations, and client's reaction.

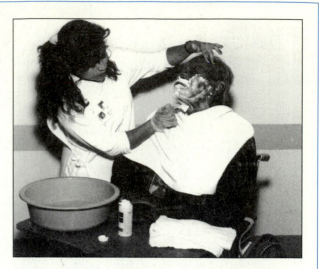

Figure 29-3D Shave area under the client's chin.

Client Care Procedure 30:
Dressing and Undressing the Client

Purpose

- To keep the client clean and comfortable
- To increase client's self-image and well-being
- To reduce client's discomfort and reduce client's risk of strain or injury

NOTE: Do not allow client to remain in nightclothes during the day (unless case manager states it is all right). The client needs to know that it is daytime and needs to dress accordingly.

Procedure

1. Wash your hands and tell client what you plan to do.
2. Assemble clean clothing.

   undergarments
   outergarments—let client select if
     possible
   stockings and shoes

3. If client is able, help the client to sit at the edge of the bed and dangle the legs. If the client is too weak to sit up, have client lie flat on the bed. Place a sheet or robe over client to avoid embarrassing or chilling the client.
4. Assist the client to put on undergarments. If client has weak leg, place weak leg in first, then the other leg. Then put on outergarments in the same manner. If client can stand, pull the pants or slacks up to the waist. If the client must remain on the bed, ask the client to press the heels into the bed and raise the buttocks. While the client is in this position, quickly slide the pants or slacks up to the waist. Assist the client as necessary. Slacks with elastic waist are preferred as they go on easier than pants with zippers and buttons. Cotton jogging suits are becoming a very popular option for the disabled or elderly clients. They are warm, easy to get off and on, and attractive. They also launder easily.

5. To dress the client in a shirt, slip, or dress, help the client place the weak arm into the sleeve first, Figure 29-4A, then the strong arm. If dress or shirt needs to go over head, help client place both arms into armholes and then slip the neck of the garment over the client's head.

6. To put on socks or stockings, turn each sock down to the toe end. Slide client's toe into place and, with one arm on each side of leg, pull the sock or stocking up, Figure 29-4B. Make sure socks are smooth over the feet and legs. Put on shoes if client is to remain out of bed. Let client assist as much as possible.

7. To undress the client simply reverse the instruction for dressing. If the client has a weak arm or leg, undress the weak limb last.

8. Wash hands.

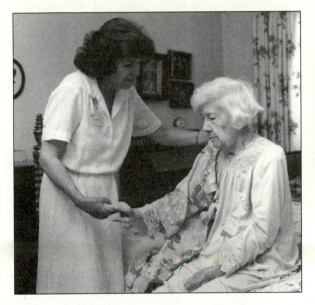

Figure 29-4A   Place sleeve over weak arm first and then over strong arm.

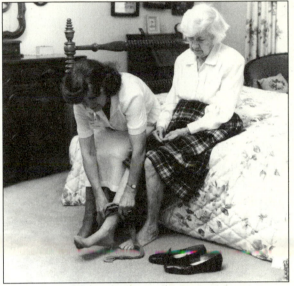

Figure 29-4B   Roll down stocking to toe and then put on foot.

Client Care Procedure 31:
Applying Elasticized Stockings

Purpose

- To prevent swelling of feet and ankles
- To prevent formation of blood clots in legs
- To increase blood circulation in the legs

NOTE: It is better to apply the elastic hose in bed rather than in the chair. Elastic hose should be removed and reapplied daily. Elastic hose come in a variety of sizes and lengths. They need to be supportive but not too tight. If they are too loose, they lose their effectiveness.

Procedure

1. Wash your hands.
2. Tell client what you plan to do.
3. With client lying down, expose one leg at a time.
4. Turn stocking inside out to heel by placing your hand inside stocking and grasping heel. Position stocking over foot and heel of client, making sure the heel is properly placed. Continue to pull the remaining part of the hose upward over the client's leg.

Continued on the following page.

5. Check to be sure stocking is applied evenly and smoothly and there are no wrinkles.
6. Repeat procedure on opposite leg.

7. Wash your hands.
8. Document time and completion of the procedure and client's reaction.

Client Care Procedure 32:
Making an Unoccupied Bed

Purpose

* To apply clean and fresh linens to bed
* To add to the client's comfort by removing wrinkled or soiled sheets

NOTE: Complete one side of the bed entirely before moving to the opposite side. If a fitted sheet for the bottom of bed is not available, and the bed is twin size, it is recommended that a full sheet be used for the bottom. The full sheet, once tucked in, will stay in place longer than a flat twin sheet. Remember to use good body mechanics when making a client's bed.

Procedure

1. Strip bed of dirty linens and place in laundry.
2. Wash hands.
3. Assemble clean linens.

   top sheet and fitted bottom sheet, if available
   pillow cases
   mattress pad, bedspread, and blankets if needed

4. Place mattress pad on bed and then put clean fitted sheet or flat sheet on bed. If flat sheet is being used, unfold the sheet with the long fold at the center of the bed. Place lower hemline even with the bottom of the mattress, Figure 29-5A.
5. Open sheet gently; do not shake. Starting at the head of the bed, miter the corner and tuck in that side of the sheet, Figures 29-5B through 29-5E and 29-6. A great

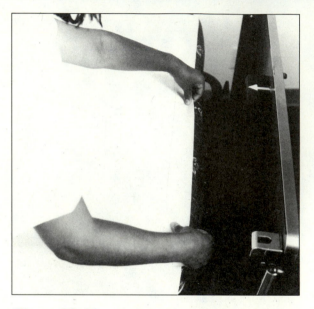

Figure 29-5A Place sheet even with end of mattress at foot of bed.

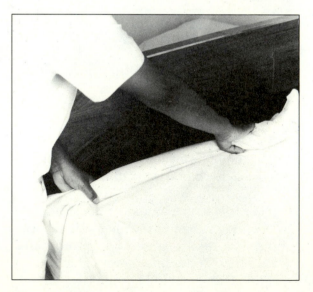

Figure 29-5B Tuck sheet under mattress at top of bed.

deal of time is saved by working on only one side of the bed at a time. Sizes of bedrooms differ greatly in clients' homes; you will need to adjust this procedure to your client's bed placement in the home.

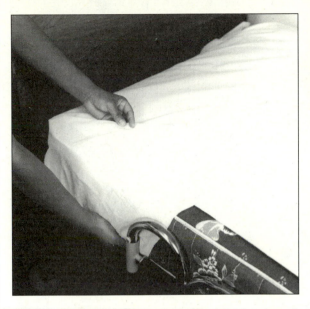

Figure 29-5C Make triangle with sheet and place on top of bed. Tuck in remaining sheet under mattress.

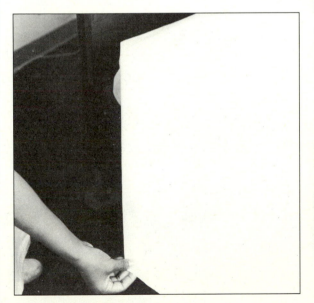

Figure 29-5D Bring triangle portion of sheet down.

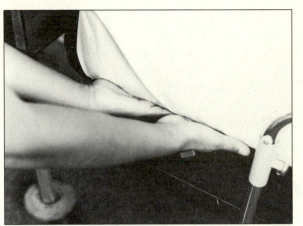

Figure 29-5E Tuck in sheet under mattress. Corner should be neat looking and tight.

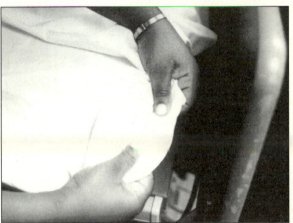

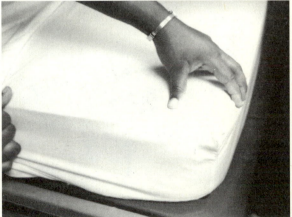

Figure 29-6 If a fitted bottom sheet is used, fit it properly and smoothly around one corner. (From Hegner and Caldwell, *Nursing Assistant, A Nursing Process Approach,* 6E, copyright 1992 by Delmar Publishers Inc.)

Continued on the following page.

6. Place top sheet over the bottom sheet wrong side up. Place hem even with the top edge of the mattress, Figure 29-7. Place the center fold at the center of the bed. Tuck in top sheet at foot of bed and make a mitered corner, Figure 29-8. (**Note:** The top sheet, blanket, and spread, if used, may be tucked under the mattress at the same time.)

7. Place the blanket back on the bed. Put the top edge 12 inches from the top of the mattress. Place bedspread on the bed.

8. Tuck the blanket and top sheet under the bottom of the mattress at the foot end of the bed. Miter the corner. Fold top sheet over the top edge of the bed.

9. Walk over to opposite side of bed and make remaining part of the bed.

10. Put pillowcases on pillows, Figure 29-9.

11. Wash your hands.

12. Document task completed.

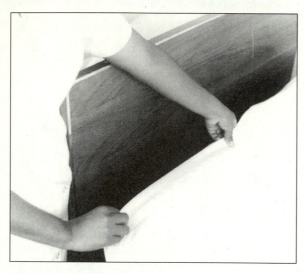

Figure 29-7　Place top sheet even with top of mattress.

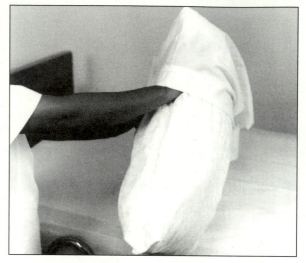

Figure 29-9　Apply clean pillow case.

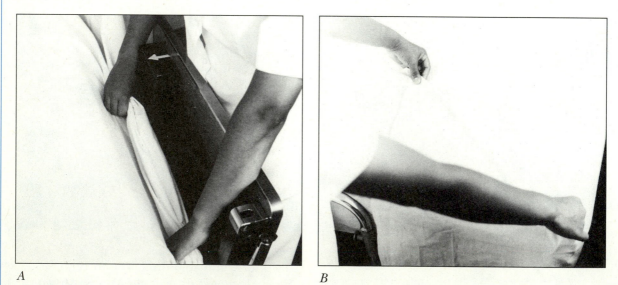

A

B

Figure 29-8　*A.* Tuck sheet in at the foot of the mattress. *B.* Miter the corner of the sheet at the foot of the bed.

Client Care Procedure 33:
Making an Occupied Bed

Purpose

- To apply clean linens while the client remains in the bed
- To add to the client's comfort by removing soiled and wrinkled sheets

Procedure

1. Wash your hands.
2. Assemble clean linens.

   flat sheet and fitted bottom (if available)
   extra flat sheet or drawsheet if used by client
   pillow cases
   large plastic bag (for soiled linens)

3. Tell client what you plan to do and provide for the client's privacy by closing the bedroom door.
4. Place clean linen on a clean chair or table in room in the order you plan to use them.
5. Loosen bedding from under mattress by lifting the mattress with one hand as you pull out bedding with the other hand.
6. Remove top covers one at a time, folding each to the foot of the bed.
7. Leave top sheet covering the client to prevent chilling and afford privacy.
8. Place two straight chairs against one side of the bed. This helps protect the client from falling out of bed. If the bed has side rails this is not necessary. Simply raise the side rail on the opposite side of the bed.
9. Assist the client to turn on the side facing the chairs or side rail. Assist the client to move near the edge of the bed by the chairs. Stand at the other side of the bed.
10. Roll or fanfold (fold in pleats) the soiled bottom sheet to the center of the bed beside the client's back.
11. Fold the clean bottom sheet lengthwise and place the fold at the center of the bed. Fanfold half the clean sheet next to the soiled sheet. Tuck the other half under the mattress. Make a mitered corner at the top. Tuck from the top or head of bed and move toward the foot of the bed.
12. Help client turn toward you onto the clean sheet. Bring the chairs to the other side of the bed for the client's protection (or raise the side rail).
13. Go to the other side and remove soiled sheet. Place dirty linen into large plastic bag.
14. Pull clean sheet across bed and tuck under mattress. Miter corner at top and tuck along side from head to foot of bed. Make certain the sheet is tight and wrinkle free.
15. Turn client onto the back in center of the bed. Place clean top sheet over the soiled top sheet. Slide the soiled sheet out from under the clean sheet. Have client hold fresh top sheet in place.
16. Place soiled sheet in large plastic bag.
17. Unfold blankets and place over top sheet.
18. Tuck in the bottoms of the sheet, blanket, and bedspread at the foot of the bed. Miter the two corners; leave extra room for foot and toe movement.
19. Change the pillow cases and replace pillows under client's head. Put soiled cases in large plastic bag.
20. Be sure client is comfortable and that the room is neat. Remove soiled linens from room.
21. Wash your hands.
22. Document procedure completed.

Client Care Procedure 34: Giving Nail Care

Purpose

- To keep the client's nails clean and well groomed
- To observe for signs of irritation

NOTE: You never cut a diabetic client's toenails or fingernails. Nail care is usually given at bath time or when there is a need because of a broken nail or hangnail. A manicure may be done to make the client feel more attractive. In the elderly, you might note very thick toenails, which require special clippers to cut; this usually is done by a podiatrist (foot doctor).

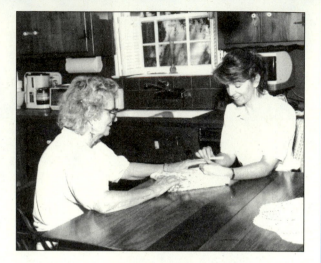

Figure 29-10 File fingernails smoothly.

Procedure

1. Assemble supplies.

   soap, water, and basin
   nail brush
   towel and lotion, preferably lanolin
     lotion
   small scissors or clippers
   emery board or nail file and orange stick

2. Wash your hands.
3. Tell client what you plan to do.
4. Soak toenails or fingernails in soap and water for 10 minutes.
5. Brush nails with nail brush. Clean under nails. Rinse well. Dry hands and nails.
6. Wear gloves if clipping nails/toenails.
7. If nails are too long, make a straight cut for toenails and a curve cut for fingernails. Check to make sure that you are allowed to cut nails.
8. Use file or emery board and smooth edges of nails, Figure 29-10.
9. Massage lotion on the hands or feet.
10. If you accidently cut a client's skin while cutting nails, remember to use universal precautions. Report the cut to your supervisor.
11. Clean the basin, brush, and scissors or clippers. Return equipment to proper place.
12. Wash your hands.
13. Document procedure, any observations, and client's reaction.

Client Care Procedure 35: Shampooing the Client's Hair in Bed

Purpose

- To clean the hair and scalp
- To stimulate circulation in the scalp
- To make the client feel and look better
- To prevent accumulation of dandruff or formation of scalp crusts

NOTE: A plastic shampoo tray may be used in a client's home, if available. Occasionally your agency may supply you with this shampoo tray. The shampoo tray is used in place of a rubber sheet or plastic bag and is easy to use.

Procedure

1. Assemble equipment.

   shampoo and hair conditioner or rinse
      (optional)
   3 or 4 towels
   large plastic garbage bags or rubber sheet
   large empty container or large waste-
      paper basket or bucket
   large pitcher for warm water
   comb and brush
   disposable gloves
   newspapers

2. Wash your hands. If client has sores or lesions of the scalp, wear gloves.
3. Tell client what you plan to do.
4. Position client so that the head rests over the edge of the bed. The back and shoulders should rest on the edge. (Your instructor will demonstrate this procedure.)
5. Loosen clothing from around client's neck. Roll a towel to be placed around neck, Figure 29-11A and B.
6. Spread a newspaper on a chair or on the floor and set large empty bucket or container on the newspaper. Move the chair with the basin to a position beneath the head of the client.
7. Slide a plastic bag or sheet under the client's shoulders. Let the other end of the plastic fall into the basin. This allows the water to go from the head into the catch basin or bucket.
8. With pitcher full of warm water, wet the client's hair, Figure 29-11C.
9. Apply shampoo to the head, lather well, and massage scalp with your knuckles. If nonprescription medicated shampoo is

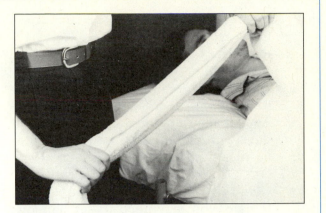

Figure 29-11A   Fold large towel into a roll lengthwise.

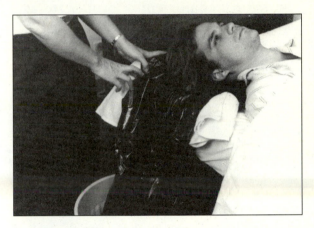

Figure 29-11B   Place towel on large piece of plastic and roll to form a trough at the top and both sides.

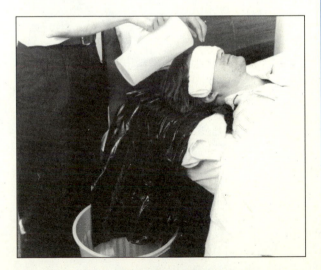

Figure 29-11C   Position client on side of bed and moisten hair with a pitcher of water. Be sure to cover client's eyes. Note placement of bucket.

Continued on the following page.

ordered, please follow any special instructions on label.

10. Rinse hair with water thoroughly, making sure to remove all traces of shampoo.

11. If necessary, reapply shampoo, lather well, and rinse thoroughly.

12. Apply hair conditioner or rinse. Follow directions on the bottle, as some need to be diluted and others do not.

13. Dry client's hair with large towel. Comb and brush hair, Figure 29-12. If female, you may need to set hair on rollers. If hair dryer is available, blow dry hair gently.

14. Return equipment to proper storage area.

15. Wash hands.

16. Document procedure completed, your observations, and client's reaction.

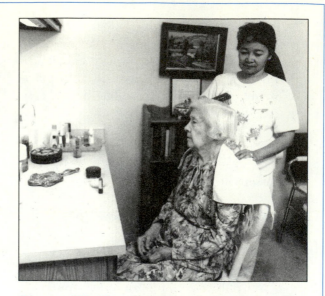

Figure 29-12   Comb and dry hair after shampoo. Before combing, be sure to place towel on shoulders to collect fallen hair.

Client Care Procedure 36:
Assisting the Client with Self-administered Medications

Purpose

- To relieve pain and other symptoms, to help the body fight infections, and to treat diseases (medications are prescribed by doctors)

- To encourage the client to take the prescribed medication at the right time, in the right dose, in the right amount, and in the right manner

- The following information should be made available to you by your nurse supervisor and clearly written down.

  name of each medicine
  what each medication is for
  description of medicine—color, form
  what time(s) of day or night when each
     medicine is to be taken
  how long the medicine should be taken
  whether the medicine should be taken
     with food or other liquid
  possible side effects

- The home health aide should be aware of common reactions to medications so the nurse supervisor can be called if symptoms appear.

NOTE: The home health aide *does not* give medications. The aide can help clients to take their own medications. The aide can remind the client when to take the prescribed medication and assist the client in checking to see if the dosage and amount of medicine are correct. In some instances the client may also take over-the-counter medications. It is a good idea to report to your nurse supervisor what over-the-counter medications your client is taking.

    The aide must take special care in assisting blind clients with their medications. Be sure that medications are coded so that the client can find the correct bottles when they are needed. Medications for the blind client must be kept in exactly the same spot so that an error will not be made. Special arrangements should be made by the pharmacist or nurse supervisor in setting up the coding.

Procedure

1. Have the nurse supervisor or pharmacist prepare a list of medications prescribed and the time they are to be given. Some medications are given 3 times a day (tid), usually before (ac) or after (pc) each meal. Others may be ordered 4 times a day (qid) or every 6 hours (q6h). A medication taken every 6 hours could be given at 6 AM, noon, 6 PM, and midnight. The pharmacist usually informs the client at which times the medications should be taken.

2. The nurse supervisor will set a schedule to be followed daily. After each medication has been taken, check it off. This informs both the aide and the client that the medicine has been taken. Refer to the schedule and remind the client when medicine is due. Your nurse supervisor may prepare your client's medication in special containers that have all the medication needed for a specific time, Figure 29-13.

3. Check with the client each time to make sure the medicine is the correct one listed on the schedule.

4. Make sure the correct method of taking the medication is followed. For example, some medicines are taken with juice or milk instead of water. Others are taken on an empty stomach, others with food.

5. Certain medications such as nitroglycerin tablets must be within the client's reach

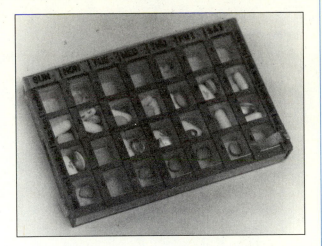

Figure 29-13   Special medication container

at all times. When the client has chest pain, the client needs to place these tablets under the tongue immediately.

6. Be sure sleeping and pain medication bottles are kept in a safe place after each use. They should only be taken as often as the doctor has ordered.

7. Review the times with the client when the prescribed medicines are to be taken. Leave the medication within easy reach of the client. Remind the client to take the nighttime dose in a well-lit room.

8. If the client has questions about the medications, encourage the client to ask the pharmacist, nurse supervisor, or doctor. The client should be knowledgeable about medications that he or she is taking.

9. As a home health aide, you are not allowed to pour the client's medication from the bottle; the client needs to do this himself/herself.

Client Care Procedure 37:
Inserting a Hearing Aid

Purpose

- To increase the hearing ability of the client
- To ensure the client's optimal use of the hearing aid

NOTE: Many types of hearing aids are on the market today. They all take special batteries. The batteries generally do not last a long time, some only 24 hours. Always check to

Continued on the following page.

see if your client has an adequate supply of batteries on hand.

Procedure

1. Wash your hands.
2. Check hearing aid appliance to see that the batteries are working and tubing is not cracked, Figure 29-14.
3. Tell the client what you plan to do. You may need to use gestures because client may not be able to hear spoken words.
4. Check inside of client's ear for wax buildup or any other abnormalities.
5. Check to make sure the hearing aid is off or the volume is turned to its lowest level.
6. Handle the hearing aid very carefully. Do not drop it or allow it to get wet. Store in a safe area when client is not wearing it. Be sure hearing aid is clean before giving it to client. Follow manufacturer's directions in cleaning your client's hearing aid.
7. Assist the client in inserting the earmold in the ear canal.

Alternate Actions

8. Place the hearing aid over the client's ear, allowing the earmold to hang free.
9. Adjust the hearing aid behind the client's ear.
10. Grasp the earmold and gently insert the tapered end into the ear canal.
11. Gently twist the earmold into the curve of the ear, pushing upward and inward on the bottom of the earmold, while pulling on the ear lobe with the other hand.
12. Let client turn on switch and adjust volume.
13. Wash hands.

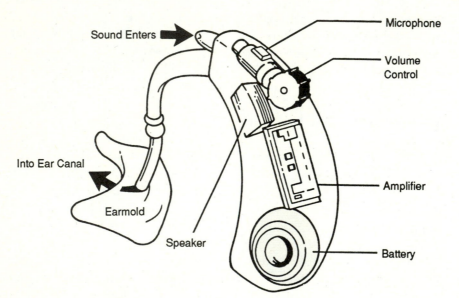

Figure 29-14 Parts of the hearing aid (From Hegner and Caldwell, *Assisting in Long-Term Care*, copyright 1988 by Delmar Publishers Inc.)

Client Care Procedure 38:
Caring for an Artificial Eye

Purpose

- To ensure proper care of client's artificial eye
- To prevent infection or irritation of the eye socket

Procedure

1. Assemble equipment.

   eyecup with gauze square (not cotton filled)
   cleansing solution, if ordered
   washcloth and basin of lukewarm water
   gloves
   cotton balls
   small plastic bag for wastes

2. Wash hands and apply gloves.
3. Tell client what you plan to do.
4. Have client lie down if possible. Position yourself and equipment to be on the same side as the client's artificial eye.
5. With moistened cotton balls clean the outside of the eye from the nose to the outside of the face. Stroke once only with each cotton ball.
6. Remove artificial eye by depressing lower eyelid with your thumb while lifting upper lid with your index finger. If client can remove artificial eye, let the client do it. Carefully take eye and place in gauze lined eyecup. Place eyecup in a very safe place nearby while you clean the outside of the eye socket.
7. Clean eye socket using warm water and cotton balls. Pat area around eye dry.

Observe area for signs of irritation or infection.

8. Carry eyecup to bathroom. Place washcloth in bottom of sink, as a precaution against breakage. Remove eye from eyecup and gently wash in sink. Remove all secretions on outside of the eye. Do not use any cleaner on eye unless specifically ordered.
9. Place clean gauze in bottom of eyecup and return to client. Assist the client to insert eye into socket. If eye is moist, it will slide in easier. You may need to depress the lower eyelid and slip gently over the eye as it slips into the socket.
10. If client does not wish to have eye inserted into socket right away, the eye needs to be stored in water in the eyecup.
11. Return equipment and wastes to correct areas.
12. If client wears glasses, clean the glasses with a cleaning solution, rinse with clear water, and dry with tissues. Handle the glasses only by the frame. Return glasses to client or place in case.
13. Remove gloves and wash hands.
14. Document procedure completion, your observations, and client's reaction.

Unit 30 Feeding and Toileting

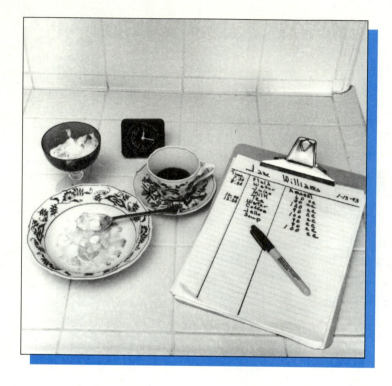

CLIENT CARE PROCEDURES

39. Feeding the Client
40. Measuring and Recording Fluid Intake and Output

41. Giving and Emptying the Bedpan
42. Giving and Emptying the Urinal

LEARNING OBJECTIVES

After studying this unit, you should be able to:

- Demonstrate clear ability to perform all procedures.
- Explain the purpose of each procedure.
- Calculate, record, and report results of all procedures.

- Encourage client to do as much as possible with remaining abilities.
- Be aware of precautions to take with every procedure.

Client Care Procedure 39:
Feeding the Client

Purpose

- To provide proper nutrition for the client who is unable to feed him/herself or needs assistance in feeding
- To provide suitable food, based on client's condition, meeting standards of the food guide pyramid
- To provide a pleasurable experience for the client
- To encourage client to use adaptive devices for feeding

NOTE: Eating for a client should be a pleasant and enjoyable experience. The foods should be served with "hot foods hot, and cold foods cold." Food should be served attractively. If possible have the client eat in a pleasant environment, Figure 30-1, and preferably not in the bedroom.

If the client needs to be fed, it is desirable that the client be sitting up in a chair, Figure 30-2. If this is not feasible, you can position the client up in bed with the use of a few pillows. The food will be digested better if the client is in a sitting position. It is recommended that the aide sit while feeding and be at the eye level of the client.

Most clients will prefer to feed themselves if possible. Many different feeding devices available today make this possible, Figure 30-3. The feeding device will need to be chosen according to the client's disability.

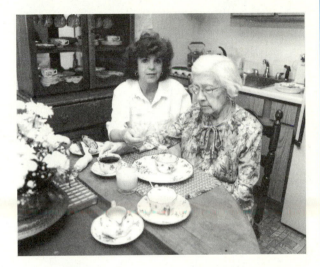

Figure 30-2   Home health aide (sitting) feeding client slowly, one food at a time. Client is holding her own coffee cup.

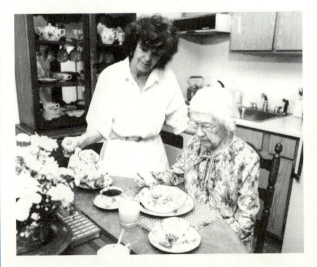

Figure 30-1   Client eating a well-balanced meal prepared by her home health aide. The environment is made as pleasant as possible to promote enjoyment of the meal.

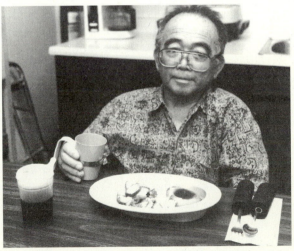

Figure 30-3   Client feeds himself using special feeding devices.

Continued on the following page.

If your client chokes easily, it may be recommended to mix a thickener in the liquid foods. Clients do choke more readily on thinner liquids than thick liquids. If the client has a poor appetite and is becoming malnourished, it is advisable to offer high-calorie and high-protein drinks often throughout the day.

Some clients are fed through a feeding tube inserted into the stomach through the nose, Figure 30-4A, or through an opening in the abdominal wall. A special control apparatus monitors the rate at which fluid nourishment is supplied to the client, Figure 30-4B. It is the nurse's responsibility to monitor tube feeding.

Procedure

1. Wash your hands.
2. Prepare the client to eat. Wash the client's face and hands. Position client in sitting position in bed or sitting up in a chair. Make environment as pleasant as possible. If necessary do mouth care before to increase the client's desire to eat. Place large napkin over client's chest.
3. Bring food to client. Tell client what foods you prepare.
4. How you feed or assist your client depends on the handicap or physical problem the client has. If the client is blind, you need to tell the client where each food is on the plate in relation to a clock. If the client has use of only one hand, a suction plate or plate guard may be used. If the client cannot chew food, the food will need to be soft in consistency.
   Caution: The client should never be given cause to be embarrassed because of any physical disability.
5. Ask the client which food is desired first. (Getting the client's cooperation and participation is important.)
6. If the client must be fed by the aide, remember:

   • Check to see if dentures are in place.
   • Feed slowly; let the client set the pace.

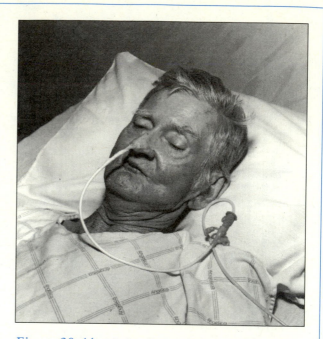

Figure 30-4A A feeding tube may be inserted into a client's stomach through the nose to maintain proper nutrition, if the client is unable to eat. The nurse inserts the feeding tube into the client's stomach.

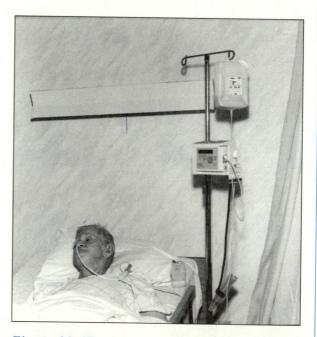

Figure 30-4B The tube feeding is regulated with a special monitor placed on a pole. It is the nurse's responsibility to set the monitor at a specific rate and to replace the special nourishment in the container.

- Thermal bowls and cups will assist in keeping foods at proper temperature.
- Feed small amounts of food at a time.
- Make sure the consistency of the food is appropriate.

- Do not use a syringe to feed the client. A child's feeder cup or plastic glass works well in this situation.
- If possible, have client hold finger foods or bread.

Client Care Procedure 40:
Measuring and Recording Fluid Intake and Output

Purpose

- To identify food items that need to be measured for fluid intake
- To measure and record fluid intake and output accurately

NOTE: Intake is a measure of all the fluids or semiliquids that a person drinks. Output is all the fluid that passes out of the body. The abbreviation for measuring fluid intake and output is I&O. Figure 30-5 shows the fluids that should be included in the measurement of intake and output.

MEASURE FOR INTAKE	
ice	water
juices	pop
coffee	ice cream
yogurt	soup
jello	pudding
any other food that is liquid at room temperature	

MEASURE FOR OUTPUT	
vomitus (emesis)	liquid stools
urine	
blood or drainage from wounds	

Figure 30-5 Various fluids and substances are measured and recorded as intake and output.

Procedure

1. Assemble supplies.

   measuring cup or container for intake
   large measuring container for output

2. Wash hands and apply gloves if measuring output.
3. Measure and record all liquids taken by the client, Figure 30-6. This includes all fluids taken with meals and between meals: coffee, milk, fruit juices, beer, and water. Liquids are recorded in cubic centimeters, abbreviated cc, Figure 30-7. You need to remember that 30 cc equals 1 ounce. Example: If a client drank a can of pop that is 12 ounces, you need to multiply 12 by 30, which equals 360 cc.
4. Ask the client to use a urinal or bedpan for all voiding. If the client can use the toilet, a special plastic hat can be placed in the toilet to collect the urine, Figure

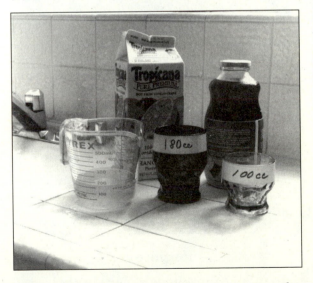

Figure 30-6 It is a good idea to measure the cubic centimeter (cc) capacity of commonly used glasses and cups. This will be helpful in recording the intake of a client.

Continued on the following page.

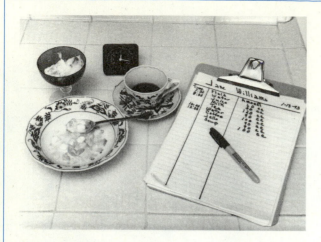

Figure 30-7 Intake is recorded in cubic centimeters (cc) after the client has drunk the liquid.

30-8. All urine must be collected so that it can be measured.

5. Pour urine from bedpan or urinal into a measuring device, Figure 30-9. Record the amount. Always record output in cc.
6. Be sure to explain to the client how to keep exact records. The client will need to record the fluids at times when the aide is off duty.
7. Clean equipment after each use.
8. Remove gloves and wash hands.

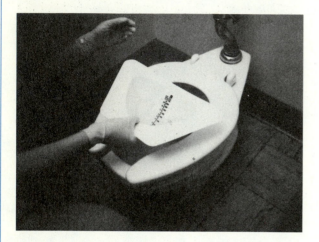

Figure 30-8 If a client's urine needs to be measured, a special toilet insert (potty hat) may be used to collect the urine. (From Hegner and Caldwell, *Nursing Assistant, A Nursing Process Approach,* 6E, copyright 1992 by Delmar Publishers Inc.)

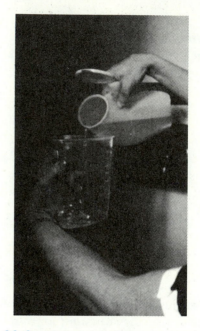

Figure 30-9 Urine can be measured with a special plastic container or a large measuring cup. (From Hegner and Caldwell, *Nursing Assistant, A Nursing Process Approach,* 6E, copyright 1992 by Delmar Publishers Inc.)

Client Care Procedure 41:
Giving and Emptying the Bedpan

Purpose

- To provide for routine elimination of bladder and bowels
- To observe or measure urinary or fecal output

NOTE: The bedpan is used for clients who are confined to bed. The bedpan should be given whenever the client requests it. The client may be undergoing retraining to establish bowel and bladder continence. The aide should follow a regular schedule of offering the bedpan or urinal. If the client does not remember to ask, the home health aide should offer to bring the bedpan or urinal. The aide can politely remind the client by asking, "Do you need to use the bedpan or urinal?"

A female client will use the bedpan for both urinating and defecating, Figure 30-10. A male client will need a urinal if he needs to urinate, Figure 30-11. If the client is very small or has a body cast on, a smaller bedpan or fracture pan can be used.

Procedure

1. Assemble equipment and supplies needed.

   bedpan and bedpan cover
   toilet tissue
   moistened washcloth

2. Wash hands and apply gloves.
3. Tell client what you plan to do.
4. If a metal bedpan is used, first warm it by running hot water over the rim. Dry the rim and sprinkle it with powder if available. The powder prevents the client's buttocks from sticking to the bedpan.
5. Place bedpan near the bed. Put toilet tissue near the client's hand.
6. Fold top blanket and sheet at an angle. Remove the client's bottom clothing.
7. To raise the buttocks, have the client bend knees and push on the heels. As the client lifts, place your hand under the small of the client's back. The aide holds the bedpan in place when the client is lying on his/her backside and then turns the client.
8. Lift gently and slowly with one hand. Slide the bedpan under the hips with the other hand. The client's buttocks should rest on the rounded shelf of the bedpan. The narrow end should face the foot of the bed. If the client cannot assist, turn the client to one side and position the bedpan over the buttocks, Figure 30-12. Roll the client onto the bedpan. Make sure the client's head is elevated.

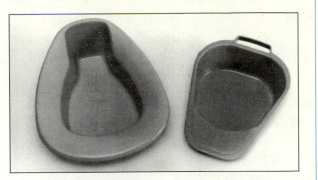

Figure 30-10   Regular bedpan (*left*) and fracture bedpan (*right*)

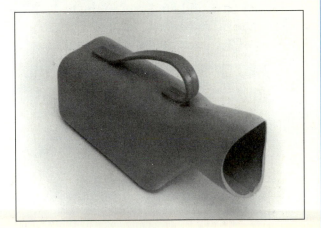

Figure 30-11   Male urinal

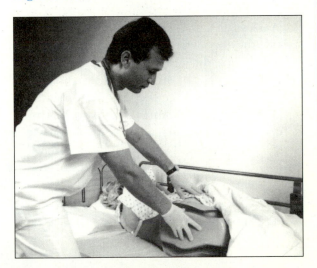

Figure 30-12   Roll client away from you while supporting client with one hand on client's hip and arm. Place bedpan with the other hand. Then roll client back onto bedpan. (From Hegner and Caldwell, *Nursing Assistant, A Nursing Process Approach*, 6E, copyright 1992 by Delmar Publishers Inc.)

Continued on the following page.

9. Pull sheet over the client for added privacy. Make sure the client is as comfortable as possible. An extra pillow under the head may be used.
10. While client is using the bedpan, the aide can be moistening the washcloth.
11. Remove the bedpan when the client is finished using it. Do not leave the client sitting on the bedpan for longer than 15 minutes. Remove the bedpan by having the client bend the knees and push on the heels. Place one hand under small of client's back and lift. Remove the bedpan with the other hand.
12. If possible, have clients wipe. If they are not able to do this, the aide must wipe the client. Discard tissues in the bedpan.
13. Replace the client's clothing. Give client washcloth to wipe hands.
14. Take bedpan to toilet, observe contents and measure if necessary. Empty contents into toilet. Flush. Fill bedpan with cold water and empty. Clean bedpan by using warm soapy water and the toilet brush. Empty water into toilet and rinse bedpan. Dry well.
15. Return bedpan to proper storage area.
16. Remove gloves and wash hands.
17. Record amount of urine; color, amount, and consistency of stool.

Client Care Procedure 42:
Giving and Emptying the Urinal

Purpose

- To provide for routine elimination of urine

Procedure

1. Wash your hands and apply gloves.
2. Lift the top bedcovers and place the urinal under the covers so that the client can grasp the handle. If he cannot do this, you must place the urinal in position and ensure the penis is placed in the opening of the urinal. If possible, assist the client to stand when using the urinal.
3. Remove gloves and dispose of them properly. Leave client alone if possible. You may give the client a bell to ring when he is done.
4. Put on gloves and remove urinal once client is done using it.
5. Take the urinal to the bathroom and observe contents. Measure if required. Empty the urinal. Rinse with cold water and clean with soapy water. Rinse with disinfectant or water, dry, store properly.
6. Remove gloves and wash hands.
7. Record amount and color of urine, as required.

Unit 31 Collecting Specimens and Catheter Care

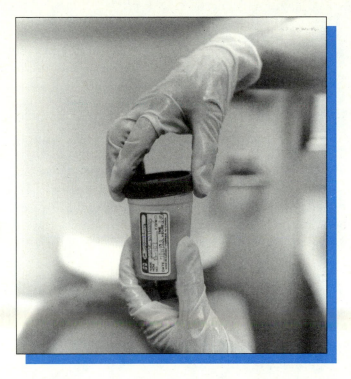

CLIENT CARE PROCEDURES

43. Collecting a Clean-catch Urine Specimen
44. Caring for a Urinary Catheter
45. Connecting the Leg Bag
46. Emptying a Drainage Unit
47. Retraining the Bladder
48. Collecting a Sputum Specimen

NOTE: All procedures are not allowed in all states. Make sure you are aware of limits as outlined by state guidelines.

LEARNING OBJECTIVES

After studying this unit, you should be able to:

- Demonstrate clear ability to perform all the procedures.
- Explain the purpose of each procedure.
- Use universal precautions when handling body substances.
- Recognize abnormal conditions.
- Report and record observations.

Client Care Procedure 43:
Collecting a Clean-catch Urine Specimen

Purpose

- To provide a urine sample for a diagnostic test

NOTE: A clean-catch specimen is requested to obtain a urine sample that is as free of contamination as possible. This is required to make the test results as accurate as possible.

Procedure

1. Assemble needed supplies.

   sterile urine specimen container with completed label
   plastic or zip-lock bag and paper bag
   gloves
   clean bedpan or urinal
   antiseptic soaked wipes

2. Wash hands and apply gloves.
3. Inform client of what you plan to do.
4. Wash the client's genital area or have the client do so, if able. It is especially important for the urinary opening to be cleansed.
5. Give the client a labeled specimen container.
6. Explain the procedure to the client.
7. Have the client begin to void into the bedpan, urinal, or toilet. After a small amount of urine has been voided, have the client catch some of the urine in midstream in the sterile specimen container. You will only need 2 ounces or 60 cc.

After the specimen has been collected, the client can resume voiding into the bedpan, urinal, or toilet.

8. Immediately place the sterile cap on the specimen container, Figure 31-1, so the specimen will not become contaminated.
9. Remove bedpan and wipe client.
10. Place labeled specimen container inside a plastic bag or zip-lock bag, then put this bag inside a paper bag with completed label.
11. Remove gloves and wash hands.
12. Place specimen bag in refrigerator until time to take to local laboratory.
13. Document time of collection and type of specimen.

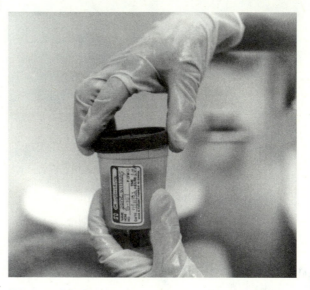

Figure 31-1   Screw top on securely. Wipe outside of container with paper towel.

Client Care Procedure 44:
Caring for a Urinary Catheter

Purpose

- To clean the area around where the catheter enters the body
- To prevent infection of the urinary tract
- To decrease odors and make the client comfortable
- To maintain closed drainage system correctly

NOTE: A urinary catheter is a tube inserted into the bladder to drain urine. Germs can easily enter the bladder while the catheter is in place. Therefore, cleaning around the urinary opening is important. The catheter is inserted by the nurse. The catheter is replaced weekly or once a month.

The collection bag, tubing, and catheter are referred to as the *closed drainage system*, Figure 31-2. The system should never be disconnected. The reason the system should not be opened is to prevent germs from entering the system, Figure 31-3. You should never raise the collection bag higher than the client's bladder. Always check to see if the tubing is lying in correct position and not kinked. Always cover bag with a cloth to prevent embarrassment of your client.

Procedure

1. Assemble supplies.

gloves	plastic bag for waste
antiseptic wipes	cotton-tipped
basin of warm water	applicators

2. Wash your hands and apply gloves.
3. Tell client what you plan to do.
4. Position client on his/her back. Expose only a small area where the catheter enters the body. Using soap and warm water or antiseptic wipes, wash area surrounding the catheter.
5. Using antiseptic wipes or gauze pads dipped in warm water, wipe the catheter

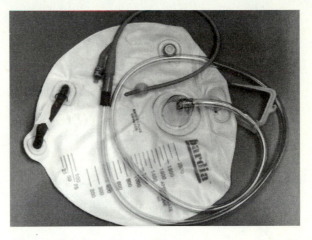

Figure 31-2 Closed drainage system. Note tubing, urine collection bag, and indwelling catheter with bulb inflated.

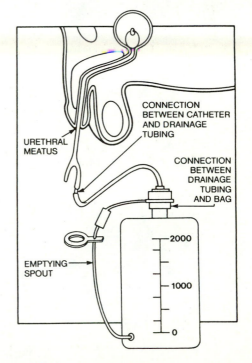

Figure 31-3 Special care must be taken to protect the possible sites of contamination in the closed urinary drainage system. (From Hegner and Caldwell, *Nursing Assistant, A Nursing Process Approach,* 6E, copyright 1992 by Delmar Publishers Inc.)

Continued on the following page.

tube. Make only one stroke with each swab or pad. Discard each wipe after one stroke. Start at the urinary opening and wipe *away* from it. Be careful not to dislodge the catheter. Clean the catheter up to the connection of the drainage tubing.

6. Remove gloves and discard into plastic bag.
7. Check to be sure tubing is coiled on bed, Figure 31-4, and hanging straight down into the drainage container. Check level of urine in the collection bag. Tubing should not be below the collection bag, Figure 31-5. Do not raise collection bag above the level of the client's bladder.
8. Cover client and discard wastes properly.
9. Wash hands.
10. Document procedure and time, your observations, and client's reaction.

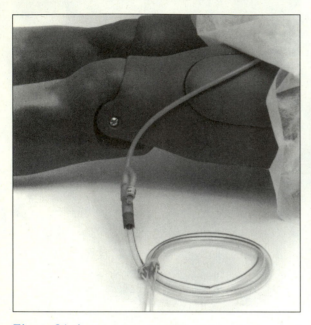

Figure 31-4 Tubing should be placed on top of the leg. The excess tubing should be coiled on the bed.

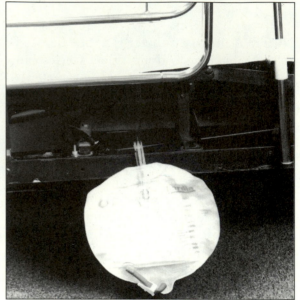

Figure 31-5 The urinary collection bag should be attached to the bed frame. Check to see that the tubing does not fall below the level of the collection bag.

Client Care Procedure 45:
Connecting the Leg Bag

Purpose

* To provide a smaller collection bag for client when client is out of bed

NOTE: The leg urinary collection bag is smaller than the bedside urinary collection bag. The leg bag is attached to the client's thigh (upper leg). The leg bag allows for greater mobility for the client, but must be emptied more frequently. A client may use the leg bag while up in the wheelchair or ambulating and can be connected to the bedside drainage bag when in bed for the night. The leg bag must be rinsed according to agency policy and hung in the bathroom or drain (over bathtub towel bar). A clean cap or stopper must be used at the end of the tubing while the bedside urinary collection bag is not in use.

Procedure

1. Assemble needed equipment.

leg bag	paper towels
alcohol wipes	gloves

2. Wash your hands and apply gloves.
3. Tell client what you plan to do.
4. Place paper towel underneath catheter connection area.
5. Use alcohol to disinfect area to be disconnected.
6. Disconnect catheter from tubing. Wipe end of catheter with alcohol, Figure 31-6. Remove cap from end of leg bag and connect leg bag to catheter. Place cap on end of closed drainage system.
7. Attach leg straps and bag to leg of client, Figure 31-7. Check to see if the part marked "top" of bag is in the correct position.
8. Empty and measure urine from bedside collection bag.
9. Remove gloves and wash hands.
10. Document procedure completed.

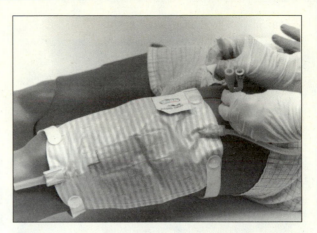

Figure 31-6   Wipe end of catheter with alcohol before connecting leg bag.

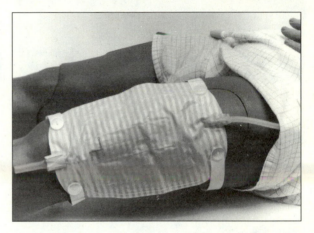

Figure 31-7   Apply leg bag to client's upper leg. Be sure the straps are smooth and not too tight.

Client Care Procedure 46:
Emptying a Drainage Unit

Purpose

• To empty urinary collection bag

Procedure

1. Assemble equipment.

   gloves
   alcohol wipes
   measuring device
   paper towel

2. Wash hands and apply gloves.
3. Tell client what you plan to do.
4. Place paper towel and measuring device on floor below drainage bag.
5. Open drain or spout and allow the urine to drain into measuring device, Figure 31-8. Do not allow the tip of tubing to touch sides of the measuring device.
6. Close the drain and wipe it with the alcohol wipe. Replace it in the holder on the bag.

Continued on the following page.

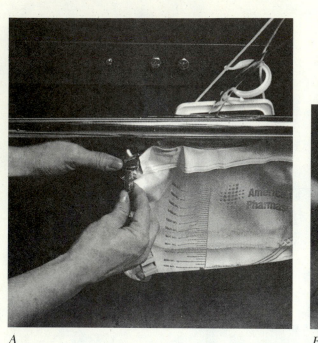

7. Note the amount and color of urine. Empty urine into toilet. Wash and rinse measuring device.
8. Remove gloves and wash hands.
9. Document amount.

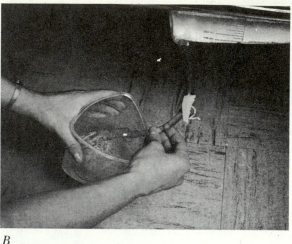

A   B

Figure 31-8   A. Open the drain on the bottom of the collection bag. B. Allow the urine to drain into the graduate. Note that the end of the drain is not touching the sides of the container. Wipe the drain off with alcohol before replacing. It is a good idea to place paper towels under the graduate, just in case some urine is spilled. (From Hegner and Caldwell, *Nursing Assistant, A Nursing Process Approach,* 6E, copyright 1992 by Delmar Publishers Inc.)

Client Care Procedure 47:
Retraining the Bladder

Purpose

- To regain bladder control

Procedure

A home health aide will need to keep a record of how often and how much the client voids throughout the day and night for a few days. Once the client's voiding pattern is known, the nurse supervisor can analyze the client's voiding record and formulate a schedule for the aide to follow. The schedule developed by the nurse will include regularly scheduled times for the aide to have the client drink a measured amount of fluid.

After the client has drunk the liquid, the aide notes the time and then 30 minutes later the aide will toilet the client. The aide will need to encourage the client to void each time the client is positioned on the commode or toilet. It is helpful at times to run water from the faucet to give the client an urge to void. Other methods of encouraging the client to void are to have the client apply light pressure to the bladder area to stimulate the urge to empty the bladder; or have the client lean forward on the toilet to stimulate emptying the bladder. Remember that the client needs to be toileted at regular intervals to prevent accidents. The client will need consistent positive reinforcement to remain dry. At first it may be necessary to take the client to the bathroom every 2 hours; intervals may be lengthened as control is gained. A common cause of incontinence is delay in getting the client to the bathroom. It is of utmost importance to take the client to the bathroom on a *regular* time schedule. The plan will also call for the aide to maintain the client's fluid intake at about 2500 cc/day. The aide should encourage the client to wear regular underwear to enhance the client's self-esteem and to help the client from reverting back to the previous incontinence habit.

Client Care Procedure 48:
Collecting a Sputum Specimen

Purpose

- To provide a sputum specimen for a diagnostic test
- To monitor the client's ongoing condition

Procedure

1. Assemble supplies.

   specimen container, cover with label
      completed
   tissues
   gloves
   moisture-proof plastic bag
   mask (optional)

2. Wash hands and apply gloves. Wear a mask if client has an infectious disease.
3. Ask client to cough deeply and bring up sputum from the lungs. Have client expectorate (spit) into the container. Collect 1 to 2 tablespoons of sputum unless otherwise directed. Be sure to have client cover mouth with tissue to prevent the spread of infections. If excess sputum contaminates the outside of the container, wipe off right away. Cover specimen container and place in moisture-proof bag.
4. Remove gloves and wash hands.
5. Document collection of sputum and when transported to laboratory.

Unit **32** Vital Signs and Measurement

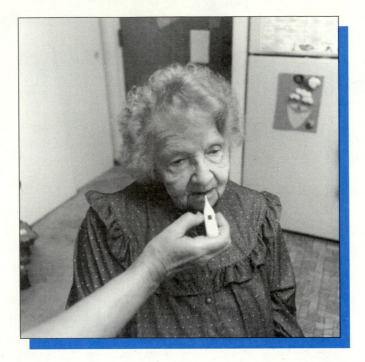

CLIENT CARE PROCEDURES

49. Taking an Oral Temperature
50. Taking a Rectal Temperature
51. Taking an Axillary Temperature
52. Taking the Radial and Apical Pulse

53. Counting Respirations
54. Taking a Blood Pressure
55. Measuring Weight and Height

NOTE: All procedures are not allowed in all states. Make sure you are aware of limits as outlined by state guidelines.

LEARNING OBJECTIVES

After studying this unit, you should be able to:

- Demonstrate clear ability to perform all the procedures.
- Explain the purpose of each procedure.
- State when the procedures should and should not be done.

- Identify precautions to be taken for each procedure.
- Recognize abnormal readings.
- Record vital signs properly.

Client Care Procedure 49:
Taking an Oral Temperature

Purpose

- To measure the client's body temperature in the most appropriate way
- To routinely check the temperature to note any significant change

NOTE: Using an oral thermometer is the most convenient way to obtain a person's temperature. However, it is not the most accurate method. If the client has taken a cold or hot drink within 15 to 20 minutes, the temperature of the mouth changes. In addition to accuracy, the aide must consider safety as it is possible that the thermometer might break in the client's mouth. **Caution:** the oral thermometer can only be used when the client is able to hold it in the mouth properly. If for any reason the client cannot keep the thermometer in the mouth, call the supervisor for instructions. In some of these cases, a rectal temperature may need to be taken with a rectal thermometer.

Procedure

1. Ask the client not to drink any liquids or smoke 15 minutes before the temperature is taken. Otherwise an inaccurate reading could result.
2. Gather the equipment needed.

   oral thermometer, Figure 32-1
   tissues
   pad and pencil
   watch with second hand
   alcohol
   gloves

3. Wash your hands thoroughly and put on gloves.
4. Ask the client to find a comfortable position, either in a chair or in a bed.
5. Hold thermometer by stem end and read mercury column. It should register

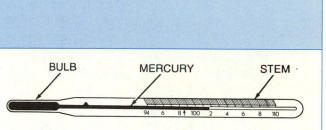

Figure 32-1A   Glass thermometer for oral use (From Hegner and Caldwell, *Nursing Assistant, A Nursing Process Approach,* 6E, copyright 1992 by Delmar Publishers Inc.)

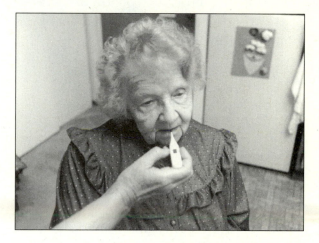

Figure 32-1B   Inexpensive digital thermometer may be used instead of a glass thermometer.

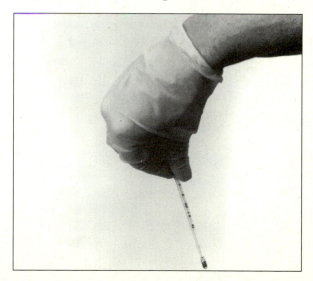

Figure 32-2   Shake mercury down in column by holding thermometer by the stem and snapping the wrist. Check the reading. Repeat until the reading is below 96°F.

Continued on the following page.

96°F or lower (35.5°C). If it does not, shake down the thermometer with a snap of the wrist, Figure 32-2. Shake the thermometer down until it reads 94°F (34.4°C).

6. Insert bulb end of thermometer under client's tongue, Figure 32-3. Slant it toward the side of the mouth. Ask the client to close the mouth and place the thermometer under the tongue.

7. Be sure the client holds the thermometer under the tongue for a minimum of 3 minutes and then remove the thermometer.

8. Gently wipe the thermometer with a tissue from the stem to the bulb end, Figure 32-4. Discard the contaminated tissue. If using a cover, discard it.

9. Hold the thermometer at eye level, Figure 32-5, and record the measurement. Normal oral temperature is 98.6°F (37°C). Mark down the time the reading was made and the temperature reading. Report any temperature which reads above 101°F (38°C).

10. Clean the thermometer by washing it with a small amount of soap and cold water. Rinse all soap from the thermometer. A tissue wet in alcohol may also be used to clean the thermometer. Wipe from stem end to the front, bulb end (clean to dirty).

11. The client may have an electric thermometer with a digital readout, see Figure 32-1B.

12. Return thermometer to the proper storage place.

13. Remove gloves and wash your hands after the procedure.

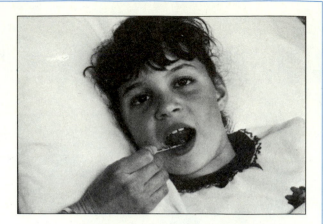

Figure 32-3 The bulb end of the thermometer is inserted under the tongue, left 3 minutes, then removed. (From Hegner and Caldwell, *Nursing Assistant, A Nursing Process Approach*, 6E, copyright 1992 by Delmar Publishers Inc.)

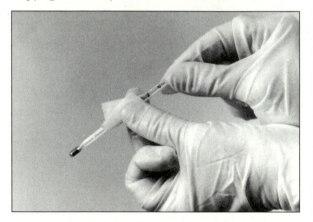

Figure 32-4 Wipe thermometer after removing it from client's mouth. Always wipe from stem to bulb.

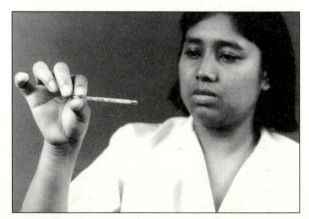

Figure 32-5 Hold the thermometer at eye level. Locate the column of mercury and read closest line.

Client Care Procedure 50:
Taking a Rectal Temperature

Purpose

- To obtain the most accurate measure of the client's temperature
- To obtain the temperature of a person who cannot hold an oral thermometer in the mouth
- To routinely check the temperature to note any significant change

NOTE: A rectal temperature is sometimes taken instead of an oral temperature. At times this is done because the rectal temperature is more accurate. If a person breathes through the mouth or uses oxygen, an oral temperature would not give an accurate reading. Drinking fluids or smoking before a reading also alters it. In these situations clients must have rectal temperatures taken. A rectal temperature is necessary for those who cannot hold a thermometer in the mouth. Infants, small children, and adults who are seriously ill or mentally confused cannot hold a thermometer properly. In addition, rectal temperatures are taken for any person with a history of convulsions.

The rectal thermometer is shaped differently than the oral thermometer. The bulb end of the rectal thermometer is thicker and more rounded. This shape adds to the safety and comfort of the client. The normal rectal temperature (99.6°F) is 1° higher than the normal oral temperature (98.6°F).

Procedure

1. Gather the equipment needed.

   rectal thermometer
   lubricant
   tissues
   pad and pencil
   watch with second hand

   alcohol
   gloves

2. Wash your hands thoroughly and apply gloves.
3. Tell the client that you plan to take a rectal temperature. Provide for privacy. Do not expose the client unnecessarily.
4. Shake down the thermometer to 96°F (35.5°C).
5. Position client on left side, Sims' position. Cover the client with a sheet or blanket and remove the client's clothing from the rectal area of the body.
6. Lubricate the bulb tip of the thermometer with a water-soluble jelly and a tissue. This makes insertion easier and more comfortable.
7. Fold back the sheet or blanket to expose the client's buttocks. Raise top buttock with your hand and, with the other hand, gently insert bulb end of thermometer into the client's rectum about 1 to 1½ inches, Figure 32-6.

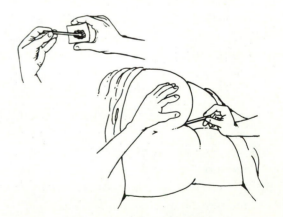

Figure 32-6   The rectal thermometer is lubricated and then inserted 1½ inches into the rectum. (From Hegner and Caldwell, *Nursing Assistant, A Nursing Process Approach*, 6E, copyright 1992 by Delmar Publishers Inc.)

Continued on the following page.

8. Redrape the client and hold the thermometer in place for 3 to 5 minutes. **Caution:** Do not let go of the rectal thermometer.
9. Remove the thermometer; wipe it from stem to bulb end (clean to dirty).
10. Discard contaminated tissue.
11. Read the thermometer and record the temperature. Record the time and place the letter *R* (rectal) beside the temperature reading.
12. Return the client to a comfortable position.
13. Clean the thermometer using soap and cold water or alcohol. Rinse it thoroughly. Store properly.
14. Remove gloves and wash your hands thoroughly after the procedure.

Client Care Procedure 51:
Taking an Axillary Temperature

Purpose

- To obtain the client's temperature reading when a rectal or oral reading is not possible.

NOTE: The axillary temperature is not the most accurate method of taking a temperature. However, it may be ordered by the nurse supervisor when an oral reading is not possible. Taking an axillary temperature is more convenient than taking a rectal temperature and is less embarrassing for the client. An axillary temperature is usually 0.5° to 1.0°F (0.28° to 0.56°C) lower than an oral temperature.

Procedure

1. Wash your hands before beginning the procedure.
2. Rinse the thermometer in cold water and wipe it dry with a tissue.
3. Shake down the thermometer so the mercury is below 96°F (35.6°C).
4. Dry the client's armpit with a tissue.
5. Place the thermometer in the center of the client's axilla (armpit) with the bulb end toward the client's head, Figure 32-7.

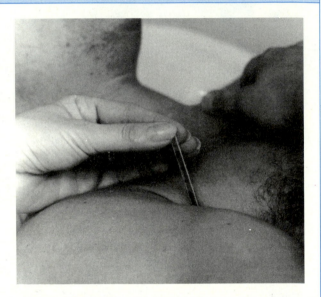

Figure 32-7   To take an axillary temperature, place glass thermometer in center of the client's axilla.

This position rests the bulb end against the blood vessel and a more accurate reading can be obtained.

6. Position the client's arm close to the body and place the client's forearm over the client's chest. This position enables the arm to hold the thermometer in place.

7. Leave the thermometer in place for 10 minutes.
8. Remove the thermometer and wipe it clean of any perspiration.
9. Read the temperature indicated on the thermometer. (A normal axillary temperature is 97.6°F.)

10. Record the temperature. An axillary temperature is recorded with an *Ax* beside the number, e.g., 97.6°F Ax.
11. Shake down the thermometer, clean it, and return it to its proper place.
12. Wash your hands following the procedure.

Client Care Procedure 52:
Taking the Radial and Apical Pulse

Purpose

- To measure, record, and observe the character of the client's pulse rate with confidence and accuracy
- To report changes or abnormal rates to the supervisor, nurse, or doctor

NOTE: A pulse is taken to determine its regularity, strength, and rate. Regularity is described as either regular or irregular. An irregular pulse may indicate skipped heartbeats or changing rhythm patterns. An irregular pulse should always be recorded.

Strength is described as bounding, strong, weak, or thready. If the strength has changed, the aide should call the supervisor.

Pulse rate is described as the number of beats per minute. The age, size, and sex of the client may influence the rate. Normal ranges in pulse rates are:

60–100 adults
70–90 children over 6 years of age
80–100 children under 6 years of age
100–130 infants

Procedure for Determining Pulse Rate

1. Gather the equipment needed.

wrist watch with a second hand
note pad and pen or pencil

2. Wash your hands before beginning the procedure.
3. Tell the client that you are going to check the pulse rate. Ask the client to help by remaining quiet and still while you are counting.
4. Have the client sit in a comfortable chair or lie in bed with arms resting gently on the chest.
5. Place the tips of your first two fingers on the pulse site. The radial pulse on the inner wrist is most often used, Figure 32-8. **Caution:** Do not use your thumb to

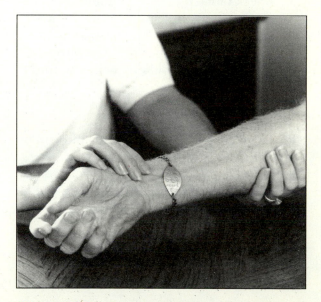

Figure 32-8 Locate the pulse on the thumb side of the wrist with the tips of your fingers.

Continued on the following page.

feel the client's artery. Using the thumb can result in an inaccurate reading.

6. Count the pulse beats for 1 full minute.
7. Record the pulse rate, regularity, and strength. Also record the time the pulse was taken. If irregular, take apical for 1 minute and record apical pulse.

Procedure for Taking Apical Pulse

1. Assemble equipment.

   stethoscope
   watch with second hand

2. Tell client what you plan to do.
3. Clean stethoscope earpieces and bell with disinfectant, Figure 32-9.
4. Place stethoscope earpieces in your ears.
5. Place the stethoscope diaphragm or bell over the apex of the client's heart, 2 to 3 inches to the left of the breastbone, below the left nipple.
6. Listen carefully for the heart beat. It will sound like "lub-dub."
7. Count the louder sound for 1 complete minute.
8. Check radial pulse for 1 minute. The best way to obtain these numbers is to have an aide count the apical pulse. Another aide may take the radial pulse at the same time the apical pulse is being counted, Figure 32-10.
9. Compare the results and note the numbers on a pad.
10. Clean earpieces and bell or diaphragm of stethoscope with alcohol wipe.
11. Document both pulse rates, i.e.,

    apical pulse = A 100 @10:00 AM
    radial pulse = R 92
    Pulse deficit: 8 (100 − 92 = 8)

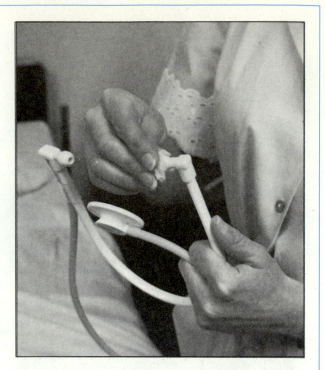

Figure 32-9   Carefully clean earpieces of the stethoscope before use. (From Hegner and Caldwell, *Nursing Assistant, A Nursing Process Approach,* 6E, copyright 1992 by Delmar Publishers Inc.)

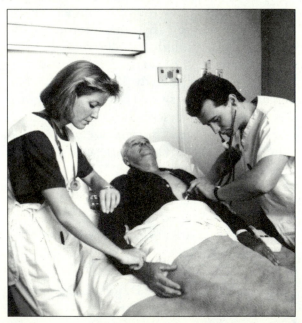

Figure 32-10   If another aide is present, it is better to take the apical and radial pulses at the same time. (From Hegner and Caldwell, *Nursing Assistant, A Nursing Process Approach,* 6E, copyright 1992 by Delmar Publishers Inc.)

Client Care Procedure 53:
Counting Respirations

Purpose

- To count the rate and observe the character of respirations

NOTE: Character of respirations is described as regular or irregular; labored, difficult, shallow, or deep; and noisy or quiet.

Normal respiration rate for adults is 16 to 20 breaths per minute.

Procedure

1. Gather equipment needed.

   wrist watch with a second hand
   note pad and pen or pencil

2. After client's pulse has been taken, leave the fingers in position on the wrist. By doing this, the client is not aware that you are counting respirations.

3. One rise and fall of the chest counts as one respiration. Count the number of respirations during a full 1-minute period.

4. Note how deeply the client breathes. Also check the regularity of the rhythm pattern. Note the sound of the breathing.

5. Record the number of respirations occurring in 1 minute. Record the character of the client's breathing.

6. Report changes from the client's usual way of breathing. Report any difficulty in breathing to the supervisor at once.

7. Wash your hands following the procedure.

Client Care Procedure 54:
Taking a Blood Pressure

Purpose

- To take blood pressure correctly
- To accurately report blood pressure readings to the case manager, nurse, or doctor

NOTE: Blood pressure is taken by the use of a sphygmomanometer (an instrument with a cuff, rubber bulb, and dial gauge for recording pressure) and a stethoscope (a listening device that magnifies sound).

Two readings are recorded: the systolic pressure is recorded first. This is the pressure that is felt in the artery when the heart contracts. The diastolic pressure is recorded second. This is the pressure that is felt in the artery when the heart is in the relaxation stage. The systolic rate is always higher than the diastolic rate. Normal blood pressure for an adult is about 120/80, although it may vary depending on age, sex, emotional state, exercise, and weight.

The cuff should be the right size for the client's arm; otherwise an incorrect reading may be obtained. Cuffs come in various sizes: child, normal adult, and extra large. It is important to read the mercury at eye level; therefore, it is best to take the readings while you are sitting down, next to the client.

Procedure

1. Gather equipment needed.

   sphygmomanometer
   stethoscope
   alcohol sponges or cotton balls

Continued on the following page.

2. Wash your hands before beginning the procedure.

3. Explain to the client what you plan to do. Have the client sit or lie in a comfortable position with one arm extended at the same level as the heart. The palm should be upward. Arm should be in resting position. Locate brachial pulse.

4. Pick up the stethoscope. Wipe the earpieces. Place the stethoscope around your neck.

5. Pick up the cuff and wrap it securely around the client's arm, about 1 inch above the elbow, Figure 32-11. Fasten. (Some cuffs have a Velcro fastener; others have hooks at the end of the cuff.) The center of the rubber bladder should be directly over the brachial artery. If the cuff is marked with an arrow, place cuff so that the arrow points over the brachial artery.

6. Attach the manometer (the dial gauge) to the top of the cuff so you can read it, Figure 32-12.

7. Tighten the small round valve that is located along the side of the rubber bulb. (This valve controls the pumping you will do later.)

8. With the tips of your fingers, locate the artery on the inside of the client's elbow, Figure 32-13. When you feel a throbbing beat, you have located the artery. Keep your fingers on the spot. Never use your thumb since it, too, has a pulse beat.

9. Place the round disk of the stethoscope over the artery you located on the client (slipping your fingers to hold it in place), Figure 32-14. With your other hand, insert the earpieces in your ear.

10. Take the rubber bulb in your hand. Look at the dial gauge while you pump air into the cuff by squeezing the bulb. Pump until the reading on the dial gauge is about 180 to 200.

11. Listen with the stethoscope placed in your ears and the disk over the artery. You should not hear any sound.

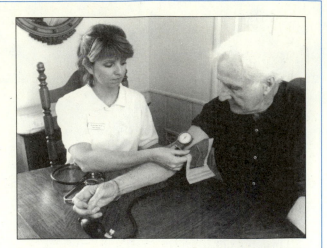

Figure 32-11 Apply cuff snuggly to arm at least 1 inch above the elbow.

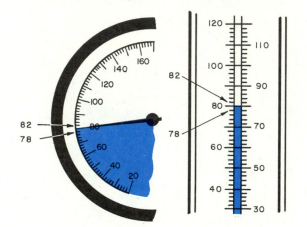

Figure 32-12 The aneroid gauge (*left*) and the mercury gravity gauge (*right*). Take reading at the closest line. (From Hegner and Caldwell, *Nursing Assistant, A Nursing Process Approach*, 6E, copyright 1992 by Delmar Publishers Inc.)

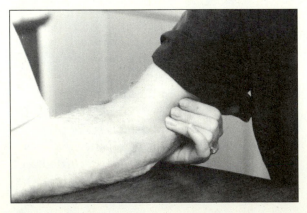

Figure 32-13 Locate and feel the brachial pulse.

12. While listening, slowly release the air by opening the valve located beside the bulb, using the thumb and forefinger. (This will cause air to escape from the cuff and the reading on the manometer will drop.) You may have to tighten the bulb valve if the air escapes too fast.

13. Listen carefully. When the first sound is heard, remember the number seen on the dial gauge. This is the systolic pressure.

14. Watch the dial continue to fall as the air escapes. When the thumping sound becomes a muffled sound, remember the number. This is the diastolic pressure.

15. Release the remainder of the air from the cuff and remove it, leaving the valve open.

16. Record the two readings, Figure 32-15. Blood pressure reading is written as a fraction with the systolic (top) listed first and the diastolic (bottom) written under the line; for example,

$$BP \frac{120 \text{ (systolic pressure)}}{80 \text{ (diastolic pressure)}}$$

17. **Caution:** Be careful not to pump the pressure too high. Remember that the pressure of the cuff can cause the client discomfort so it is important to release the air and work quickly when taking the blood pressure. If it is necessary to repeat the procedure, wait a few minutes before inflating the cuff; this allows the circulation to return to normal.

18. If you are unsuccessful in obtaining a blood pressure reading after three attempts, move to the client's other arm and try again, repeating the same procedure. (A reading taken after three attempts would probably be inaccurate and the client would become uncomfortable.) Never guess. If a blood pressure is hard to take or you are not sure, tell the nurse. Record reading.

19. Wash your hands following the procedure.

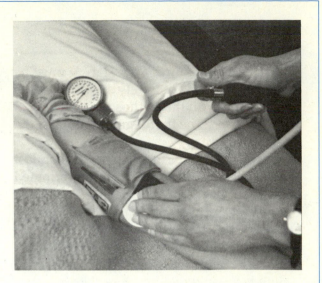

Figure 32-14   Place stethoscope diaphragm or bell right over the brachial artery. (From Hegner and Caldwell, *Nursing Assistant, A Nursing Process Approach,* 6E, copyright 1992 by Delmar Publishers Inc.)

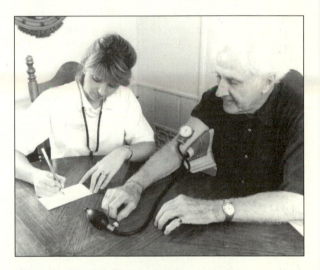

Figure 32-15   Record your reading right away. If repeat procedure is necessary, wait at least 1 minute.

Precautions
• If you are taking the blood pressure of a stroke client, use the unaffected arm only.
• If your client is having home dialysis (as part of a kidney treatment), or is receiving intravenous (IV) fluids, take the blood pressure on the unaffected arm.
• Do not inflate cuff unnecessarily high.

Client Care Procedure 55:
Measuring Weight and Height

Purpose

- To determine if unusual weight gain or loss has occurred
- To routinely check height

NOTE: Weight changes can make a difference in medical prescriptions and should be reported to the case manager. For instance, some medication amounts are determined by the weight of a client and a sudden or gross weight loss would require a lesser dosage.

Procedure

If the client is bedbound and cannot stand to be weighed, the case manager can bring a chair scale into the house. If the client is mobile, weight can be checked daily or weekly on a bathroom scale, Figure 32-16. Guidelines to follow:

1. Client should be weighed at the same time of day.
2. Client should be wearing the same amount of clothing each time.
3. Scale should be checked to see if it is balanced correctly.
4. Record and document weight.

NOTE: Height is not a common measurement for the elderly. As individuals age, there is some "settling" and a loss in height of perhaps an inch or two. If you need to take a height of an immobile client, you need a tape measure and a pad and pencil.

Procedure

1. Have client positioned in bed flat on his back with arms and legs straight.
2. Make a small pencil mark at the top of the client's head on the sheet.
3. Make a second pencil mark even with the feet.
4. Using the tape measure, measure the distance between the two marks.
5. Record the height on the paper and record in client's record.
6. If client can stand, have the client stand with his back to the wall. Mark the wall with a small pencil mark on top of client's head. Client is not to wear shoes.
7. Measure from floor to small pencil mark with tape measure.
8. Record on paper and then on client's chart.

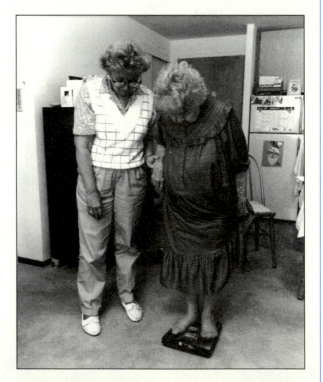

Figure 32-16   Weighing client using a portable bathroom scale

Unit 33 Hot and Cold Applications

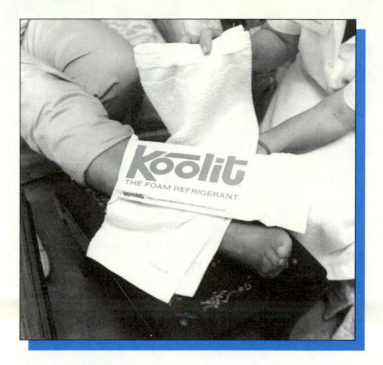

CLIENT CARE PROCEDURES

56. Applying an Ice Bag, Cap, or Collar
57. Applying a K-Pad—Moist or Dry

58. Performing a Warm Foot Soak

NOTE: All procedures are not allowed in all states. Make sure you are aware of limits as outlined by state guidelines.

LEARNING OBJECTIVES

After studying this unit, you should be able to:

- Demonstrate clear ability to perform all procedures.
- Explain the purpose of each procedure.
- State when the procedures should and should not be done.

- Identify precautions to be taken for each procedure.
- Recognize signs of client discomfort.
- Follow all rules of client safety when doing the procedures.

Client Care Procedure 56:
Applying an Ice Bag, Cap, or Collar

Purpose

- To ease pain or decrease swelling of localized area

NOTE: Cold applications such as an ice bag, ice cap, or collar should NOT be applied without a doctor's order. The supervisor will tell the aide when to apply ice and how to do it.

All ice applications must be covered with a cloth. Never apply ice or the cap, bag, or collar directly to the skin. A towel, face cloth, or fitted cover should be used against the skin.

Procedure

1. Wash your hands before beginning the procedure.
2. Fill an ice bag, cap, or collar with ice cubes or crushed ice. Use a spoon to transfer the ice. Fill the container half full so that its weight will not be uncomfortable for the client, Figure 33-1.
3. Place the bag on a flat surface with the top in place but not tightened. Hold the neck of the bag upright. Gently press the bag from the bottom to the opening in order to expel the air.
4. Secure lid firmly and wipe dry with paper towels. Periodically test for leakage.
5. Wrap ice bag in towel or soft cloth. Covering it protects the client's skin from direct contact. A disposable cold pack can also be used, Figure 33-2.
6. Apply to affected body area. Make sure that any metal parts face away from the skin. Place an extra towel around the bag if the skin appears sensitive to the cold.
7. Check the client's skin every 5 minutes. Look for signs of redness, whiteness, or cyanosis (blue color). If these signs appear, call the supervisor for instructions.

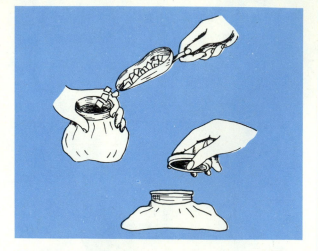

Figure 33-1   An ice bag should be half filled so it can lie flat against the client's body and not cause discomfort due to its weight.

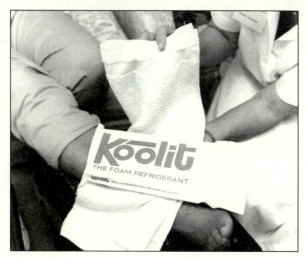

Figure 33-2   A disposable ice pack can be applied readily to a client's swollen ankle.

8. If ice melts, replace with fresh ice and continue treatment.
9. Remove ice bag after 20 minutes.
10. Empty bag, allow it to dry. Store it properly.
11. Return client to a comfortable position.
12. Wash your hands following the procedure.

Client Care Procedure 57:
Applying a K-Pad—Moist or Dry

Purpose

- To increase circulation to a body part
- To relax tension and relieve pain

Procedure

1. Assemble supplies.

    K-Pad and control unit
    distilled water
    cover for pad (a pillow case can be used)
    warm wet towel (if moist application)
    large plastic bag—optional

2. Wash your hands.
3. Tell client what you plan to do.
4. Place the control unit close to the client on a stand, Figure 33-3.
5. Remove the cover and fill the unit with distilled water to the fill line.
6. Screw the cover in place and loosen it one-quarter turn.
7. The temperature, usually 95°F to 100°F, is set by a key. Turn unit on and let the pad warm up a few minutes.
8. Cover pad and place it on the client. Secure the pad if necessary with tape. Never use pins. Be sure that the tubing is coiled on the bed or chair to facilitate the flow of water inside the pad. Do not let the tubing hang down below the chair or bed.
9. If the application is to be a moist application, warm a towel under hot water and wring out excess water. Wrap plastic bag and take to client. Apply moist towel, then K-pad and if necessary wrap with

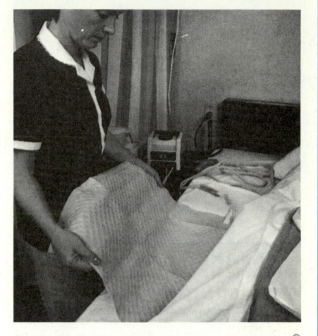

Figure 33-3 The disposable Aquamatic K-Pad® and control unit maintain an even temperature. (From Hegner and Caldwell, *Nursing Assistant, A Nursing Process Approach*, 6E, copyright 1992 by Delmar Publishers Inc.)

   plastic bag or linen protector to keep area around the moist application dry.
10. Note time of application. Follow orders on length of time the treatment should last.
11. Check the control unit periodically. Refill as needed.
12. Wash hands.
13. Document completion of the procedure, your observations, and client's reaction.

Client Care Procedure 58:
Performing a Warm Foot Soak

Purpose

- To stimulate circulation in a client's feet
- To relieve pain or discomfort
- To soften the toenails to make them easier to cut

NOTE: Never cut toenails unless supervisor directed and follow agency policies.

Procedure

1. Assemble equipment.

    large basin—plastic oblong dishpan
    warm water—100° to 110°F
    large plastic garbage bag or sheet of
       plastic
    small thin blanket
    2 towels

2. Wash hands and apply gloves.
3. Tell client what you plan to do.
4. Have client sit in comfortable chair if possible.
5. Place plastic bag on floor and place basin of water on top of plastic covering.
6. Remove client's shoes and socks and slowly place client's feet in basin of warm water, Figure 33-4. Be sure to follow any special instructions for special soaps or solutions that might be ordered.
7. Place thin blanket over the client's legs and feet.
8. Replenish water as necessary to maintain proper temperature.

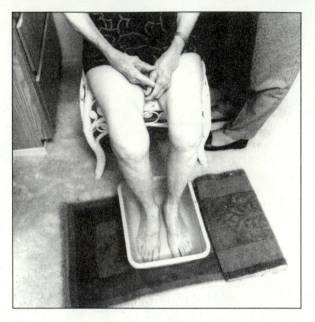

Figure 33-4   Client is sitting in comfortable chair while she soaks her feet.

9. Discontinue treatment in 20 to 30 minutes.
10. Remove feet from the basin and pat dry. Be sure to dry well in between toes. When feet are dry, massage lotion on both feet. Put shoes and socks on client's feet.
11. Clean up equipment and return to storage area.
12. Wash hands.
13. Document completion of procedure, your observations, and client's reaction.

Unit 34 Rectal Care

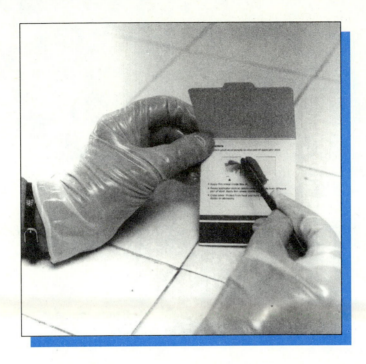

CLIENT CARE PROCEDURES

59. Giving a Commercial Enema
60. Giving a Rectal Suppository
61. Training and Retraining Bowels

62. Applying Adult Briefs
63. Collecting a Stool Specimen

NOTE: All procedures are not allowed in all states. Make sure you are aware of limits as outlined by state guidelines.

LEARNING OBJECTIVES

After studying this unit, you should be able to:

- Demonstrate clear ability to perform all the procedures.
- Explain the purpose of each procedure.
- State when the procedures should and should not be done.

- Demonstrate universal precautions when doing the procedures.
- Record and report results of all procedures.

Client Care Procedure 59:
Giving a Commercial Enema

Purpose

- To relieve the client of constipation
- To prepare client for diagnostic tests
- To make the client more comfortable

NOTE: An enema is the technique of introducing fluid into the rectum to remove feces and flatus (gas) from the rectum and colon.

Because enemas distend or dilate the rectum, the client may experience a feeling of urgency in the bowel, that is, a very strong need to empty the bowel as soon as possible.

Enemas can only be given on a doctor's orders.

The two commercially prepared enemas are the chemical (often referred to as Fleets) and oil retention enemas. Oil retention enemas are given to soften hard feces in the rectum and are usually followed by a soap solution enema.

Procedure

1. Assemble supplies, Figure 34-1.

   gloves
   commercial prepackaged enema
   protective pad
   bedpan (if client is bedridden)
   toilet paper
   lubrication jelly

2. Wash hands and put on gloves.
3. Tell client what you plan to do.
4. Provide for the client's comfort and privacy.
5. Have client turn to left side. Turn covers back to expose only the buttocks.
6. Remove cover on tip of enema. Apply extra lubricant to tip to ensure easy insertion.
7. Place protective pad underneath the client's buttocks.

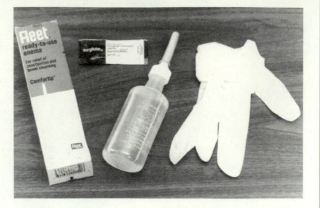

Figure 34-1   Equipment needed to give a commercial enema

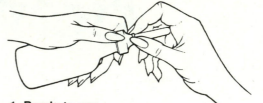

1. Ready to use

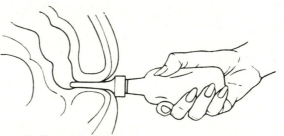

2. Easy to administer

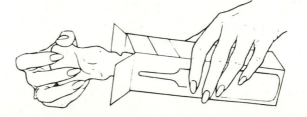

3. Disposable

Figure 34-2   Administering a commercial enema (Courtesy of C.B. Fleet Co., Inc. From Hegner and Caldwell, *Nursing Assistant, A Nursing Process Approach*, 6E, copyright 1992 by Delmar Publishers Inc.)

8. Separate the buttocks and insert tip into rectum for at least 3 inches. Tell client to take a deep breath and hold the solution as long as possible. Slowly squeeze the flexible plastic tube, Figure 34-2. This forces the solution to flow evenly into the rectum.

9. Remove enema tip while holding the client's buttocks together.

10. Position client on bedpan, commode, or toilet.

11. After client has expelled feces and enema solution, assist the client in cleaning area around anus and buttocks.

12. Return client to comfortable position. It may be necessary to leave the protective pad in place until the effects of the enema are complete.

13. Remove gloves and wash hands.

14. Record results of enema—color, amount, consistency—10:00 AM, Fleets enema given, good results—large, brown, formed stool.

Client Care Procedure 60:
Giving a Rectal Suppository

Purpose

• To relieve a client of constipation
• To make the client more comfortable

NOTE: A rectal suppository is a cone-shaped, easily melted, medicated mass that can readily be inserted into a client's rectum. Suppositories are usually stored in the client's refrigerator and are wrapped in foil. The suppository will melt once inserted into the warm environment of the rectum and colon. The suppository contains ingredients that once absorbed by the lining of the colon will give a stimulus to the colon to evacuate stool. It will take the suppository at least 5 to 10 minutes to melt. It is important that the aide inform the client to wait a few minutes after the suppository is inserted before trying to have a bowel movement.

Procedure

1. Assemble supplies.

   rectal suppository
   gloves
   lubricant
   protective pad or paper towels

2. Wash hands and apply gloves.
3. Tell client what you plan to do.

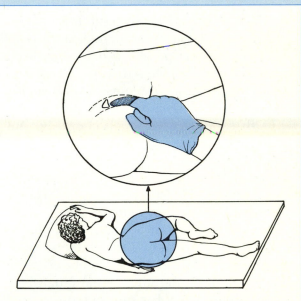

Figure 34-3 Carefully place the rectal suppository into the rectum about 3 inches for adult clients.

4. Open foil-wrapped suppository. Turn client to one side.

5. Lubricate gloved finger and insert suppository into rectum, Figure 34-3. Push the suppository along the lining of the rectum with your index finger as far as your finger allows. Be careful not to insert suppository into the feces. The suppository needs to be next to the lining of the colon for it to be effective.

Continued on the following page.

6. After 10 minutes has passed, assist the client to the toilet or commode.
7. After client has had a bowel movement, assist client back to bed or chair.

8. Observe results of elimination.
9. Remove gloves and wash hands.
10. Record results. It is important to note color, consistency, and amount.

Client Care Procedure 61:
Training and Retraining Bowels

Purpose

- To train a client to be continent of bowel movement
- To regulate a client to have regular bowel movement

NOTE: Constipation can result from illness, poor eating habits, drug therapy, and lack of exercise. Constipation causes the client added discomfort when it occurs in addition to other physical problems. An individualized bowel program is designed by the health care team for each client. For instance, one client can regulate the bowels by adding prune juice to the diet twice a day. Another client may need to drink daily prune juice but also needs a daily laxative and stool softener by mouth.

Older clients can become overly "bowel conscious" and have a misconception of what normal elimination should be. The frequency of bowel movements may range from three times a day for one person to only once every 2 or 3 days for another. Therefore, the term constipation should not be used to describe a missed movement or two, but only the unusual retention of fecal matter along with infrequent or difficult passage of stony, hard stool.

Among the elderly, constipation is very often encountered. If a client is unable to exercise and move about regularly, bowel action becomes sluggish. Sometimes medications, especially painkillers, can cause constipation. If a client has hemorrhoids,

there may be a fear of pain and so the client avoids trying to have a bowel movement. If a client does not have a bowel movement for a few days, the client may develop an impaction. An impaction is a large amount of hard stool in the lower colon or rectum. This is a very painful condition. If a client does develop an impaction, the nurse will need to remove it manually.

Procedure

1. Health care team assesses prior habits of client. If client always had a bowel movement early in the morning, this would be important to know in planning the client's retraining program.
2. A plan is designed and implemented. Important elements of the plan are:

   - high intake of fiber foods
   - adequate intake of liquids
   - regular exercise
   - toileting client at regular intervals
   - praise by aide of slightest progress of client
   - less reliance on laxatives and enemas
   - privacy for client for bowel movements

3. Follow bowel retraining program developed by the health care team. If plan does appear to be working, note success of program. If plan does not work, report. It is also important to give some suggestions to the health care team of possible solutions for retraining of the client.

Client Care Procedure 62:
Applying Adult Briefs

Purpose

- To keep incontinent client dry
- To minimize embarrassment to the client
- To reduce chance of urinary infections and reduce odor
- To minimize chance of pressure sore formation

NOTE: While bed pads are used to keep the sheets from becoming wet or soiled, special supplies can be used for both men and women. The adult brief comes in various styles and sizes. One design may be an insert to go inside a specially designed brief. Another popular type is a "wrap-around brief" fastened with Velcro-like tabs, Figure 34-4. It is important to have the correct size for your client to ensure their effectiveness. It is also important to read the instructions on the package on how to apply each particular style of brief. Many briefs do have a tab on them that changes color when the brief needs to be changed. The brief should be checked at regular intervals and changed as needed. Do not apply powder to the client's perineal area when adult briefs are used. Many of the briefs have special treated wipes to use to clean the client's perineal area

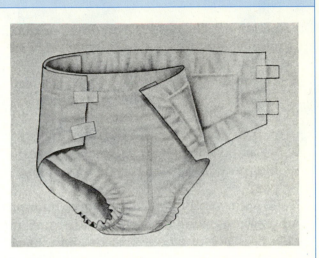

Figure 34-4 Wings® contoured incontinence briefs (*Wings® is a registered trademark of Professional Medical Products, Inc.* From Hegner and Caldwell, *Nursing Assistant, A Nursing Process Approach*, 6E, copyright 1992 by Delmar Publishers Inc.)

when changing the briefs. They are very reasonable in cost and are recommended over soap and water. If a certain brief does not appear to be working, report this to your case manager. There are many different types on the market, and some work better on some clients than others.

Client Care Procedure 63:
Collecting a Stool Specimen

Purpose

- To provide a stool sample for a diagnostic test

Procedure

1. Assemble needed supplies.

gloves
bedpan
specimen container or hemoccult slide packet with label completed

2. Inform client of need for specimen.

Continued on the following page.

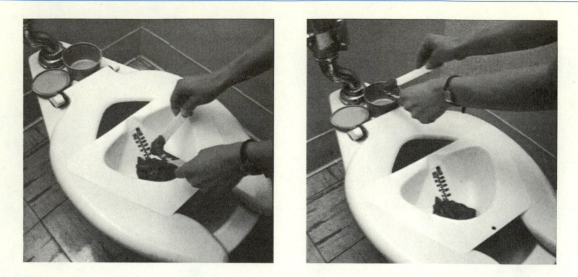

Figure 34-5   Use tongue blades to transfer the stool specimen from the collection container to the specimen container. (From Hegner and Caldwell, *Nursing Assistant, A Nursing Process Approach,* 6E, copyright 1992 by Delmar Publishers Inc.)

3. After client has defecated in bedpan, apply gloves and with wood applicator remove stool, Figure 34-5. If specimen is to be collected in specimen container, place small amount (approximately 1 tablespoon) of stool in container. If the test is for occult blood or guaiac, place small amount of stool on hemoccult blood card, Figure 34-6.
4. Place specimen in proper storage place. Be sure the specimen is sent to laboratory as directed by your supervisor.
5. Remove gloves and wash hands.
6. Document stool specimen collection.

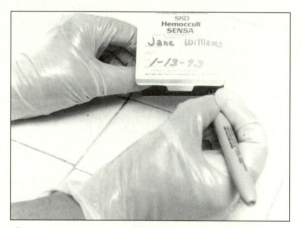

A

Figure 34-6   A. Fill in label on specimen card. B. Open card and apply a small sample of stool on the special area on the card for occult blood test.

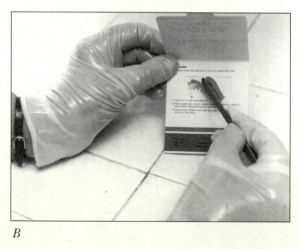

B

Unit *35* Special Treatment

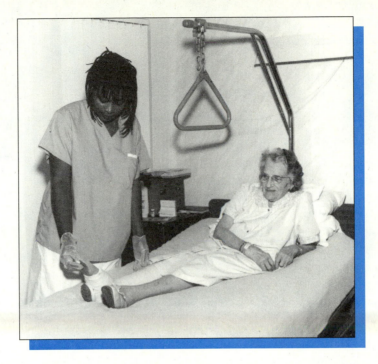

CLIENT CARE PROCEDURES

64. Applying Unsterile Dressing and Ointment to Unbroken Skin
65. Caring for Casts
66. Assisting with Changing an Ostomy Bag
67. Assisting the Client with Oxygen Therapy
68. Assisting with Cough and Deep Breathing Exercises

NOTE: All procedures are not allowed in all states. Make sure you are aware of limits as outlined by state guidelines.

LEARNING OBJECTIVES

After studying this unit, you should be able to:

- Demonstrate clear ability to perform all procedures.
- Explain the purpose of each procedure.
- State when the procedures should and should not be done.
- Be aware of precautions to take with each procedure.
- Report and record unusual different signs and symptoms that you observe.

Client Care Procedure 64:
Applying Unsterile Dressing and Ointment to Unbroken Skin

Purpose

- To absorb drainage from wound or incision area
- To protect area from contamination and irritation
- To reduce odor and keep client comfortable

NOTE: Most dressings will be changed as indicated by the nurse. On occasion when the dressing change is done by the home health aide, the aide should observe and record the color, amount, and consistency of the drainage; the progress of the healing; and the surrounding skin condition. **Caution:** Before changing dressings, the aide must have approval of the nurse supervisor.

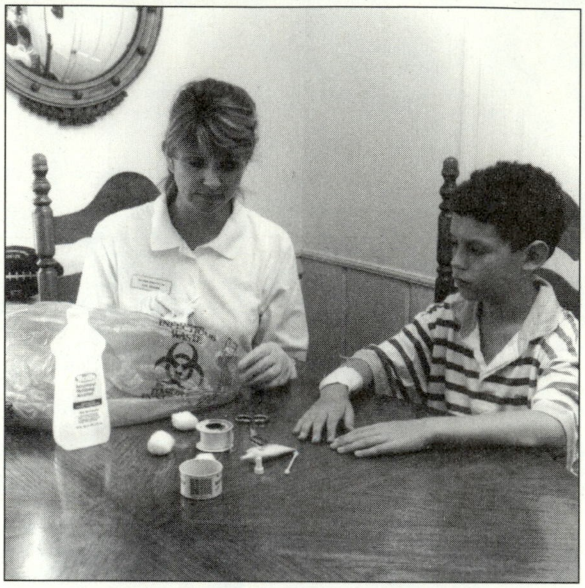

Procedure

1. Assemble supplies.

   two or more 4 × 4 gauze pads prepackaged
   gloves
   over-the-counter ointment (if ordered)
   receptacle for wastes, i.e., plastic bag
   tape and scissors

2. Wash your hands and apply gloves.
3. Tell client what you plan to do.
4. Position client so area with dressing is accessible while maintaining client comfort, Figure 35-1.
5. Remove old dressing. If the dressing does not lift off easily, pour hydrogen peroxide over it to loosen it. Discard used dressing in open waste receptacle (plastic bag). Note color, amount of drainage, and condition of surrounding skin.
6. Open the package of gauze pads without touching the pads, Figure 35-2. Be care-

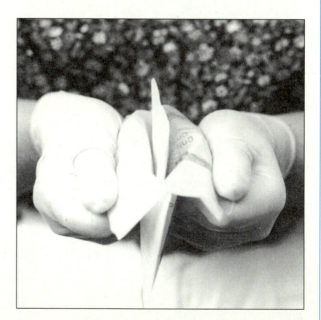

Figure 35-1 Assemble supplies and position client so area of dressing is accessible.

Figure 35-2 Correct method of opening dressing

ful not to have dressing touch bed linens or client's clothing. Cut tape. Apply ointment if ordered. Apply dressing. Do not touch center of dressing. Hold all dressings on the corners only. Apply tape correctly, Figures 35-3 and 35-4.

7. Position client comfortably.
8. Discard wastes and return supplies to storage. Be sure to follow universal precautions throughout this procedure.
9. Remove gloves and wash hands.
10. Record observations of the wound and skin condition. Report signs of redness, swelling, heat, foul odor, or amount of drainage. Document dressing was changed. In addition, report client complaints of pain around the wound.

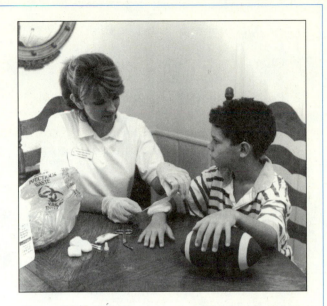

Figure 35-3   Apply tape correctly over dressing.

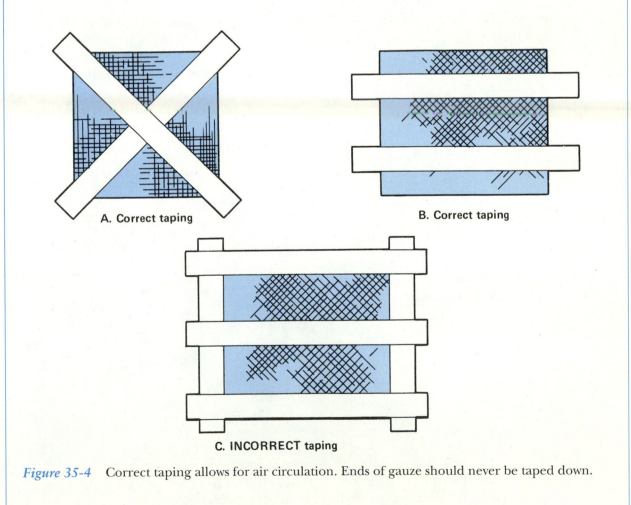

A. Correct taping

B. Correct taping

C. INCORRECT taping

Figure 35-4   Correct taping allows for air circulation. Ends of gauze should never be taped down.

Continued on the following page.

Topical Applications to Unbroken Skin

1. Obtain correct topical medication. Check label of medication with nursing care plan.
2. Position client so area is accessible, while maintaining client comfort.
3. Wash hands and apply gloves.
4. Apply medication in a thin layer to affected area only. Note color and appearance of skin.
5. Remove gloves and reposition client.
6. Wash hands.
7. Return medication to correct storage area.
8. Chart treatment and appearance of skin.

Client Care Procedure 65:
Caring for Casts

Casts are used to immobilize extremity or joint following trauma or fractures or to correct a body bone/joint defect. Casts may be applied to an extremity or to the entire body. Casts may be made of plaster of Paris, fiberglass, or polyester.

Purpose

- Promote healing of injured area that is casted
- Provide comfort to the client
- Prevent skin irritations and possible skin breakdown

Procedure

1. Observe the new cast every 2 to 3 hours for the first 2 days and then 4 times daily.

   - Note the color of the skin at the farthest end of cast—normal pink, warm to touch, and movable toes or fingers, Figure 35-5.
   - Look for edema at both ends of the cast; report and record this information.
   - Observe for response to touch (that is the response of the nerves to stimulation); report and record this information.

2. Observe the cast daily for roughness around the edges. This may cause skin irritation and may be filed or covered with soft padding. These rough edges can be covered with plain white tape. This is called petaling and can be done by the nurse.

3. Observe the cast itself, noting any redness that may indicate bleeding or drainage from under the cast. Circle the area with a magic marker, noting the date and time that you first notice the marking. Also note any unusual odor. Record and report immediately.

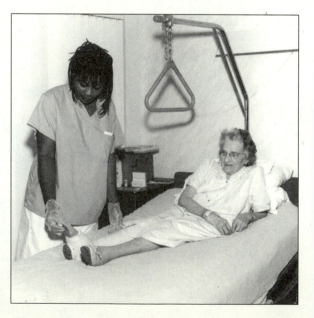

Figure 35-5   Frequently check the client's toes for warmth, color, and response to touch.

4. Observe the cast constantly for any cracks. Cracks are unsafe and you should notify your nurse supervisor of the crack. You must state the exact location and length of the crack as well as the depth of it.

5. When the cast is near the perineal area, protect it from moisture. Ask your case manager for special instruction on what waterproof or protective device to use. Protect the cast and skin by preventing any dirt, sand, or small articles from getting inside the cast, which could cause an infection under the cast. Note that plaster of Paris cast tends to crumble and become soft when moist; therefore, this type of cast must always be kept dry.

6. Ask the client if he/she has pain in any particular area under the cast. This may indicate a pressure point and skin breakdown under the cast. Note this area. Report and record immediately. Be sure to position your client correctly. Figure 35-6 shows several types of casts commonly applied.

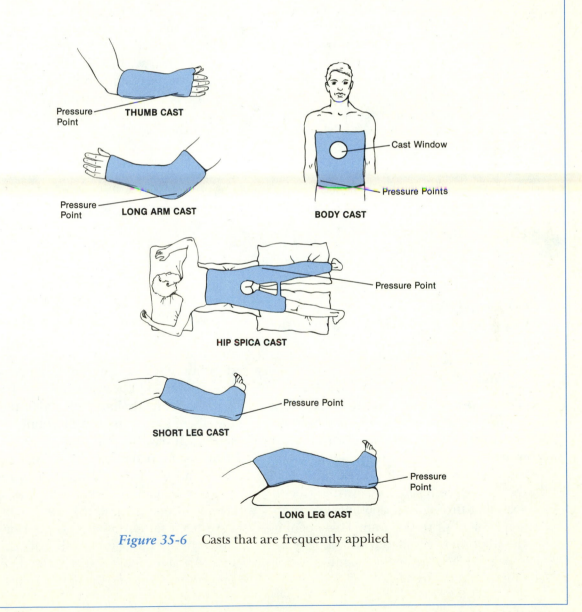

Figure 35-6   Casts that are frequently applied

Continued on the following page.

Safety for Client with a Cast

1. Check the house for throw rugs or objects on the floor. Remove any hazard that may cause the client to fall. Remind client to leave a night-light on to prevent a fall in the middle of the night.
2. Remember that at first the client may not have a good sense of balance and may be unsteady in walking. Arrange the furniture so that the client may hold on to furniture or handrails while walking.
3. Assist the client in making changes in eating, dressing, writing, toileting, and walking.
4. Ask the case manager for specific orders for passive range of motion exercises. A physical therapist or occupational therapist may come to assist the client with specific exercises. A home health aide may not perform these exercises without orders and direct supervision.
5. Determine the composition of the cast by asking the case manager. Plaster of Paris casts take at least 24 hours to dry, while polyester or fiberglass casting tape takes 5 to 15 minutes to dry. Be sure you do not touch the wet cast because fingers may leave dents in the cast. Do not allow cast to dry on hard surface, as this will flatten the cast. Do place entire new cast on pillows and expose to air. Do not allow client to put anything between the cast and the skin if the skin under the cast starts to itch. If itching becomes unbearable, air can be blown in by use of a hair dryer, if the nurse supervisor gives you permission to do this. When positioning a client with an extremity cast, elevate the cast on pillows. Generally it is not allowable to have the client lie on the injured side. Instruct the client to wiggle toes or fingers frequently on cast extremity. Do not cover cast extremity because air needs to be allowed to circulate inside the cast.

Client Care Procedure 66:
Assisting with Changing an Ostomy Bag

Purpose

- To keep the client clean
- To prevent skin breakdown around the stoma
- To regulate and establish a daily routine for removing wastes

NOTE: An ostomy bag is sometimes called a stoma bag. It is used for clients who have had a surgical operation called a colostomy or an ileostomy. In these operations, the intestine is cut and brought to the outside of the body, Figure 35-7. Body wastes (feces) are expelled through an opening in the abdomen instead of the rectum. This opening on the abdomen is called a **stoma.** The ostomy bag is placed over the opening to collect the wastes, Figure 35-8.

Until a client has adjusted to using the ostomy bag there may be strong feelings of embarrassment. The home health aide can help the client accept the inconvenience by being understanding. The aide should not show displeasure in assisting the client. An ostomy bag should be changed when it becomes one-third or one-half full. Once regulated the client can change it at about the same time each day. In some cases, the client may wear a gauze pad instead of a bag or pouch.

In addition to changing the bag, the client may need to wash out the intestines. If the client needs to do this, the client would have been taught at the hospital or by the nurse how to irrigate (wash out) the intestine. An aide may assist the client with this procedure. However, the aide may not do the

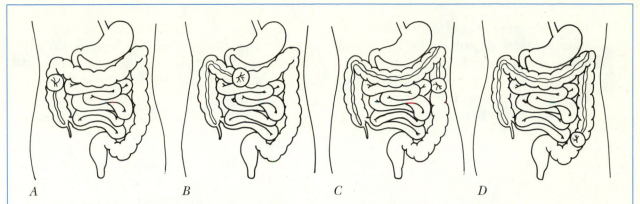

Figure 35-7   Colostomy sites vary depending upon the part of the bowel that needs to be removed. *A.* Assending colostomy. *B.* Transverse colostomy. *C.* Descending colostomy. *D.* Sigmoid colostomy. (From Hegner and Caldwell, *Nursing Assistant, A Nursing Process Approach,* 6E, copyright 1992 by Delmar Publishers Inc.)

procedure unless advanced training in the procedure has been learned and the agency requirements have been met.

The bags and attachments come in many styles today. They are lighter, odor proof, and fit more tightly. Many types of bags and appliances are available; a few require a belt to attach the appliance, others do not require a belt. Colostomy bags can be in one-piece disposable pouches or two-piece disposable pouches. A popular method of attachment is with a synthetic preparation resembling real skin that is attached to the area around the stoma. This artificial skin can stay on indefinitely. On this artificial skin is a raised seal that the colostomy bag may attach to. This artificial skin protects the real skin from irritation and contamination with the client's feces and also serves as a place where the colostomy bag can be put on and taken off. Another popular method of attaching a colostomy bag is with a brown colored gum-type substance called Karaya, which does not irritate the client's skin and prevents skin breakdown. Your nurse will give you special instructions on the type of skin attachment and bag the client is using.

Procedure

1. Assemble supplies.

   basin of warm water and soap

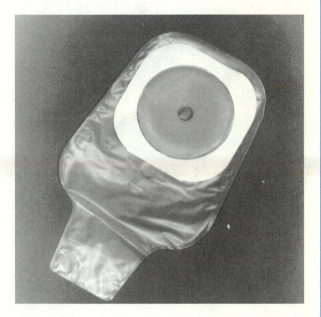

Figure 35-8   Stoma protector and drainage bag

   clean ostomy bag
   double bags
   gloves
   skin ointment (if ordered)
   toilet tissue

2. Wash your hands and apply gloves.
3. Tell client what you plan to do.
4. Gently remove soiled colostomy bag from the stoma. Place in double-bagged receptacle. In a few instances, the colostomy bag can be washed and reused.

Continued on the following page.

5. If there is stool on the skin remove with toilet tissue. Wash area around the stoma with mild soap and water. Pat the area dry. Occasionally a special substance may be applied to assist the new colostomy bag to adhere better.
6. Apply ointment if ordered. Observe area around the stoma for redness or open areas.
7. Apply client's pouch.

   • If one-piece pouch or bag is being used, remove self-stick backing from new ostomy appliance. Press the new bag to the area around the stoma, being sure to seal tightly.
   • If two-piece pouch is being used, be sure to cut opening to the correct size. (A few bags are premeasured and this step is not necessary.) Remove adhesive backing on face plate. Firmly apply face plate to client's skin around stoma, working from the stoma outward. Then apply the bag to this face plate. Let your client assist you as much as possible. Be sure to follow any special manufacturer's instruction in application of appliance.

8. Assist the client to connect belt to appliance, if client is using this type of appliance.
9. Remove wastes. Observe stool for color, amount, and consistency. If necessary spray the room with deodorizer.
10. Remove gloves and wash hands.
11. Document procedure and time, your observations, and client's reaction.

Client Care Procedure 67:
Assisting the Client with Oxygen Therapy

Purpose

• To assist the client to receive correct amount of oxygen ordered
• To avoid misuse of oxygen equipment and careless practices that risk causing fires, explosions, or injury
• To describe two devices used to administer oxygen
• To assist with special mouth care for client receiving oxygen therapy

Procedure

1. Check the meter of the oxygen tank or reservoir. If low, check to see if there is a spare tank. If there is not a spare tank, call for a replacement.
2. Wash your hands before beginning the procedure.

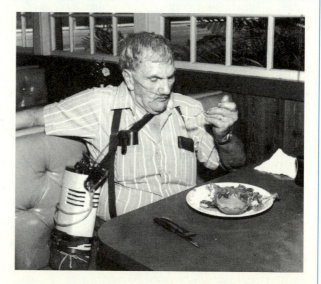

Figure 35-9   Client is receiving oxygen through a nasal cannula.

3. Check to see if the client oxygen mask or cannula is placed properly, Figure 35-9. The straps on the cannula should be secure but not too tight. Check top of ears for signs of irritation. Check for signs of irritation where the prongs touch the client's nose. Be sure both prongs are in the client's nose.

   If a mask is being used, check to see whether the mask is over both nose and mouth. If inside of mask is wet, remove and dry inside.

4. Check the gauge to see if the oxygen is being given at correct amount of liter flow, Figures 35-10 and 35-11. (Oxygen therapy is delivered in liters.) The client's care plan should state the liter flow to be administered to the client. Follow any special instructions that the respiratory therapist may prescribe.

5. Check the client position. If in bed, elevate the head with three pillows to assist the client in breathing, Figure 35-12.

6. Check to see if there is an adequate water supply for the humidifier, Figure 35-13. If

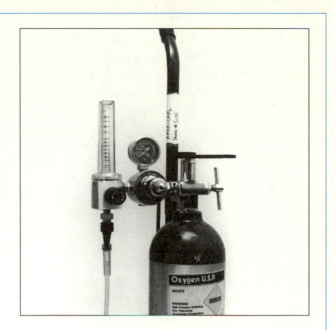

Figure 35-11   No. 1 gauge notes the liter flow. No. 2 gauge notes the amount of oxygen left in the tank.

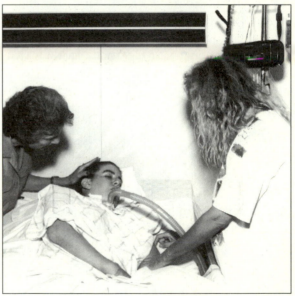

Figure 35-12   This young client is receiving oxygen through her tracheotomy.

you need to refill the humidifier, it is best to use distilled water. Humidification means adding moisture to oxygen. Oxygen is dry and can be irritating if used alone. Use of a humidifier with oxygen therapy is optional; some individuals do

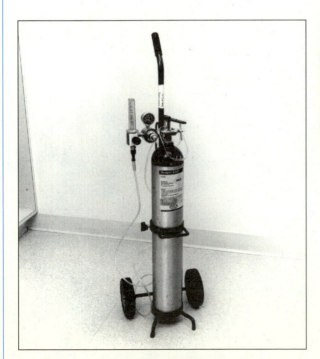

Figure 35-10   Portable oxygen tank

Continued on the following page.

not require it. The respiratory therapist will instruct you on proper procedure on how to refill the humidifier on the oxygen tank your client has.

7. Do frequent mouth care for clients receiving oxygen therapy. Client's mouth can become dry and have an unpleasant taste. Apply lubricant to lips, if permitted, if they become dry.

8. Check that all safety precautions are being observed.

- Do not smoke in room where client is receiving oxygen. Post "No Smoking" sign, if necessary, to warn visitors not to smoke.
- Do not use matches, candles, or open flames where oxygen is used or stored.
- Do not use electrical appliances during oxygen therapy. Avoid sparks. If you need to shave the client, turn off the oxygen while using the electric razor.
- Avoid use of woolen blankets, which may create static electricity sparks.

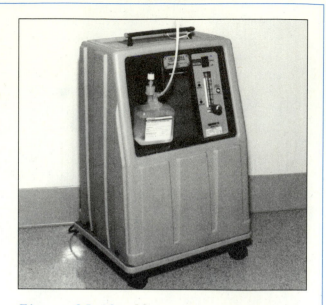

Figure 35-13   Many types of portable oxygen devices are available. This type can be readily moved from one room to another in a client's home.

9. Wash your hands.
10. Document the liter flow and the device being used, your observations, and client's reaction.

Client Care Procedure 68:
Assisting with Cough and Deep Breathing Exercises

Purpose

- To prevent congestion or infections in the client's lungs
- To expand the lungs

Procedure

1. Wash your hands.
2. Tell client what you plan to do and ask for cooperation, Figure 35-14.
3. Assemble equipment needed.

gloves—optional
pillow case-covered pillow
tissues
small basin or receptacle

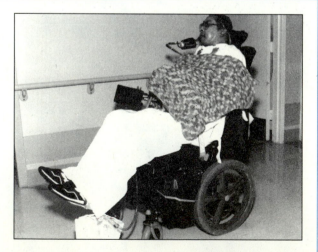

Figure 35-14   This client is a quadriplegic and needs to be encouraged to cough and deep breathe to prevent upper respiratory infections.

4. Have client sit up if possible.
5. Have client place hands on either side of rib cage or operative site.

   A pillow over operative site may be used to support incision during the breathing exercises.
6. Ask client to take as deep a breath through the nose as possible and hold it for 5 to 7 seconds and then exhale slowly through pursed lips.
7. Repeat this exercise about five times unless the client is too tired.
8. Give client tissues and instruct client to take a deep breath and cough forcefully twice with mouth open. Collecting any secretions that are brought up in tissues. Protect yourself from secretions and droplets.
9. Put on gloves if you will be touching or handling the tissues.
10. Dispose of tissues in plastic bag and assist client to comfortable position.
11. Remove gloves and wash hands.
12. Document procedure completed, your observations, and client's reaction.

Unit 36 Infant Care

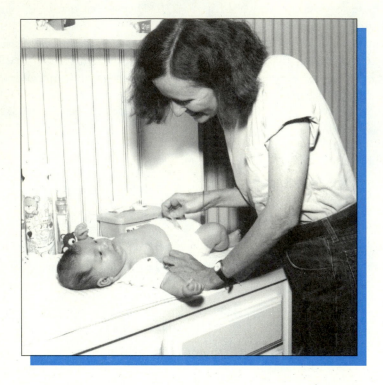

CLIENT CARE PROCEDURES

69. Assisting with Breast-feeding and Breast Care

70. Giving the Infant a Sponge Bath

71. Bottle-feeding the Infant

NOTE: All procedures are not allowed in all states. Make sure you are aware of limits as outlined by state guidelines.

LEARNING OBJECTIVES

After studying this unit, you should be able to:

- Demonstrate clear ability to perform all procedures.
- Explain the purpose of each procedure.
- State when the procedures should and should not be done.
- Identify precautions to be taken with each procedure.

Client Care Procedure 69:
Assisting with Breast-feeding and Breast Care

Purpose

- To provide for cleanliness and prevention of infection to the breasts
- To prevent breasts from sagging and losing muscle tone
- To protect the nipples and observe for cracking or signs of soreness
- To protect the infant from bacterial infection
- To provide for the mother's comfort before, during, and after nursing the child
- To nourish infant
- To promote mother–child interaction

Procedure*

1. Provide supplies.

   mild soap
   warm water in basin
   clean washcloth and towel
   clean nursing bra (or well-fitting support bra)
   nursing pads
   cotton balls
   rinse water in basin (at feeding time)
   clock or watch to time nursing period

2. Wash your hands thoroughly before beginning the procedure.
3. Help the mother to wash her hands before handling the breasts.
4. Help the mother open the front of her dress or shirt top, if needed. Have mother wash nipples in warm water and mild soap using a circular motion, washing from the nipple outward. Rinse and dry the breasts thoroughly.
5. Have mother sit in comfortable position in a rocking chair with armrest and foot-

stool to support the feet. If mother is still on bed rest, help her lie on one side.
6. Change infant's diaper; wash your hands thoroughly after the diaper change.
7. Bring child to mother. Make sure infant's nose is not pressed against the mother's breast. The nostrils must be free so the infant can breathe as it nurses. Follow procedure as taught in hospital unless unsuccessful.
8. The nursing period is gradually built up from just a few minutes to a maximum of 20 minutes. Some mothers prefer to let baby nurse at both breasts (one at a time) during one feeding period. Others will feed the infant only at one breast for each 20-minute feeding period. They alternate breasts at different feedings.
9. To remove the baby's mouth from the breast, have mother press on two sides of nipple to release the suction.
10. At the end of the feeding period, return baby to crib. Make sure baby has been burped before it is laid down. Change diaper if necessary.
11. Wash your hands before continuing with the procedure.
12. Help the mother with her bra, putting fresh nursing pads over the nipples to absorb any leakage. If nipples are sore or cracked, have the mother contact the nurse. An ointment or medication may be prescribed. Report these problems to the case manager.
13. Return supplies to storage.
14. Wash your hands following the procedure.

*La Leche League suggests that washing the nipple before each feeding can lead to drying and cracking and should be avoided. Consult your physician.

Client Care Procedure 70:
Giving the Infant a Sponge Bath

Purpose

- To clean and refresh infant
- To observe skin tone, activity, and signs of abnormality or unusual changes in behavior

Procedure

1. Bring needed supplies to kitchen table or baby's bath table.

   warm water in basin (test temperature)
   towel and washcloth
   bath sheets
   diapers (cloth or disposable paper)
   bath oil
   baby lotion
   baby shampoo
   change of clothing (undershirt, gown, etc.)
   mild soap

2. Wash your hands thoroughly before beginning the procedure.
3. Lower siderail of crib. Keep the rail raised to its highest position whenever infant is in crib. Bring infant to bathing area.
4. Place infant on bath sheet and undress, Figure 36-1. Drop soiled diaper into diaper pail. Close diaper pins and keep out of baby's reach. **Caution:** NEVER leave the baby unattended while it is on the bath table.
5. Place infant in bath basin, Figure 36-2. Wash the infant's face with warm water only. Do not use soap on the face. Pat face dry. Make sure ears are carefully dried. Wash neck and pat dry. Rub in small amount of lotion around creases in baby's neck.
6. Gently apply a small amount of soap over baby's head and lather well to remove crust, Figure 36-3. Rinse soap away by

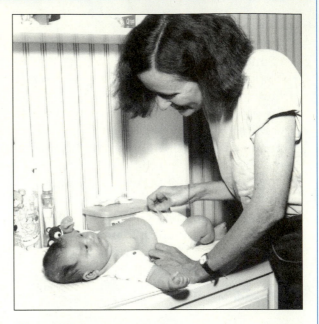

Figure 36-1   Undress infant. Note home health aide is talking to infant.

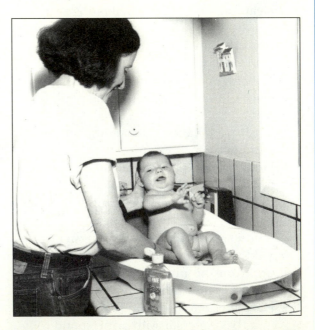

Figure 36-2   Slowly place infant into basin. Be sure to test temperature of water before placing infant in the basin.

holding head over basin as you repeatedly wipe head with wet washcloth. Keep soap out of infant's eyes. If soap is left on scalp, it will cause scales to crust and collect. Dry scalp carefully. Rub on baby oil.

7. Lather your hands and apply soap to the infant's hands, arms, and chest. Rinse completely with washcloth.

8. Apply soap to abdomen and legs and lather well. Rinse with washcloth.

9. Turn infant on the stomach and lather the infant's back; rinse and dry.

10. Wash, rinse, and dry genital (perineal) area last, Figure 36-4. Uncircumcised males should have the foreskin pushed back gently and the area washed with water only. Wash the penis and folds of the scrotum. Dry infant, Figure 36-5.

11. Dress infant, Figure 36-6. Return to crib or playpen.

12. Return supplies to storage. Clean up area where bath was given.

13. Wash your hands following the procedure.

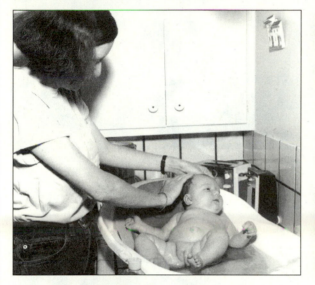

Figure 36-3   Massage scalp gently.

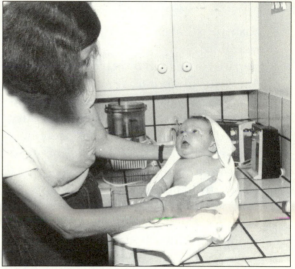

Figure 36-5   Dry infant with large, soft towel.

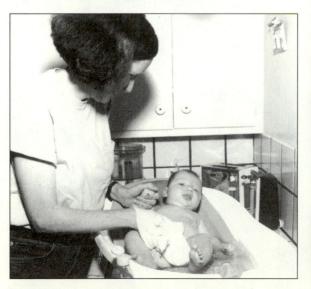

Figure 36-4   Wash, rinse, and dry genital area.

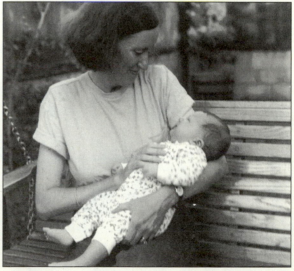

Figure 36-6   Dress infant. Talk and play with infant if time allows.

Client Care Procedure 71:
Bottle-feeding the Infant

Purpose

- To provide nutrition
- To give infant the security of being held, cuddled, and bonded
- To provide opportunity to observe infant's responses, color, skin condition, etc.

Procedure

1. Wash your hands before beginning the procedure.
2. Prepare formula as directed, Figure 36-7. Pour into baby bottle, Figure 36-8.
3. Change infant's diaper, if necessary, so infant will be comfortable, clean, and dry while eating. Wrap infant loosely in a clean receiving blanket. Leave infant in crib with side rails up.
4. Wash your hands.
5. Bring warm bottle to table next to a comfortable rocker or armchair.
6. Support infant's head and back when picking it up from the crib. Sit comfortably in chair, holding child securely in a comfortable position for taking nipple; start to feed the infant. Do not prop bottle, Figure 36-9.

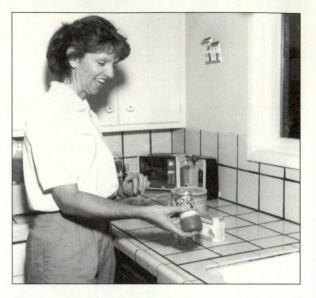

Figure 36-8 Gently shake the water and powdered formula well.

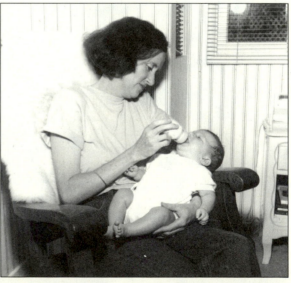

Figure 36-9 Sit in comfortable chair to feed the infant, preferably a rocking chair.

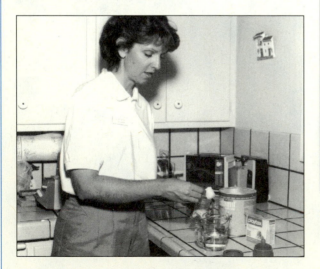

Figure 36-7 Prepare formula as directed.

7. When infant has had 2 to 3 ounces, either sit the infant upright on your lap and gently pat back, Figure 36-10, or hold the infant over your shoulder and pat its back until the infant burps.

8. Continue feeding and burping, Figure 36-11, until infant is finished or shows no interest in eating. Do not force infant to take more than it wants.

9. When the baby is finished, burp it once more then place it in the crib lying it on its side or stomach. DO NOT PLACE THE INFANT ON BACK. If infant should regurgitate, there would be a possibility of causing serious health hazard.

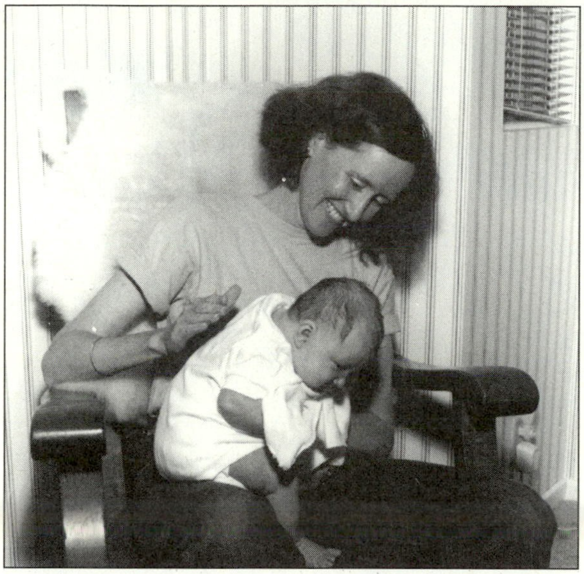

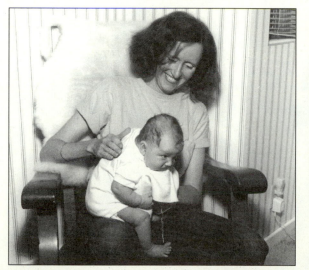

Figure 36-10 Burp the infant after every 2 to 3 ounces.

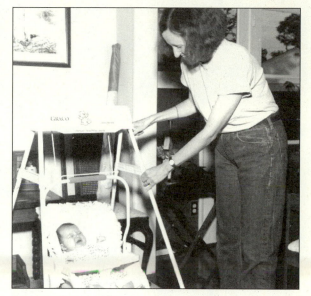

Figure 36-12 An infant may be placed in a musical swing at periodical intervals during the day.

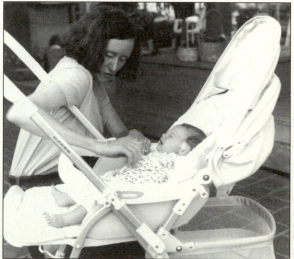

Figure 36-11 When done feeding infant, rub the infant's back a few seconds. An infant can also be burped in this position.

Figure 36-13 Infants do enjoy a short ride in a baby stroller.

Continued on the following page.

10. Wash your hands following the procedure.

Caution: Do not put infant to bed with bottle and do not prop bottle.

Spend as much time as you can with the infant and interact with the infant, Figures 36-12 through 36-14.

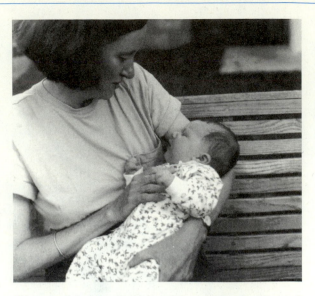

Figure 36-14   Infants like to be held and talked to.

Section 8

Employment

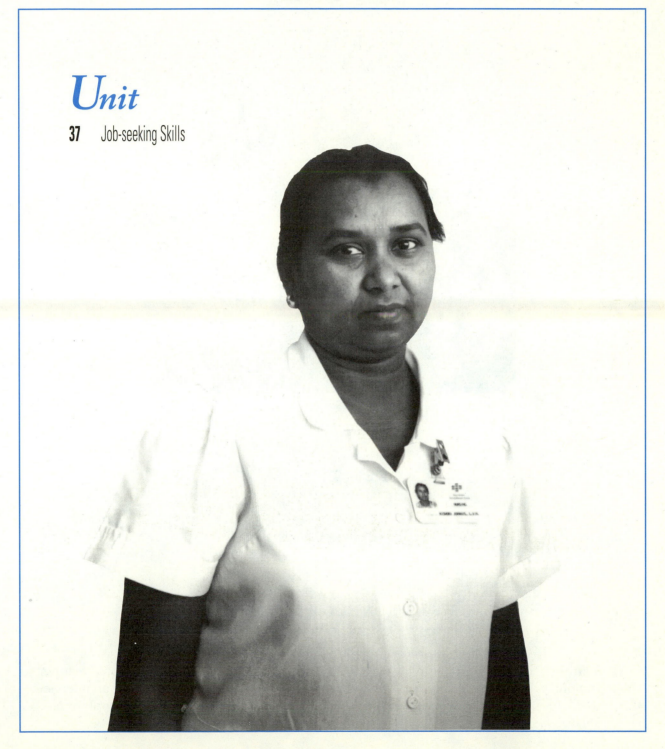

Unit

37 Job-seeking Skills

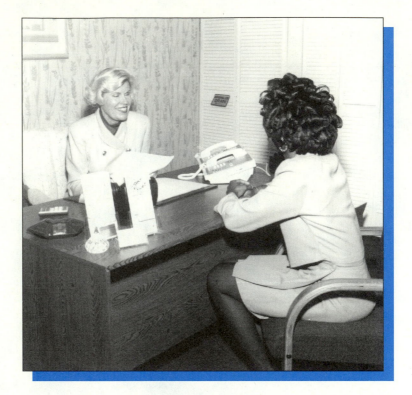

KEY TERMS

. . . .

diagnosis related groups
infraction

misconduct
personal reference

registry service

LEARNING OBJECTIVES

. . . .

After studying this unit, you should be able to:

- Accurately fill out an employment application.
- Prepare a resume and/or personal information sheet.

- Present yourself in a professional manner to a prospective employer during an interview.
- Select an agency to apply for employment.

One of the more difficult tasks faced by anyone is entering a new situation. As a student, you were probably afraid you would not be able to pass the tests, recite in class, or demonstrate a skill to the teacher in front of the other students. However, if you have passed your course for home health aide, you have already met these challenges. Now as a graduate, you are facing a new challenge—putting your new-found skills to work.

Until now, you have been guided by your instructor(s) and for the most part have worked in a team situation with your fellow students. Now you are on your own. You must "sell" yourself and your skills to an employer.

You must make your own decisions as to what kind of clients you would rather work with. Do you want part-time or full-time work? Do you want a sleep-in job? Would you rather work with elderly clients who mainly need companionship and minimal care, or do you want to use all your skills and deal with complex medical problems? Do you prefer working with children or are you willing to take whatever jobs are open?

Trends Affecting Employment

Knowledge about home care has become increasingly important in recent years. Since October 1983, Diagnosis Related Groups system for reimbursing hospitals has encouraged early discharge of patients and treating patients more on an outpatient basis in order to control costs. The most recent Medicare data show that the average annual cost per Medicare beneficiary receiving inpatient hospital care was $5360, nursing home care ranged between $15,000 to $30,000 per year, home health care range was $50–$200 per day. Medicaid is currently paying 44% of the cost of nursing home care. What this means to you is more and more people are going to choose home care for economic reasons.

Another trend occurring is the change of focus of hospitals to a more community concept approach rather than providing only acute care services for the patient. A few hospitals are now offering or sponsoring Adult Day Care and Continuing care retirement communities. Other housing arrangements are also becoming popular that allow the person to remain at home and maintain independence. A few examples of these options are: house sharing, where two or more unrelated people live together in a combination of shared and common space; board and care homes that provide a room and 3 meals a day and personal care services; congregate housing facilities that offer independent living with central dining and social and recreational programs.

Government programs are also providing funds for home-delivered meals, friendly visits, telephone reassurance and chore services. (Chore services done by the chore aide usually include services such as shopping, marketing, transportation, and heavy cleaning.) These services may be offered free of charge or on a sliding scale fee basis. In some cases, both cost savings and increased independence can be achieved by using various home health care services plus housing options instead of nursing homes. These different housing options provide a variety of employment opportunities for the home health aide.

The demand for health care and assistance with activities of daily living by the young as well as the old will continue to increase. Americans age 85 and older—those most at risk—are the fastest growing segment of our population, and 49% of these individuals will need some assistance in their personal care needs. The rise in the number of individuals with AIDS will also increase the need for additional home health aides. Health care services rank in the top five in the nation as far as job opportunities are concerned.

Contacting Prospective Employers

Your first step toward finding a job is to know where to look. There are local and national agencies in most areas that are listed in the telephone book. Your instructor may also be able to give you a list of addresses and phone numbers. You can look in the employment section of your local newspaper; you can contact your local department of social services; and you can see if your hospitals have a **registry service** where you may apply. Some medical groups also have lists of clients who need home health aides.

Make a list of those places you plan to contact; then keep a record of the date you called and any appointments you may set up. Remember, you may register at several agencies and you may work for more than one agency on a part-time basis. When you phone for an appointment, know what you want to say. "I am a graduate of the ABC home health program, and I am looking for work. May I have an appointment?"

The Job Interview and Application Form

When you go to your appointment remember that personal appearance is very important. Dress neatly and look your very best.

It is better to go alone to the interview. Bringing someone with you to the interview may give the impression that you are not able to make decisions alone.

Before you go to the interview, learn all you can about the agency. (Check in the yellow pages to see what services they offer, ask employees about what type of clients they serve, etc.). It is also good to familiarize yourself with typical questions and decide how you will answer them. Determine what you will wear. Dress neatly and conservatively—remember you only have one chance to make a first impression.

Arrive at least 15 minutes early and alone. This will tell your prospective employer that you are prepared to arrive on time for your assignments if you are hired.

Introduce yourself to the interviewer by name, with a smile and *firm* handshake and eye contact. Always be polite, speak clearly, sit or stand straight, and use correct grammar—no slang. Do not chew gum or smoke during the interview. Answer all questions truthfully and with more than one word. Be ready to talk about the training and experiences you have had. Be positive about former employers and working conditions. Be honest about the kind of cases you prefer. Take a copy of certification, Social Security card, and also an official ID. Be

prepared with questions that will help you make a sound decision about accepting the position if offered. Suggested questions are:

- How far will I need to travel to and from each client? Is public transportation available or will I need to have an automobile?
- What are the fringe benefits? Is health insurance available and for what cost? Do I get holiday or vacation pay? Do I get sick days? Is there a pension plan available?
- Is child care available? If so, at what times and what is the cost? Do they take infants?
- What shift or shifts will I be expected to work?
- If the position is part-time, is there a possibility of a full-time position soon?
- Is there a mechanism in place for advancement or additional training?
- If traveling is required between clients, is mileage paid? If so, how much per mile?

Listen carefully to your interviewer. Do not immediately ask about salary unless the employer brings it up first. This information is usually supplied by the interviewer toward the end of the interview. If you are unclear about information on the position, ask questions.

You should not anticipate receiving a definite indication of a job offer or rejection at the end of the interview. The interviewer will usually let you know when you will be contacted. Be sure to thank the interviewer as you leave.

After the interview has taken place, send a thank-you letter and again express an interest in the position. Try to evaluate the interview to discover ways to improve on the next one. It is all right to call the agency in a few days to inquire about the status of the position.

The Application Form

Have an information sheet with you listing some facts that usually appear on an application form. This will save you time and you won't make foolish errors when you fill out the application. Some of the facts that you should have on your information sheet are listed in Figure 37-1.

CUSHMAN MANAGEMENT ASSOCIATES

EMPLOYER:

APPLICATION FOR EMPLOYMENT

We are an equal opportunity employer. Federal and state laws prohibit discrimination in employment practices based on race, color, religion, sex, age, handicap, disability, or national origin. No question on this application is asked for the purpose of limiting or excluding any applicant's consideration for employment because of his or her race, color, religion, sex, age, handicap, disability, or national origin.

Name: Last	First	Middle	Social Security No.	Telephone No.

Address: Street	City	State	Zip Code	Licensed Nurses Only	
				Mass. Reg. No.	Date Granted:
If your records may be under a name other than indicated above, please specify:				Last Renewal:	Expiration Date:

Are you a citizen of the United States? ☐ yes ☐ no

If you are not a U.S. Citizen, do you have the legal right to remain permanently in the United States? ☐ yes ☐ no

Explain

Are you between the ages of 18 and 70? ☐ yes ☐ no

Do you know of any fact that would limit or impair your ability to perform the functions of the job you are applying for? ☐ yes ☐ no

Describe

Date of last Physical Examination:

Family Physician:

I authorize my doctor to release to you the results of my pre-employment and subsequent medical examinations, and to discuss those results with you. ☐ yes ☐ no

Position desired:

Hours desired:

Salary expected:

Specialized training or experience not shown on other side of form:

Where now employed?

Reason for desiring change:

Have you ever pleaded guilty or been convicted of a felony? ☐ yes ☐ no

If yes to either, please explain:

or a misdemeanor other than a first conviction for drunkenness, simple assault, speeding, minor traffic violations, affray, or disturbance of the peace within the past 5 years? ☐ yes ☐ no

In case of emergency notify	name	relationship
	address	telephone

*I authorize the schools, employers, and individuals listed in this application to release any information regarding my previous employment, character, general reputation and personal characteristics.   ☐ yes ☐ no

I certify that the statements I have made in this application are true and hereby grant the employer permission to verify the accuracy and completeness of this information and to investigate all references and educational records. I understand that any false or misleading statements made by me on this application or in conjunction with my physical examination will be sufficient cause for the rejection of this application or for immediate dismissal if such false or misleading information is discovered after my employment. If I am accepted for employment, I agree to abide by the rules and regulations of the employer.

Signed ————————————

Date ————————————

E-2   "It is unlawful in Massachusetts to require or administer a lie detector test as a condition of employment or continued employment. An employer who violates this law shall be subject to criminal penalities and civil liability".

Figure 37-1   On application forms, answer all questions to the best of your ability. Be sure the information is accurate. (Form courtesy of Danvers Twin Oaks Nursing Home. From Hegner and Caldwell, *Nursing Assistant, A Nursing Process Approach,* 6E, copyright 1992 by Delmar Publishers Inc.)

TO THE PHYSICIAN: Please fill out the following medical form as completely as possible. State law requires that our employees have a completed physical on file with a yearly update. Please forward this form immediately upon completion of examination. Pending test results will be followed up by our office. Information required is indicated by a check mark.

NAME OF PATIENT: _____ AGE: _____

ADDRESS: _____
Street No.   Town (City)   State   Zip Code

PHYSICAL FINDINGS:

BP:_____ Pulse:_____ Resp:_____ Height:_____ Weight:_____

____ Cardiovascular   ____ Gastrointestinal   ____ Musculoskeletal
____ Respiratory   ____ Genitourinary   ____ Nervous

____ Above physical findings essentially normal.
____ Abnormal findings/limitations: _____

_____

HISTORY

Habituation/Addiction
____ Alcohol   ____ Depressants   ____ Stimulants   ____ Narcotics   ____ Other: _____
If any, please explain: _____

Illness/Injury — please indicate any past or present condition that would result in physical, mental or behavioral limitations in normal functioning: _____

MANDATORY IMMUNIZATIONS/TESTS:

DIPHTHERIA/TETANUS — should have booster every ten years.
Date of Last Immunization: _____

RUBELLA — MUST show proof of immunity through direct immunization or *positive* antibody titer test.
Date of immunization: _____ Date of Antibody Titer Test: _____
Results: _____

TUBERCULOSIS — MUST have Mantoux (ppd) skin test every year and follow-up chest X ray if test
results positive.
                                            Follow-up Chest
Date of Mantoux: _____ Results: _____ X ray date: _____
Hepatitis B Vaccine: _____   Pos.   Neg.

ENTERIC PATHOGENS — stool examination and/or culture (only if indicated by check mark)
Date of Examination/Culture: _____ Results: _____

This person (is is not) physically and mentally capable of performing the functions of an aide in the home setting, and is free from any condition which would endanger his/her safety or the safety and well-being of the clients to be cared for.

DATE: _____ PHYSICIAN'S SIGNATURE: _____

ADDRESS: _____
Street No.   City   State   Zip Code
PHONE NO.: _____

Figure 37-2   Some agencies have their own forms for physical examination.

If you do not have a telephone, you should leave the number of a neighbor or friend who has agreed to take messages for you. **Personal references** may not be relatives, but may include your minister, doctor, or instructor(s). Be sure that you have permission from those people you list as references to use their names. If possible, obtain letters of recommendation from these people before you go for a job interview. This will save time for the agency, and the person who is giving the recommendation only has to write one letter of reference. The agency can then make a copy of your letters of reference and confirm them by phone.

Each agency will have its own application form, but if you are prepared with the sample in Figure 37-1, you should not have any difficulty completing the agency application form. It is always a good idea to read the application form carefully before completing it. It may include special instructions, such as asking the applicant to type or print all information. Fill out each item neatly and completely. Do not leave any items blank; if the item does not apply to you, write "N.A." (not applicable). Take care to spell words and to punctuate sentences carefully. Do not write in spaces marked "office use only." Review your application before submitting it to the employer.

You should have with you your Social Security card, your alien green card, a driver's license, your certificate, and, if at all possible, a copy of your most recent physical examination showing your immunizations, including hepatitis B, the results of a TB test, and other facts about your personal physical condition. Some agencies will have their own form to be given to the examining physician, Figure 37-2. Remember to take your own pen.

The Interview

After the application has been filled out, you will probably be interviewed by the case manager or personnel manager. Make sure that you know the correct date and exact time of your interview as well as the name of the person who will be interviewing you. Check to make sure that you know how to get to the appropriate location, or ask for specific directions.

Dress neatly and conservatively, Figure 37-3. Make sure that your clothes are clean and well pressed. Avoid excessive jewelry or makeup. Observe the personal hygiene rules discussed in Unit 2 of this text.

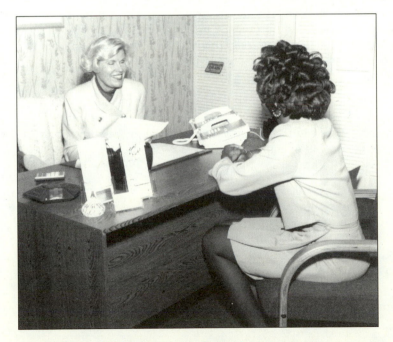

Figure 37-3   Dress neatly for the job interview.

If you are offered the job, you have the choice of accepting the agency's terms or looking elsewhere for a position. Once you have accepted a position with an agency, be realistic in your goals. As in any kind of employment, this is a system of progression where the new employees must prove themselves. It is possible that an agency may test you by calling you for weekend or holiday part-time work. Many employers think it is a sign of dedication if you accept the assignments offered. After you have worked for a while, the agency will have a better idea of your abilities and strengths and will work you into a regular schedule.

When you are employed by an agency, you may be asked to sign a document similar to the

---

TO THE EMPLOYEE

Because you are important to us, we want to help you develop a good work record. If we feel that you are violating any of our rules and policies, or that you have misunderstood the terms of employment, we will hold a conference with you. Continued *infractions* will cause your immediate dismissal. PLEASE READ THE FOLLOWING CAREFULLY.

1. *Attendance and tardiness record:* Recurring cancellations of promised scheduled workdays may result in dismissal. Absence without call in may result in immediate termination. No pay raises will be granted if attendance and tardiness records are unsatisfactory. We must be able to depend on you. You must call in if you are unable to meet your assignment.

2. *Unbecoming conduct:* Any of the following are considered to be gross *misconduct:* carelessness and inattention to client care; failure to perform duties; violation of safe practices; inefficiency and wasting of materials; refusal to obey direct orders; insubordination; rude, discourteous or uncivil behavior; intoxication, drinking or possession of intoxicating beverages while on duty; gambling on duty; sleeping on duty; unauthorized absence from assignment or leaving early without permission; failure to report an injury or accident concerning an employee or client; soliciting tips from clients or families; sale of services to clients or families; divulging confidential information about client and family; theft and/or dishonesty; *pilferage* of drugs or violation of any law on drug use including use or sale of same; damaging, defacing or mishandling equipment or property; interfering with work performance of another employee; falsifying client or personnel records or any form of misrepresentation.

Employee's statement:

I have read the above rules and regulations and understand my responsibilities to the agency and client. I agree to abide by these terms of employment.

_____   _____
Employee Signature   Date

_____   _____
Supervisor's Signature   Date

Figure 37-4 Once you have decided to accept a position with an agency, you may be asked to sign a document that states that you have read and understood the rules of the agency.

one presented in Figure 37-4. This document will indicate the policies and rules of your agency. You should read it carefully and be willing to accept and abide by the conditions included in it.

New York state has recently implemented a new and very restrictive code for agencies providing home health care. To be qualified to operate, agencies must meet exacting standards set by both the Department of Health and the Department of Social Services. Included in the standards required by New York state are:

- A grievance procedure for an agency's employees
- A patient's bill of rights which MUST be explained to the client (or client's family) in the presence of a witness

- Documentation of certification of all employees
- Proof of an annual physical examination by employees
- Proof of employee's attendance at a minimum number of in-service programs each year
- Proof of citizenship and/or verified alien registration
- Satisfactory completion of an approved home health aide course of study
- No legal record of client abuse or misuses of client's property in a caregiver's situation
- Proof of being on the state registry for home health aide in the state in which you are applying for a position

SUMMARY

If you have successfully completed the home health aide program and have a certificate, and are on the state registry, you should have no trouble finding employment. When you go to an agency or prospective employer, be on time, dress neatly, and be prepared to talk about your training and experience. Do not chew gum or smoke during the interview. Fill out the application form neatly and completely.

Appendices

A   Temperature Conversion Chart   415

B   Sample of Weekly Time Sheet   416

C   Daily and Weekly Scheduling Chart   417

D   Living Will and Durable Power of Attorney   418

E   Prefixes and Suffixes Commonly Used in Medical Terminology   422

NOTE: The following table is provided as an aid for study and comparison of temperatures. Some homemaking duties and client care procedures refer to temperatures in Fahrenheit or Celsius.

DEGREES FAHRENHEIT TO DEGREES CELSIUS AND VICE VERSA											
°F	°C	°F	°C	°F	°C	°F	°C	°F	°C	°F	°C
96	35.6	118	47.8	140	60	162	72.2	184	84.4	206.6	97
96.8	36	118.4	48	141	60.6	163	72.8	185	85	207	97.2
97	36.1	119	48.3	141.8	61	163.4	73	186	85.6	208	97.8
98	36.7	120	48.9	142	61.1	164	73.3	186.8	86	208.4	98
98.6	37	120.2	49	143	61.7	165	73.9	187	86.1	209	98.3
99	37.2	121	49.4	143.6	62	165.2	74	188	86.7	210	98.9
100	37.8	122	50	144	62.2	166	74.4	188.6	87	210.2	99
100.4	38	123	50.6	145	62.8	167	75	189	87.2	211	99.4
101	38.3	123.8	51	145.4	63	168	75.6	190	87.8	212	100
102	38.9	124	51.1	146	63.3	168.8	76	190.4	88	213	100.6
102.2	39	125	51.7	147	63.9	169	76.1	191	88.3	213.8	101
103	39.4	125.6	52	147.2	64	170	76.7	192	88.9	214	101.1
104	40	126	52.2	148	64.4	170.6	77	192.2	89	215	101.7
105	40.6	127	52.8	149	65	171	77.2	193	89.4	215.6	102
105.8	41	127.4	53	150	65.6	172	77.8	194	90	216	102.2
106	41.1	128	53.3	150.8	66	172.4	78	195	90.6	217	102.8
107	41.7	129	53.9	151	66.1	173	78.3	195.8	91	217.4	103
107.6	42	129.2	54	152	66.7	174	78.9	196	91.1	218	103.3
108	42.2	130	54.4	152.6	67	174.2	79	197	91.7	219	103.9
109	42.8	131	55	153	67.2	175	79.4	197.6	92	219.2	104
109.4	43	132	55.6	154	67.8	176	80	198	92.2	220	104.4
110	43.3	132.8	56	154.4	68	177	80.6	199	92.8	221	105
111	43.9	133	56.1	155	68.3	177.8	81	199.4	93	225	107.2
111.2	44	134	56.7	156	68.9	178	81.1	200	93.3	230	110
112	44.4	134.6	57	156.2	69	179	81.7	201	93.9	235	112.8
113	45	135	57.2	157	69.4	179.6	82	201.2	94	239	115
114	45.6	136	57.8	158	70	180	82.2	202	94.4	240	115.6
114.8	46	136.4	58	159	70.6	181	82.8	203	95	245	118.3
115	46.1	137	58.3	159.8	71	181.4	83	204	95.6	248	120
116	46.7	138	58.9	160	71.1	182	83.3	204.8	96	250	121.1
116.6	47	138.2	59	161	71.7	183	83.9	205	96.1	255	123.9
117	47.2	139	59.4	161.6	72	183.2	84	206	96.7	257	125

Appendix B Sample of Weekly Time Sheet

064-40-0878 Name: Judy Goldstein W/E **9-11-93**
SS # Month - Day - Year

PRINT THIS TIME SHEET   USE A SEPARATE LINE FOR EACH CASE   SKIP A LINE BETWEEN DAYS

Agency	Case #	CLIENT Last Name–First initial	DATE Mo.	Day	Travel to 1st Case Hr.	Min.	Mi.	Fare	Arrived Hr.	Min.	Left Hr.	Min.	Svce. Hrs.	Miles on Case	Travel to next case Hr.	Min.	Mi.	Fare	Travel to Home Hr.	Min.	Mi.	Fare	Other Exp.	Signature
VNA	2303	Brown, J.	9	6		25	6		9	00	12	00	3							25	6		.10	*J. Brown*
		Holiday	9	7																				
ERDS·C	1963	Casillio, P.	9	8		20	8		8	30	12	30	4	6		30	10							*P. Casillio*
SOC.SERV	2036	Williams, S.	9	8					1	00	4	00	3							35	12		.30	*Sam Williams*
V.A.	1845	Kelly, A.	9	9		20	8		9	00	5	00	8	28						25				*A. Kelly*
VNA	2306	Garcia, M.	9	10		40	15		8	30	12	30	4											*M. Garcia*
SOC.SERV	1495	Garcia, M.	9	10		20	8		12	30	4	30	4							45	15			*M. Garcia*

Appendix C Daily and Weekly Scheduling Chart

Daily and Weekly Scheduling

As a beginning home health aide, you may have some difficulty in scheduling your activities. The authors have prepared a time checklist, which they recommend be used until you have established a pattern of work. It provides a reminder of what is expected. An individual notebook, detailing the procedures done and the time required for each, can be kept instead of a checklist.

You should become accustomed to making a working schedule and putting it into practice. Post conferences with your instructor may be quite helpful in recognizing areas in which you can make adjustments leading to greater efficiency and ease of accomplishing goals. The need for personal flexibility should be stressed. You should be flexible to meet client needs and still maintain the home within reasonable bounds.

As each procedure is completed, note the time required. At the end of the day make a note of undone tasks, and see if the time spent could have been used more effectively.

Daily Checklist

DUTIES	COMPLETED	TIME REQUIRED
AM client care	_____	_____
Client unit—bedroom/bath	_____	_____
Breakfast made/served	_____	_____
Kitchen clean up	_____	_____
Shopping	_____	_____
House cleaned	_____	_____
Lunch made/served	_____	_____
Aide's lunch period	_____	_____
Kitchen clean up	_____	_____
Laundry/ironing	_____	_____
Major job—clean oven	_____	_____
refrigerator		
mop floor		
vacuum		
Other client care	_____	_____
List procedures		
_____	_____	_____
_____	_____	_____
_____	_____	_____
PM client care	_____	_____

Observations by home health aide _____

_____

_____

Appendix **D** Living Will and Durable Power of Attorney

In 1991, the United States government mandated that individuals seeking health care complete an advanced directives statement. The two common types of advanced directives are living wills and durable power of attorney. One of these forms should be completed before the client's care is started and while the client is mentally competent.

Form A245 Living Will

LIVING WILL

    DIRECTIVE MADE this   day of   , 19   , to my physicians, my attorneys, my clergyman, my family or others responsible for my health, welfare or affairs.

    BE IT KNOWN, that I,   , of   State of   , being of sound mind, willfully and voluntarily make known my desire that my life shall not be artificially prolonged under the circumstances set forth below and do hereby declare that, if at any time I should have an incurable injury, disease or illness certified to be a terminal condition by two physicians and where the application of life-sustaining procedures would serve only to artificially prolong the moment of my death and where my physician determines that my death is imminent or needlessly prolonged whether or not life-sustaining procedures are utilized, I direct that such procedures be withheld or withdrawn and that I be permitted to die naturally with only the merciful administration of medication to eliminate or reduce pain to my mind and body or the performance of any medical procedure deemed necessary to provide me with comfort care. In the absence of my ability to give directions regarding the use of such life-sustaining procedures, it is my intention that this directive shall be honored by my family and physician(s) as the final expression of my legal right to refuse medical or surgical treatment and I accept the consequences from such refusal. If I have bequeathed organs, I ask that I be kept alive for a sufficient time to enable the proper withdrawal and transplant of said organs.

    Special provisions:

As a witness to this act I state the declarer has been personally known to me and I believe said declarer to be of sound mind.

Signed in the presence of:

_____   _____

Witness   Address

_____   _____

Witness   Address

State of

County of   SS.   , 19

BE IT KNOWN, that the above named   ,
personally known to me as the same person described in and who executed the within Living Will acknowledged to me that said instrument was freely and voluntarily executed for the purposes therein expressed, and that said Living Will was duly executed in my presence.

_____

Notary Public

My Commission Expires:

c. E-Z Legal Forms

Living Will   *(Continued)*

Form A175 Durable Power of Attorney
For Health Care

DURABLE POWER OF ATTORNEY
FOR HEALTH CARE

BE IT KNOWN, that
of   , the
undersigned Grantor, does hereby grant a durable power of attorney for health care to
, of
, as my attorney-in-fact and Agent.

I hereby grant to my Agent full power and authority to make health care decisions for me to the same extent that I could make such decisions for myself if I had the capacity to do so. In exercising this authority, my Agent shall make health care decisions that are consistent with my desires as stated in this document or otherwise made known to my Agent, including, but not limited to, my desires concerning obtaining or refusing or withdrawing life prolonging care, treatment, services, and procedures.

I hereby authorize all physicians and psychiatrists who have treated me, and all other providers of health care, including hospitals, to release to my Agent all information contained in my medical records which my Agent may request. I hereby waive all privileges attached to physician-patient relationship and to any communication, verbal or written, arising out of such a relationship. My Agent is authorized to request, receive and review any information, verbal or written, pertaining to my physical or mental health, including medical and hospital records, and to execute any releases, waivers or other documents that may be required in order to obtain such information, and to disclose such information to such persons, organizations and health care providers as my Agent shall deem appropriate. My Agent is authorized to employ and discharge health care providers including physicians, psychiatrists, dentists, nurses, and therapists as my Agent shall deem appropriate for my physical, mental and emotional well-being. My Agent is also authorized to pay reasonable fees and expenses for such services contracted.

My Agent is authorized to apply for my admission to a medical, nursing, residential or other similar facility, execute any consent or admission forms required by such facility and enter into agreements for my care at such facility or elsewhere during my lifetime. My Agent is authorized to arrange for and consent to medical, therapeutical and surgical procedures for me including the administration of drugs. The power to make health care decisions for me shall include the power to give consent, refuse consent, or withdraw consent to any care, treatment, service, or procedure to maintain, diagnose, or treat a physical or mental condition.

I reserve unto myself the right to revoke the authority granted to my Agent hereunder to make health care decisions for me by notifying the treating physician, hospital, or other health care provider orally or in writing. Notwithstanding any provision herein to the contrary, I retain the right to make medical and other health care decisions for myself so long as I am able to give informed consent with respect to a particular decision. In addition, no treatment may be given to me over my objection, and health care necessary to keep me alive may not be stopped if I object.

This power of attorney shall not be affected by subsequent disability or incapacity of the principal. Notwithstanding any provision herein to the contrary, my Agent shall take no action under this instrument unless I am deemed to be disabled or incapacitated as defined herein. My incapacity shall be deemed to exist when so certified in writing by two licensed physicians not related by blood or marriage to either me or to my Agent. The said certificate shall state that I am incapable of caring for myself and that I am physically and mentally incapable of managing my financial affairs. The certificate of the physicians described above shall be attached to the original of this instrument and if this instrument is filed or recorded among public records, then such certificate shall also be similarly filed or recorded if permitted by applicable law. To the extent permitted by law, I herewith nominate, constitute and appoint my Agent to serve as my guardian, conservator and/or in any similar representative capacity, and, if I am not permitted by law to so nominate, constitute and appoint, then I request any court of competent jurisdiction which may be petitioned by any person to appoint a guardian, conservator or similar representative for me to give due consideration to my request.

Signed this   day of   , 19   .

Signed in the presence of:

_____   _____

State of   , 19

County of   SS.

        Then personally appeared the foregoing   ,   as
Grantor, who known to me acknowledged the foregoing to be his or her free act and deed, before me.

                                                        _____
                                                        Notary Public
                                                        My Commission Expires:

                                                                    c. E-Z Legal Forms

Durable Power of Attorney for Health Care   (Continued)

Appendix E Prefixes and Suffixes Commonly Used in Medical Terminology

a-, an-: without, not
ab-: from, away
ad-: to, toward
adeno-, aden-: gland, glandular
-algia: pain
ambi-: both
angio-: vessel, duct
ante-, pre-: before
anti-, contra-: against
audio-: sound, hearing, dealing with the ear
auto-: self

bi-, bis-: twice, double
bio-: life
brady-: slow
bronch-, bronchi-: air tubes in the lungs, bronchi

cardi-, cardia-, cardio-: pertaining to the heart
-cide: causing death
crani-, cranio-: pertaining to the skull
cyst-, cysto-, cysti-: bladder, bag
-cyte, cyt-: cell

derm-, derma-, dermo-, dermat-: pertaining to skin
dia-: through, between, apart
dorsi-, dorso-: to the back, back
dys-: difficult, painful

ecto-, ex-, exo-: outside of, external
-ectomy: surgical removal of
endo-: within, innermost
entero-: intestine, pertaining to the intestine

gastro-, gasti-: stomach
-genetic, -genic: origin, producing
genito-: organs of reproduction
glyco-, gly-: sugar
gyn-, gyno-: women, female

hemi-: half
hema-, hem-, hemo- hemato-: blood
hepato-: liver

hetero-: other, unlike, different
homo-, homeo-: same, like
hydro-: water
hyper-: over, increased, high
hypo-: under, decreased, low
hystero-, hyster-: uterus

inter-: between, among
intra-: within, into
-itis: inflammation, inflammation of

leuko-, leuco-: white
-logy, -ology: study of, science of

mal-: bad, abnormal, disordered
mast-, masto-: breast
micro-: small
mono-: one, single
multi-: many, much, a large amount
myo-: muscle

neph-, nephro-, ren-: kidney
neuro-, neur-: nerve or nervous system

-ology: study of a science
ophthalm-, ophthalmo-: eye
-ostomy: creation of an opening by surgery
ot-, oto-: ear
-otomy: cutting into

path-, patho-, -pathy, -pathia: disease, abnormal condition
ped-, pedia-: child
peri-: around
-plegia: paralysis
pnea-: respiration/breathing
pneum-: lung, pertaining to the lungs
post-: after
proct-, procto-: rectum, rectal
pseudo-: false
psych-, psycho-: pertaining to the mind

sep-, septic-: poison, rot
sub-: less, under, below
super-, supra-: above, upon, over

tachy-: fast
therm-, thermo-: heat

-toxic, -tox: poison
tracho-: trachea, windpipe

uria-: urine

Glossary

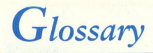

abbreviations—shortened forms of written words.

abortion—interruption of pregnancy before delivery date; may be natural or medically induced by the physician.

abuse—treatment that reasonably could cause physical pain, physical injury, mental anguish, or fear.

accelerated—speeded up; rapid.

acidosis—a condition in which the balance of acids and bases in the body is disturbed because of loss of salts, sodium and potassium or the accumulation of acids.

activities of daily living—the activities necessary for the client to fulfill basic human needs, i.e., dressing, eating, and toileting.

acute—begins suddenly and usually severe.

acute illness—a change from normal body functioning to a sudden pathological condition requiring immediate care.

addiction—a dependency on a drug or substance such as alcohol, cocaine, methadone, or cigarettes that blocks normal habits and body functions of everyday living.

adjustment—changes a person makes in behavior in order to deal with a situation.

adolescence—the period of physical and emotional development from early teens to young adulthood (usually between the ages of 13 to 18).

advanced directives—documents specifying the type of treatment individuals want or do not want under serious medical conditions in which they may be unable to communicate their wishes. Generally two forms: living will or durable power of attorney.

agitator—the spindle in a washing machine which rotates and forces the dirt out of clothes by forcing water and soap through the fabrics.

AIDS (acquired immune deficiency syndrome)—a crippling and fatal disease. It was first diagnosed in 1981. The disease breaks down the body's natural immune system so that its victims are vulnerable to almost any infection.

airborne—transmitted through the air. Sneezing and coughing are examples of pathogens being transmitted through the air.

Al-Anon—a support group for the spouses of alcoholics. The group meets regularly to learn how to work and live with a family member who is an alcoholic.

Alateen—a support group for children of alcoholic parent(s). The children meet with a counselor and learn to recognize shared problems and how to deal with them on a daily basis.

Alcoholics Anonymous—a support group that provides help for the alcoholic based on getting through one day at a time without taking an alcoholic drink.

alcoholism—an addiction to alcohol leading to physical and social breakdown; generally considered to be an illness caused by the body's inability to metabolize alcohol.

allergy—a heightened sensitivity to a substance such as food, pollen, or dust that causes a physical reaction such as sneezing, runny nose, hives, etc. Allergies can often be relieved by a series of injections or avoidance of the substance bringing on an attack.

Alzheimer's disease—a progressive, degenerative illness causing loss of memory and mental incapacity.

ambulation—walking.

amputation—the surgical procedure in which a limb or part of a limb is removed.

anemia—deficiency of quality or quantity of red blood cells in the blood.

aneurysm—localized enlargement of a blood vessel; may be due to a congenital defect or weakness of the vessel's wall.

angina pectoris—mild heart condition that may cause pain in the chest region. Pain is usually relieved with a drug called nitroglycerin.

anorexia—loss of appetite.

anticoagulant—a drug that delays or prevents the formation of blood clots within the circulatory system. Anticoagulants are not effective in dissolving clots that have already formed.

antiseptic—a product or technique preventing the growth of microorganisms or stopping and slowing the growth of pathogens.

anuria—no urinary output as a result of kidney failure.

anxiety—an unpleasant emotional or psychological state of constant fear or apprehension.

aphasia—impaired or lost ability to communicate through speech due to dysfunction of brain centers. There can be a loss of verbal understanding, word blindness, inability to understand the meaning of spoken or written words, or speaking in meaningless phrases.

apical pulse—pulse rate taken by placing the stethoscope over the tip of the heart.

apnea—absence of breathing or respirations.

ARC (AIDS-related complex)—conditions suffered by persons who are HIV positive before true onset of AIDS.

arteriogram—series of x-ray pictures that show the flow of blood in the arteries after the injection of dye or contrast substance into the artery.

arteriosclerosis—a condition in which the arteries become hard and lose the elasticity needed for good blood circulation.

arthritis—inflammation of the joints causing pain, swelling and enlargement of the joints. Usually associated with aging but can attack young people as well.

articulates—utter intelligible sounds; speaks.

ascites—the collection of fluid in the abdomen or peritoneal cavity, characterized by a swollen abdomen that feels hard to the touch.

asepsis—techniques to rid the environment of microorganisms and provide a sterile area.

assault—attempt or threat to do violence to another.

assistive devices—equipment used to help clients be more effective in their physical activities.

asthma—a disorder of the respiratory system. Symptoms may include labored breathing, wheezing, coughing. There may be a secretion of fluid from the bronchials. Condition may be caused by pollutants, infection, emotional stress, and allergies.

atherosclerosis—fatty tissue (lipid) collected within or beneath the surface of blood vessels causing impaired circulation. Common cause of arterial occlusion (blocking).

atrophy—shrinking or wasting away of tissues.

attention span—increasing your ability and time to study with comprehension of the assigned reading material.

attitude—state of mind, behavior, or conduct about a particular matter.

auditory—relating to hearing.

automatic speech—continuous repetition of phrases or words with no meaning.

axillary—the triangular space at the underside of the shoulder between the upper part of the arm and the side of the chest commonly called the armpit.

AZT—drug used in the treatment of AIDS.

bacteria—one-celled microorganisms that are round, rod-shaped or spiral in form. They can cause infections in the body or in the environment.

behavior—how an individual responds to a given situation.

benign tumor—noncancerous tumor.

bile—a yellowish green product of the liver which is manufactured and stored in the gallbladder. Bile is used by the body to metabolize fat in the small intestine.

biopsy—The surgical technique in which a sample of tissue is removed from an area where cellular change is suspected and examined under the microscope for signs of cancer.

bland diet—food prepared with no spices featuring easily digested items that are soothing to the digestive tract.

blended family—merging of two (2) families after their parents remarry.

blood lancet—small pointed surgical instrument used to pierce the skin to obtain a blood sample.

blood pressure—the force exerted by the blood on the walls of the blood vessels.

body language—a form of communication using gestures and facial expressions instead of words.

body mechanics—the techniques used to get the most effective and least taxing body movements. Bending the knees when lifting to avoid unnecessary strain to the back and legs is an example of good body mechanics.

bonding—a process of attachment of mother, father and infant happening immediately after birth. Infant is placed on mother's abdomen and father feels and touches infant.

bony prominences—areas of the body where bones protrude, e.g., the elbows, wrists, knees, pelvic bones, spinal column. Such bones have little natural padding and are areas where pressure sores can easily form.

brachial—relating to the arm; commonly referred to when taking the blood pressure and checking the brachial artery or taking the brachial pulse.

bradycardia—an extremely slow heartbeat.

brooding—an emotional response to depression characterized by sadness and lack of communication.

bulk—roughage foods needed by the body to prevent constipation and to keep the stool soft. High-bulk foods are fruits, green leafy vegetables, potatoes, and whole-grain cereals.

cachexia—state of malnutrition and debility, usually seen in long illness.

calorie-controlled diet—calorie count of diet is adjusted to either high for a malnourished client or low for an obese client.

cancer—a disease characterized by rapid growth of abnormal cells that form a tumor; it often spreads to other sites.

capillaries—the tiny vessels joining arteries and veins within the circulatory system.

carcinogen—a substance or agent which produces cancer; may be related to environment or heredity.

cardiac—anything related to the heart and the disorders associated with the heart.

cardiac arrest—heart stops beating.

cardinal sign—those signs which quickly indicate the status of a person's life functions. Cardinal signs include pulse, temperature, respirations, and blood pressure; these signs are often referred to as vital signs.

cardiopulmonary resuscitation—the restoring of respirations and heart beat by artificial means. It is performed by an individual following standard procedures which include establishing a clear airway for the victim, breathing into the victim's mouth, and compressing the victim's chest in order to restore breathing.

career—profession or occupation which one has been educated for.

care plan—nursing plan for care of client in the home.

carotid—pertaining to the main arteries at the side of the neck which provide the main supply of blood to the neck and head area.

case manager—member of the health care team who coordinates all the services the client may require in the home. Usually is a social worker or registered nurse.

catastrophic reaction—severe and unpredictable violent behavior of a person with dementia.

catheter—plastic or rubber tube inserted in the body to release or introduce fluids, e.g., dyes are introduced during heart catheterization, urine is released by use of the Foley catheter.

catheterization—thin tube is introduced into the artery or vein and passed through the heart. Diagnostic test used to diagnose heart abnormalities.

cerebral hemorrhage—blood vessel burst in the brain. Common cause of a stroke.

cerebral infarction—the condition in which a portion of the brain dies when an artery becomes blocked and blood is prevented from reaching that part of the brain.

cerebral palsy—condition where there is impaired muscular power and coordination due to lack of oxygen to the brain before or during birth.

cerebral vascular accident—a disorder of the blood vessels of the brain due to a blockage caused by an embolus or hemorrhage.

certified—meeting a specified standard. One who has special training in a particular subject as required by state law is said to be certified.

cesarean section—surgical abdominal delivery of a fetus; performed when normal birth canal delivery would be dangerous to the mother or fetus.

challenge—an invitation to participate in a competition.

CHAP—Community Health Accreditation Program, Inc.—accreditation body for home health agencies.

chemotherapy—a treatment for cancer in which chemicals are used to destroy or slow the growth of cancerous cells.

Cheyne-Stokes respirations—term used to describe respirations: periods of apnea followed by periods of dyspnea.

child abuse—emotional or physical abuse of an individual under the age of 18 by an adult.

chore services—shopping, transportation, heavy cleaning, yard work or other similar services available alone or in combination of home health care.

chronic—lasts a long time.

chronic illness—a long-term condition.

chronological—according to or related to the age of an individual.

civilized—meeting standards of refinement; the act of being polite.

clear liquid diet—a special diet consisting of only liquids that one can see through, i.e., apple juice, tea, broth, gelatin.

clinical—relating to a clinic; procedures such as bedmaking, bathing, oral care, etc.

cognitive—relates to thinking.

collateral circulation—when small blood vessels take over the circulation from near-by damaged or scarred blood vessels. These vessels enlarge themselves to carry the blood to the body parts.

colon—the large intestine which is divided in three parts—the ascending, transverse, and descending.

colostomy—the removal of the diseased area of the gastrointestinal tract and making an external opening on the abdomen called a stoma. In some cases this may be a temporary solution and at a later date the intestine can be reattached to the bowel. Other colostomies may be permanent.

coma—a state of unconsciousness in which there is little or no eye movement, diminished response to external stimuli, and the inability to talk or communicate.

communication—the sending and receiving of messages; may be verbal or nonverbal.

compensation—making up for a weakness by becoming very good in some other area.

complication—the worsening of a body condition due to added factors.

components—the separate parts of a machine or a procedure which make up the whole.

conception—occurs when a female egg is fertilized by the male sperm; a zygote is formed and cell growth and multiplication take place and a fetus develops.

confident—self-assured; ability to perform in an efficient manner.

confidentiality—keeping a client's personal affairs private. A home health aide must not give out information about the client except to the nursing supervisor or doctor.

confined—restricted to a certain location or area.

congestive heart failure—a condition in which the heart cannot pump enough blood to the body. This can start as an acute problem which leads to a chronic condition with slow deterioration and the possibility of complications to other body systems.

consciousness—a normal state of awareness and responsiveness during the waking period.

constipation—infrequent or difficult bowel movements where the feces are usually hard.

constrictive—something that is tight or narrowed.

consultation—the exchange of views on a particular subject; a conference between physicians about a patient and the patient's treatment.

contagious—refers to diseases that can spread rapidly from one person to another person or place to place; a communicable disease.

contaminated—that which is dirty and contains pathogens which may lead to infection.

continent—ability to control the passage of stool and urine.

contracture—a permanent shortening of muscle tissue causing deformity or distortion.

convenience foods—prepared foods that are ready to serve or require only cooking. These foods are often more expensive and may not be as tasty as foods prepared from fresh products.

conversion reaction—a defense mechanism whereby suppressed emotion takes the form of a physical symptom.

convulsion—abnormal, involuntary series of violent muscle contractions; often associated with epilepsy.

coronary occlusion—a condition in which a blood vessel in the heart muscle closes or is blocked by a blood clot.

crisis—an unstable, critical period that can alter one's life, either for better or for worse.

crisis intervention center—specialized units often run by volunteers who give information on how to deal with a specific problem. Drug hot lines, alcohol information centers, abortion clinics, Planned Parenthood, and poison control centers could all be considered crisis intervention centers.

critical—a dangerous time; relates to a crisis period in an illness.

culture—the learning behavior patterns of a race, nation or people; the life-style standards in society.

custom—common practice among a group of individuals or within a family or community; the ordinary or usual manner of acting.

cyanosis—lack of oxygen in the blood causing the client to appear bluish; indicates improper heart/lung function.

cyanotic—a bluish skin tone due to some problem of the respiratory system preventing proper inspiration and exhalation; the result of lack of oxygen to the blood cells.

cystic fibrosis—an inherited condition that affects children's sweat glands, pancreas, and respiratory system.

cystitis—inflammation of the bladder.

dangling—sitting up with legs hanging over the edge of the bed.

DARE—Drug Awareness Resistance Education—a group organized to stop young people from getting started on illegal drugs.

debilitating—causing weakness.

defamation—something harmful to the good name or reputation of another; slander.

defense mechanism—a technique used by an individual to protect the self from unpleasantness, shame, anxiety or loss of self-esteem.

degenerative—a disease or condition causing tissues or organs to weaken and become abnormal. May be a progressive degeneration in which the condition becomes worse and worse with time.

delicatessen—a specialty store selling cheeses, coldcuts, sodas, sandwiches, and convenience foods.

dementia—progressive mental deterioration due to organic brain disease; loss of mind.

denial—refusal to accept an unpleasant fact.

depression—a mental state characterized by loss of hope, feelings of rejection, generalized sadness and, in severe cases, the inability to function.

dermis—the inner layer of skin.

developmentally disabled—a severe chronic disability of a person.

developmental tasks—in psychology, tasks that are normally carried out as steps in personality development.

diabetes—a chronic disorder related to metabolism. It is caused by the inadequate functioning of the islets of Langerhans in the pancreas which produce insulin. Insulin is needed for the proper metabolism of sugars in the body.

diabetic complications—the results of untreated or improperly treated diabetes which can lead to blindness, gangrene, heart and kidney failure.

diabetic diet—a measured and low- or no-sugar diet for diabetics.

diagnosis—the identification of a disease or condition.

diarrhea—a condition in which stools are watery and frequent.

diastolic—measurement of blood pressure when the heart is relaxing.

dietary—related to the diet or food eaten by an individual. Certain religious groups have dietary laws which prohibit the eating of certain foods.

diet modification—special diet changes required for a particular set of conditions, e.g., low-fat diet, liquid diet, diabetic diet.

digitalis—a therapeutic drug used to slow down the heart beat and to increase the force of the heart muscle contractions thus enabling the heart to pump more blood.

dilate—to enlarge.

disinfectant—a chemical substance used to kill bacteria.

disinfected—use of a medication or germ-fighting agent to destroy microorganisms.

disorganized—confused and unable to follow and plan a step-by-step practical course of action.

disoriented—confused or mixed up; loss of the sense of time, place or identity.

displacement—taking one's own anger or frustration out on someone else, e.g., yelling at a child because you are angry with another person and afraid to yell at that person.

dispute—disagreement leading to argument.

distended—to become bloated or swollen. A distended abdomen becomes hard to the touch and bulges out.

diuretic—a drug used to reduce fluid accumulation in the body. Persons taking a diuretic urinate frequently.

diversion—a change or distraction to help a person relax. Soft music, television, or talking can be diversions to keep the client from thinking about the illness.

divorce—dissolving of the marriage or marital contract.

documentation—to record on proper form your observations and actions.

doffing—removing of the prosthesis.

donning—application of the prosthesis.

DPT—a combination immunization given to infants to prevent diphtheria, pertussis (whooping cough), and tetanus.

DRGs—Diagnosis related groups—medical ailments are reimbursed according to a fixed reimbursement formula.

duct—a tube-like structure that transports fluid or air from one part to another part of the body.

ductless gland—that part of the endocrine system that releases hormones directly into the blood and lymph systems.

durable power of attorney—legal document that designates another person to act as an "agent" or a "proxy" in making medical decisions if the individual becomes unable to do so.

dyslexia—a learning disability which prevents a person from reading or understanding the written word.

dyspnea—difficult or labored respiration.

dysuria—painful urination.

early adulthood—period between 25–45 years of age.

-ectomy—a suffix which indicates removal of.

edema—the swelling of legs and/or arms or other body parts when water is being retained unnaturally.

efficient—performance of tasks without wasted time and effort and doing them well.

embalming—the process of removing blood and fluid from a dead body and replacing the fluids with a chemical preservative to keep the body from decomposing before burial.

embolus—floating blood clot.

emergency—a sudden, unexpected happening usually related to a danger.

emotion—basic feelings common to all such as love, fear, anger, sorrow and anxiety.

emotional impact—how one is affected by a situation or individual and how one responds to that situation or individual.

emotional support—the depth of understanding for the emotional needs of others and the way in which a person successfully meets those needs.

empathy—the ability to observe and share the feelings of others in a supportive manner.

emphysema—an abnormal condition of the lung tissue in which the lungs lose their normal spongy and elastic character making for a poor exchange of gases needed for normal respirations. The condition may be acute or chronic.

empty calories—foods high in carbohydrates and fats and low in proteins, minerals and vitamins; "junk" food.

empty nest syndrome—period of time in a mother's life after all her children leave when the mother needs to find things to do to occupy her time and keep herself from feeling worthless and depressed.

endocrine—a body system made up of ductless

glands which secrete hormones directly into the blood and lymph system.

environment—the sum total of the conditions surrounding an individual.

enzymes—proteins produced by the body that break down organic matter (food) within the body; necessary for digestion and metabolism.

epidermis—the outer layer of the skin.

epiglottis—thin, irregular-shaped structure located at the rear of the tongue that covers the larynx (voice box) when a person swallows. It prevents food or liquids from entering the airway.

epilepsy—an illness related to brain dysfunction that may or may not bring on convulsions. Heredity seems to play some part in the transmission of this illness; it may also result from a head injury. Medication can control the condition in many cases.

ethics—a code of behavior. Medical ethics is the standard of professional conduct by health team members.

euphoria—a state of high feeling.

evacuation—to empty or remove the contents from.

evaluation—a determination of how well a given duty or demonstration of skill is performed.

exhale—to breath out.

expectorate—to spit.

experience—knowledge, skill, or practice derived from the direct participation in events; being part of an event.

expressive aphasia—unable to correctly express oneself verbally.

extended care facility—a nursing home, residence, or hospital wing that is licensed by the state to provide long-term care.

extended family—different generations—parent, children and grandparents living together and sharing responsibilities.

external stimulus—a message or impulse sent to the nervous system from outside the body that causes a mental or physical response.

extinguish—to cause to stop burning; to quench.

false imprisonment—unlawfully restraining another person.

familiar—that which is well known.

family unit—a group of people, usually related, who may or may not live under the same roof.

fanfold—to fold in pleats.

fantasizing—daydreaming; engaging in imagination that is not real.

fecal impaction—condition in which feces are wedged tightly in the bowel.

femur—bone in thigh, going from the hip to the knee.

fermented—rotted.

fertilization—uniting of the female ova and the male sperm which starts a new being.

fetal alcohol syndrome—condition seen in infants and children due to mother's intake of alcohol during pregnancy.

fibula—secondary and smaller bone in the lower leg, next to the shin bone.

finances—related to the money earned, spent, or saved by an individual, family, or organization.

first aid—the immediate help given in case of accident or injury.

fixed income—usually refers to the sum total of money coming in to a retired, elderly, or disabled person on a regular monthly basis.

flatus—gas or air in the stomach or intestines; air or gas expelled by way of any body opening.

flexible—the ability to adapt to new situations or conditions; pliant.

Foley catheter—indwelling catheter placed in the urinary bladder to drain urine continuously.

food guide pyramid—the six food groups making up good nutritional standards for humans.

footboard—appliance placed at the foot of the bed so the feet rest firmly against it and are at right angles to the legs.

foot drop—a condition in which the muscles of the foot are out of alignment; may be due to injury or paralysis.

fracture—a break in a bone requiring an X ray to determine the type and treatment.

fraternal twins—result from the fertilization of two female eggs by two separate male sperms. The two embryos are encased in separate amniotic sacs and have separate placentas. Fraternal twins may or may not be of the same sex.

frustration—a sense of insecurity and dissatisfaction due to unfulfilled needs and/or unresolved problems.

full liquid diet—special diet that consists of foods that are liquid at room temperature, i.e., milk, pudding, ice cream.

fungi—include two groups of microorganisms that can cause diseases such as athlete's foot and vaginitis.

gait—term used for walking style.

gait deviations—any abnormalities found in a walking style.

gambling—betting on the outcome of an event; may be an addictive behavior pattern among certain individuals.

gamma globulin—an immune factor of blood plasma which can be manufactured and injected into the body to prevent or diminish the effects of diseases such as measles, polio, chicken pox, hepatitis, etc.

gangrene—the formation of large areas of dead tissue which can become a serious complication.

gas gangrene—a complication of diabetes which causes the skin to decay requiring surgical removal of a limb or body part.

germs—microorganisms capable of causing disease.

gestation period—the time required from conception until birth. In humans the gestation period is 9 months.

gestational—refers to a type of diabetes that occurs only during pregnancy.

gesture—body, hand, muscle movements; in body language, gestures are used to communicate without words.

glucometer—instrument used to measure the level of blood sugar.

glucose—a form of sugar required by the body.

glucose tolerance test—a procedure used to measure the metabolism of carbohydrates in the body; usually refers to blood and/or urine tests to diagnose and treat diabetes.

goiter—a thyroid disorder causing unnatural enlargement of the thyroid gland which is visible as a lump at the front of the neck.

gonorrhea—a venereal disease which develops within 48 hours after sexual contact with an infected person. Painful burning sensation during urination among males; females have urinary burning and vaginal discomfort. Complications can lead to reproductive disorders, liver involvement and blindness (more common among women). Immediate treatment is required.

gout—form of arthritis caused by an increased amount of uric acid in the body.

grief/grieve—the feeling of separation or loss.

hallucination—idea or perception that is not based on reality.

hazard—that which is dangerous or could cause a serious accident.

heat exhaustion—an acute response to exposure to high temperatures; often associated with an overexposure to hot sunlight.

Heimlich maneuver—technique for removing a food particle or foreign object that has become lodged in the trachea thereby preventing flow of air to the lungs. To administer the Heimlich maneuver, wrap your arms around the victim's waist from behind; make a fist with your one hand and place it against the victim's abdomen between the navel and the rib cage; grasp your fist with your other hand and press into the victim's abdomen with a quick upward thrust. Repeat if necessary.

hemiplegia—a weakness or paralysis confined to one side of the body.

hemophilia—a blood disease usually found only among males; the blood clotting factor is missing and even small injuries can cause severe blood loss that may require transfusion.

hepatitis—inflammation of the liver.

hepatitis A—an infectious disease of the liver that has a slow onset of signs and symptoms and spread through contaminated water or food.

hepatitis B—a serious form of infectious liver inflammation transmitted by blood that contains the virus. The signs and symptoms do come on suddenly.

herbs—plants having an aroma that may be used in medicines or as a seasoning for foods to enhance taste.

heredity—the passing of physical and mental traits from parents to their offspring, e.g., height, weight, general appearance, skin color, talents and intelligence.

herpes—a sexually transmitted virus for which there is no known cure.

high-bulk diet—diet including foods that are high in fiber in order to stimulate bowel action.

HIV—human immunodeficiency virus that causes AIDS.

home care aide—caregiver who works with a client with the goal of assisting the client with independent living under professional supervision.

home health aide—performs personal and nursing care skills such as bathing the client under supervision of a registered nurse.

homemaker—performs household duties such as laundry and cooking.

homemaker/home health aide—assists with general household tasks, personal care and simple nursing duties such as feeding and bathing the client.

homosexual—a person who feels sexual attraction to members of the same sex.

horizontal recumbent position—client is positioned flat on the back, arms extended by the sides, and legs extended.

hormones—products of body glands which assist in healthy body function.

hospice—group that provides specialized care for dying clients and their families. The primary concern of hospice is the quality of life and not prolonging the length of life. The goal is to keep the client as painfree and as comfortable as possible.

hygiene—personal cleanliness of the human body.

hyperglycemia—high blood sugar.

hypertension—high blood pressure.

hypoglycemia—low blood sugar.

hypotension—low blood pressure.

hysterectomy—a major surgical technique in which the uterus is removed. In the case of a panhysterectomy, all the female reproductive organs are removed.

identical twins—result from the fertilization of one female egg by one male sperm. The fertilized egg divides into two embryos encased in separate amniotic sacs that share one placenta. Identical twins are always of the same sex.

ileostomy—the surgical removal of a diseased portion of the small intestine and the preparation of an external abdominal stoma (usually permanent) from which a liquid stool is expelled.

illiterate—the inability to read due to lack of education or a learning disability.

immobilize—to hold rigidly in one position.

immune deficiency—partial or complete inability of the immune system to respond to germs.

immunity—the ability to resist a particular disease.

immunization—injections and/or oral vaccines given to prevent the onset of communicable diseases.

impacted—tightly wedged. In reference to the stool, impaction is a condition in which the feces become hardened and lodged in the lower colon or rectum.

incinerator—a furnace for burning trash and garbage.

incontinence—the loss of voluntary control of the bladder muscles causing uncontrolled voiding.

incubation period—the time between entry of germs into the body and the appearance of the first signs of the disease.

infection—invasion of pathogenic organisms causing inflammation, discomfort, or illness. Infections may be caused by viruses, bacteria, fungi, or animal parasites.

infection control—measures used in client's care to prevent the spread of contagious diseases.

infectious diseases—diseases that are readily passed from one person to another.

infraction—violation of a rule or law.

inhale—to breathe in; that part of the breathing and respiration cycle in which oxygen is drawn into the lungs.

injection—the forcing of a fluid into a blood vessel or body cavity or under the skin.

instinct—an inborn trait.

insulin—a hormone produced by the islets of Langerhans in the pancreas which is essential for the maintenance of proper blood sugar levels. Insulin can be medically prepared from animal pancreas for use in diabetes.

insulin shock—a condition in which there is too much insulin in the body resulting in abnormally low blood sugar. The condition is characterized by nervousness. dizziness, perspiration, headache, blurred vision. Immediate treatment such as eating candy or sugar or drinking orange juice is necessary.

integument—the skin.

interaction—the reciprocating actions between two people or between members of a group.

interfere—to concern oneself in the affairs of others; meddle.

intergenerational conflict—the problems occurring among individuals of differing ages living together who all have needs and desires which may cause disagreements, anger, or unhappiness.

intermittent positive pressure breathing (IPPB)—clients suffering from pulmonary disease such as emphysema breathe through a mask connected to a machine which produces intermittent positive air pressure. Increasing the air pressure inflates the lungs; when the pressure is released, the client exhales. This helps the client to breathe easier.

internal stimulus—a message or impulse from within the body that is transmitted through the nervous system and causes a mental or physical response.

interpersonal relationships—the feelings and understanding that result from the interactions between two or more persons.

interracial family—mother and father are from different races.

intrafamily—the relationships among members of a specific family or group of individuals living together as a family.

invasion—hostile entry into another area or place.

invasion of privacy—taking liberties with the person or personal rights of another.

involuntary—body responses not subject to control that occur naturally and automatically.

irrigation—the use of a fluid to cleanse an area.

ischemia—lack of blood supply.

isolation—procedure whereby the client is kept away from others to prevent the spread of a contagious disease.

-itis—a suffix which means inflammation.

jaundice—a condition in which there is a yellowish color to the skin, mucous membranes, and eyes. It is associated with liver failure when excessive amounts of bilirubin enter the blood.

jejunostomy—surgical opening of the jejunum.

job description—duties and responsibilities involved in a position.

joint inflammation—joint is swollen, red and painful especially on movement.

Judaism—the religious practices of Jews, including dietary laws, attending services on Saturday, following the teachings of the Old Testament.

juvenile diabetes—a form of diabetes occurring among persons under the age of 25; generally a condition that is hard to keep under control requiring careful medical attention—type I diabetes.

Kaposi's sarcoma—specific type of cancer that appears in clients who are HIV positive. Lesions appear on the skin and other organs.

kosher—dietary law practiced by some Jewish people. Rules include how animals are killed, what kinds of foods may be used, and keeping separate pots, pans and dishes when preparing milk and meat products or special holiday meals.

labia majora—two large, hair covered, liplike structures that are part of the vulva.

labia minora—two hairless, liplike structures found beneath the labia majora.

laryngectomy—the surgical removal of the larynx (voice box) because of disease. Laryngectomy patients can be taught to speak through an artificial airway by gulping air through the external stoma into the esophagus.

larynx—the voice box.

legal—having to do with the law and/or laws.

lesion—a well-defined abnormal change in tissue due to disease or injury. Examples of lesions are crusts, scales, scars, ulcers, chancres, raised and reddened areas, pimples, pus.

lethargy—a state of unnatural tiredness, feelings of exhaustion and sleepiness.

liability—something for which a person has a responsibility or duty.

libel—an oral or written defamation statement.

life-style choice—individuals today have choices whether to marry, remain single, return home to one's primary family or live with a group or live with individual of own sex or opposite sex without being married.

ligaments—the tough elastic fibers that hold the bones in place.

listening—hearing with thoughtful attention.

living style—way a person decides to live, i.e., living with another person, or living alone.

living will—legal document that outlines the medical care individuals want or don't want if they become unable to make their own decisions.

lobectomy—partial removal of a lung.

localized—pertaining to a specific area.

long-term care facility—facility that provides care for individuals with long-standing disabilities or chronic diseases.

low-birth-weight baby—a full-term infant weighing less than 5 pounds.

low-residue diet—diet in which only foods low in bulk are allowed; used to lessen bowel activity.

low-sodium diet—diet containing foods with low salt content; no extra salt is to be added.

LPN—licensed practical nurse; a person who has met state educational mandates, passed a state examination, and is licensed to practice in the state.

malignant—uncontrolled growth that is resistant to treatment and has a tendency to spread to surrounding areas; often said of cancerous growths.

malnutrition—a condition resulting from poor diet that lacks needed nutrients to maintain health; early signs include muscle weakness.

mammogram—X rays of the female breasts used to determine if a tumor is present in the breasts.

mandible—lower jaw bone.

manipulation—a behavior that uses insidious means to control others to one's own advantage.

mastectomy—a surgical removal of the female breast(s); may be total or partial.

masturbate—self-stimulation of the genitalia.

maxilla—upper jaw bone.

Meals-On-Wheels—prepared meals which are delivered to homebound clients or to senior citizens centers to help assure the disadvantaged, handicapped, ill, or aged have at least one meal a day that is nutritionally sound.

measles—a highly contagious viral disease characterized by the eruption of distinct red circular spots; other symptoms are fever, general malaise, sneezing, nasal congestion, and brassy cough. Children should be immunized to prevent the disease.

meatus—tubelike opening.

mechanical life support—machines used to keep the heart and lungs working when they do not function naturally, e.g., heart-lung machines or oxygen.

mechanical lift—apparatus used to assist in lifting and transferring a client.

Medicaid—federally and state funded program that pays medical costs for those whose income is below a certain level.

medical asepsis—procedures used to stop the spread of pathogens from person to person or place to place.

Medic Alert ID—a bracelet or necklace worn by individuals with specific medical problems such as allergies, diabetes, or hemophilia. In an emergency, the ID may provide information necessary to save the person's life.

medical terminology—use of special words and abbreviations that relate to medical subjects.

Medicare—federal program that assists persons over 65 years of age with hospital and medical costs.

menopause—cessation of the monthly menstrual cycle. It normally occurs during a woman's middle years (late forties to late fifties). Following menopause, reproductive ability ceases.

mental—relating to the mind; the nonphysical health condition of an individual.

mental illness—is a state of emotional impairment in which individuals cannot act normal.

metabolic rate—the speed and efficiency of the body systems in using the nutrients in the blood after digestion has taken place; related to growth, energy and waste elimination.

metastasis—spreading of cancer cells away from primary site of the cancer tumor.

metastasize—spreading of the cancer cells from the original site to one or more places elsewhere in the body.

microorganism—organism that is not visible with the naked eye such as bacterium or protozoan; some microorganisms cause serious illnesses.

middle adulthood—period of time for an individual between the ages of 45–65 years of age.

midwife—a specially educated person who cares for pregnant women and can deliver babies. In most states, it is required that a physician be available as backup in case of an emergency.

mildew—a fuzzy, grayish fungus growth that appears in damp, dark areas.

misconduct—improper behavior; mismanagement of responsibilities.

mobile—that which moves about. Pathogens are mobile and may be carried through the air. Families who move from place to place because of job changes are called mobile families.

multiple sclerosis—a progressive disease involving the nerves of the brain and spinal cord. It may start slowly and become worse throughout life or there may be periods of remission when the condition seems to stay about the same. Signs and symptoms are tremors and inability to coordinate muscles.

muscular dystrophy—a progressive degenerative disease of the muscles surrounding the skeleton; characterized by loss of strength, physical disability and deformity.

myocardial infarction—an acute coronary occlusion commonly called a heart attack.

myocardium—heart muscle.

myth—a story that is unverifiable.

nasogastric tube—soft rubber or plastic tube that is inserted through the nose and into the stomach.

necrosis—death of tissues.

negligence—failure to give care that is reasonably expected of a home health aide.

neoplasm—new growth; tumor.

neuropathy—having mainly to do with diabetic clients, but is any disease of the nerves.

nitroglycerin—medication used in treatment of heart conditions.

nitro-patch—a patch containing nitroglycerin; when placed on the chest nitroglycerin is released and absorbed into the body through the skin. The nitro-patch is a replacement for the nitroglycerin tablet which is taken sublingually.

nocturia—excessive urination at night.

nonverbal—a way of communicating without words using gestures, facial expressions or other body language.

nutrient—the usable products derived from the food eaten after the food has been acted on by the digestive juices. Nutrients are absorbed through the walls of the small intestine and carried through the body.

nutrition—the sum of those processes using food for growth, development and body maintenance.

oath—a solemn promise to do what one has said will be done.

observation—gathering information about any change in the client's condition or behavior by using any of your five senses.

occult blood—hidden blood, must be seen by a microscope; sometimes a stool is sent to the lab for occult blood testing.

occupational therapist—a professional who evaluates the client's ability to function in everyday life and recommends adaptive equipment or exercises to help the client function as independently as possible.

offensive—causing displeasure.

oliguria—lowered urinary output.

ombudsman—client's advocate.

Omnibus Budget Reconciliation Act—(OBRA)—law that regulates the education and certification of home health aides' work in home health agencies and certified hospices.

optimal health—highest point an individual can achieve mentally and physically as adapted from Abraham Maslow's hierarchy of needs.

optimist—one who expects a positive outcome to a situation.

oral hygiene—care of the gums, lips, mouth, teeth, and tongue.

osteoarthritis—degenerative joint disease caused by disintegration of the cartilage that covers the ends of the bones.

osteoporosis—loss of bone density and strength; the bones become increasingly porous and brittle which may lead to malformations such as a dowager's hump or hip fractures. Postmenopausal women are at high risk. An adequate intake of calcium helps to prevent the disease.

-otomy—suffix meaning to cut into.

otosclerosis—chronic, progressive deafness, especially to low tones.

outsider—one who is not part of an organized group.

ovulation—that time of the month when the ovum (egg) produced in the female reproductive system's ovary is released and enters the fallopian tube where it may be fertilized.

oxygen—the colorless, tasteless, odorless gaseous element in the atmosphere which is essential to breathing.

pacemaker—artificial device placed in the body to regulate the heartbeat.

Pap smear—a medical technique whereby a sample of the vaginal cells are tested for cancer; recommended for women annually to detect early signs of cancer.

paralysis—loss of sensation in a body part making it difficult or impossible to move that part of the body.

paraplegic—paralysis of the lower body involving both legs.

patella—knee cap.

patella tendon—tendon found below knee cap.

pathogens—microorganisms causing disease or infection in the body.

Patient Self-Determination Act—law that gives an individual the right to make choices regarding specific type and kind of medical care before they become seriously ill.

peer pressure—the attitudes and behavior patterns within a particular group which all group members are expected to follow. (A peer is an equal; one of same age group, rank, social status.)

perineum—in the male, the area between the anus and scrotum; in the female, the area between the anus and vagina.

perishable—likely to spoil or decay.

peristalsis—the progressive, wavelike movements that occur involuntarily to move food through the digestive system.

permanent press—fabric with combination of natural and man-made threads that requires little or no ironing.

persistent—constantly repeated; permanent, or stubborn in a course of action.

personal care worker—assists with minimal level of daily living activities such as companionship and meal preparation.

personal reference—a person, other than a member of the individual's family, who can give a prospective employer a recommendation concerning the character and ability of an individual seeking employment.

pessimist—one who expects a negative or bad outcome to a situation or who looks on the gloomy side of life.

phalanges—any bones of a finger or toe.

phantom pain—a sensation of pain felt in an amputated part. It is caused by the nerve endings that have not had time to heal from the surgery.

phlebitis—inflammation of a vein.

phlegm—mucus from the lungs.

phobia—an abnormal fear.

pilferage—to repeatedly steal in small amounts or value.

pistoning—stump slipping up and down in the prosthesis.

pitch—the high or low tone of voice with which one speaks. Pitch is related to the sound wave frequency that causes variations in sounds from high to low.

Pneumocystis carinii—protozoan frequently causing pneumonia in clients who are HIV positive.

pneumonectomy—surgical removal of the entire lung.

pneumonia—an acute inflammation of the lungs caused by bacteria, viruses or fungi; characterized by high fever, chills, headache, cough and chest pains.

podiatrist—a foot doctor.

poliomyelitis—an inflammation of the spinal cord's gray matter which can cause paralysis and respiratory problems; a communicable disease that has been almost wiped out as a result of vaccines.

polyester—a man-made fabric.

postmortem—after death.

postpartum—after childbirth.

postural drainage—technique of positioning the client to encourage drainage of different areas of the lungs.

practice—the actual performance of the procedure; the clientele of a doctor or medical practice.

prefix—series of letters placed at the beginning of a word that produces a derivative word.

premature—an infant born before full term (37 weeks gestation is considered full term among humans).

prenatal—before birth.

prescription—usually refers to medication ordered by the doctor to be used following specific instructions and in controlled dosages.

pressure sore—dermal ulcer or bedsore.

preventative health measures—use of inoculations, special diets, or other techniques to avoid illness before it starts.

priority—decision as to what items or tasks should be done first based on their importance.

privilege—a special benefit or opportunity offered to a person or group.

procedure—the steps taken to accomplish a particular task; a course or plan of action.

produce—fresh fruits and vegetables.

professional—one who is skilled or experienced in a particular area of training or learning.

prognosis—the probable outcome of an illness.

progressive degenerative disease—disease which grows worse as time goes on, often resulting in greater and greater physical loss to a particular part of the body.

projection—a defense mechanism whereby an individual blames someone else for his or her own failure.

prolonged—that which lasts over a long period of time.

pronation—placing or lying in a face downward position; applied to the hand with the palms facing backward.

prosthesis—artificial replacement for a body part.

protozoa—tiny, one-celled microscopic animals.

psychology—the study or science concerned with mental processes and behavior of an individual; the study concerned with mental health.

psychosocial—relating to both psychological and social problems/happenings in the life of an individual.

puberty—the time period following childhood when the body matures and reproduction becomes possible.

pulse—the measurement of the number of heartbeats per minute.

quadriplegic—paralysis of four extremities—arms and legs

radial artery—artery near the radius; commonly used to determine pulse.

radical mastectomy—the surgical removal of the entire breast including the underlying muscles and lymph glands under the arm. It is performed in the hope of stopping further spread of cancer cells.

rales—bubbling sound from the lungs when fluid or mucus is trapped in the air passages.

range of motion exercises—the exercises designed to prevent contractures and loss of motion and function in the joints; usually planned by a physical therapist.

rationalization—a defense mechanism whereby a person gives excuses to account for personal failings.

Reach for Recovery—a volunteer group consisting of women with breast cancer who counsel and support other women with similar problems.

reality orientation—techniques used to keep confused clients in touch with reality.

receptive aphasia—communication problem whereby a person does not understand the words someone else says.

recreation—a pleasurable activity following a period of work; distraction from normal activity in an effort to have fun or enjoy a change of pace.

rectum—the last segment of the digestive system from which feces are expelled.

registry service—an agency that employs certified individuals to give home health care.

rehabilitation—the restoring of physical and/or mental abilities following an accident or illness. Some patients can be fully restored to normal functioning; others are brought up to the best possible level through exercise and retraining.

reinforcement—the act of supporting another individual by words and actions. Reinforcement may be either positive or negative.

remedies—the methods and medications used to cure or make well.

remission—a period in an illness when the symptoms cease or become less severe.

reporting—to make a written record or oral summary of care of client.

residue—that which is left over. In nutrition, high or low residue refers to the amount of bulk and fiber food in the diet. These foods are usually low in vitamins.

respiration—the sum total of the processes by which the body exchanges oxygen and carbon dioxide in the respiratory system.

respirations—one of the vital signs in which the breaths of the person are counted. Illness can cause the respirations to fluctuate or become abnormal.

restorative care—care that emphasizes helping the person reach or maintain physical, mental, and psychological well-being.

restricted fluids—limit to the amount of fluid intake.

resumé—short account of one's career and qualifications prepared by an applicant for a position.

rheumatoid arthritis—autoimmune response that results in inflammation of the joints.

rickettsiae—microorganisms that can cause disease and lives on lice, ticks, fleas and mites.

rigidity—stiffness or inability to bend; associated with the pain and joint stiffness caused by arthritis.

RN—registered nurse; an individual who has attended nursing school or college, taken and passed state examinations, and is licensed to practice in the state.

root word—the main part of a compound word that has a prefix or suffix.

sanitary—of or relating to health and cleanliness.

satiety—the feeling of satisfaction or fullness after eating.

schedule—a plan to organize work so that everything that needs to be done can be completed within a certain time.

security—a feeling of being comfortable or safe in a given situation.

seizure—a sudden attack; a convulsion.

self-esteem—value one places on one's self as a person functioning in society.

self-scheduling—the individual plan of action that allows one to determine priorities and to work as his/her own pace in order to accomplish set goals.

self-understanding—the awareness of one's own behavior and feelings in any given situation.

semicoma—the third level of unconsciousness in which it is difficult to rouse the patient or get the patient to respond.

semi-Fowler's position—client is positioned on the back, knees are slightly flexed, and head of bed is elevated 30° to 50°.

senescence—the period of old age; the process of growing old.

senile—pertaining to old age.

senile dementia—a group of mental disorders afflicting some aging individuals.

sensitive—being aware of the physical and emotional needs of others.

sensory deficits—lack or lessening of ability to receive stimuli in a particular sense (loss of hearing, weak eyes, weakened taste buds, inability to feel heat or cold, etc.)

separation—end of contractual relationship between husband and wife by mutual agreement.

septum—divider, as seen in the division of the heart. The septum divides right side from left side.

Seventh Day Adventist—a religious sect observing the Sabbath on Saturday and following a set of standards of daily living that may be different from other religious groups.

sexuality—maleness or femaleness of an individual.

shrinking—decreased, as in swelling.

sibling rivalry—the normal jealousy and competition found between brothers and sisters in the family setting.

sickle cell anemia—a hereditary and chronic blood anemia in which the red blood cells are shaped in a crescent formation and look like a sickle. This disease occurs mainly in African Americans.

sigmoidoscopy—direct examination of the interior of the sigmoid colon.

sign—in medicine, a change in the patient that can be observed or measured.

Sims' position—client is positioned on left side with left leg extended and right leg flexed; left arm is extended and brought behind back; right arm is flexed and brought forward.

single-parent family—a family group headed by a mother or a father in which there is no other adult providing emotional and/or financial support.

sitz bath—bath providing moist heat to the genitals or anal area.

skin breakdown—any cut or scraping of the skin due to pressure or positioning too long in the same position.

slander—false statement, oral or written, that injures the reputation of another person.

social service agency—a governmental body which provides assistance in solving problems such as housing, living conditions, clothing or food stamps for those unable to find jobs or support themselves.

soft diet—diet in which soft, easily digested foods are ordered for clients recovering from surgery or who have ulcers; this diet causes little upset to the digestive system.

somnolence—a state of drowsiness and lethargy; the desire to sleep.

spasticity—increased tension in the muscles causing irregular movements of the body part involved.

specialist—one who has studied in a concentrated area and has specialized in one particular field of knowledge.

specimen—small sample of secretions taken from the body for examination, i.e., urine, stool, sputum.

sperm—the male germ cell ejaculated during intercourse that fertilizes the ovum and starts the cycle of reproduction.

sphygmomanometer—the instrument used to measure blood pressure.

sputum—matter brought up from the lungs; phlegm.

stabilized—under control and on an even course.

staple items—those foodstuffs normally kept in most homes which are used in many ways and are the basis for preparing meals, e.g., flour, sugar, spices, herbs, canned goods.

sterile—free of pathogens.

steroids—hormonal medications used to treat many conditions. Major side effects are edema, weight gain, susceptibility to infections, and elevated blood pressure.

stimuli—messages sent from the five body senses to the brain so that a response can be made. Internal stimuli start within the body; external stimuli come from outside the body.

stoic—not affected by or showing emotions.

stoma—the surgically formed opening between a body cavity or passage and the body's surface.

stressful—a situation that is filled with pressure and causes anxiety and signs of discomfort.

stump—term used for the remaining portion of the amputated limb.

subcutaneously—refers to an injection given beneath the skin.

sublingually—under the tongue.

sudden infant death syndrome—(SIDS)—the unexpected and sudden death of a healthy infant that occurs while an infant is sleeping.

suffix—series of letters placed at the end of a word that produces a derivative word.

suicide—the act of taking one's own life.

sundowning—behavior in which a person becomes more agitated and disoriented during the evening hours.

supervisor—one who is in charge of other people.

supine—lying with face upward.

suppository—medication used to help the bowels eliminate feces.

sympathetic—having concerns or sharing the feelings of others; being sensitive to the needs of others.

symptom—those changes reported by the patient such as feeling pain which may not be visible.

syphilis—an infectious, chronic venereal disease characterized by open lesions which can spread to the entire body and affect the nervous system.

system—a group of structures or organs related to each other that work together to perform certain functions.

systolic—measurement of blood pressure when the heart is contracting.

tachycardia—a very rapid heartbeat.

tact—sensitive mental perception.

technique—the way a particular task or procedure is done following acceptable guidelines.

technological—related to scientific advances that increase productivity of machines and eliminate manual operations.

TED hose—support hose.

temperament—the usual mood of an individual.

temporal—temples; that part of the face and head near and above the ears.

terminal—final; life-ending stage.

terminal asepsis—the careful cleaning of an area after a sick person has been removed from the room to destroy any pathogens that may be in the room.

theory—the practical and necessary information one must learn about a particular topic or subject.

therapeutic—pertaining to results obtained from treatment; healing agent.

therapy—treatment designated to eliminate disease or other bodily disorder.

thrombus—blood clot that forms inside an artery.

tibia—prominent bone in the lower leg (shin).

time and travel records—records kept of the time spent with clients and the distance traveled between clients.

time organization—organizing your work in order to complete the task or tasks in the allotted time period.

tissues—collection of specialized cells that perform a particular function; piece of paper used for cleansing; for example, toilet tissue, facial tissue.

tone—related to voice pitch but includes the quality and length of sound when speaking.

tophi—outpouches or protruding lesions that contain abnormal amount of uric acid. Seen in individuals with gout.

topical—pertaining to a particular area; local.

total parenteral nutrition—meeting an individual's entire nutritional needs by providing high-density nutrients directly into the bloodstream.

trachea—the main tube running from the throat to the lungs to bring air in and out of the body; the windpipe.

tracheostomy—a surgical procedure to create an opening in the trachea; an emergency operation in cases where the trachea is obstructed and the person cannot breathe.

transfer belt—gait belt that is used to assist and support clients during ambulation.

transient ischemic attack (TIA)—temporary reduction of flow of blood to the brain.

trapeze—horizontal bar suspended overhead down the length of the bed.

tremors—a spastic condition of the muscles in which a body part develops an uncontrollable shaking.

trochanter roll—rolled sheet or bath blanket placed under the client extending from waist to mid thigh; positioned against the hip to prevent lateral hip rotation.

tuberculosis—lung disease caused by a microorganism, easily transmitted to others by sneezing and coughing.

tumor—neoplasm.

turning sheet—sheet used to turn a client.

two-career family—family where both parents are employed full-time outside of the home.

ulcer—open sore caused by inadequate blood supply and broken skin.

unconscious—a state of unawareness with four possible levels—somnolence, stupor, semi-coma, and coma.

underestimate—placing too low a value on a condition or situation; to assess as being less than actual.

universal blood and body fluid precautions—techniques used to prevent transmission of microorganisms that are carried by body fluids from one person to another.

universal precautions—a system of infectious disease control which assumes that every direct contact with body fluids is infectious and requires every health care worker exposed to direct contact with body fluid or body substance to be protected.

upward mobility—moving upward.

urethra—mucus-lined tube conveying urine from the urinary bladder to the exterior of the body; in the male, the urethra also conveys the semen.

urgency—need to urinate.

urgent—requiring immediate attention.

vaccine—a manufactured product administered to develop a resistance to an infectious disease.

validation therapy—techniques used to help people feel good about themselves.

vasoconstriction—narrowing of the blood vessel.

vasodilation—widening of the blood vessel.

vegetarian—one who does not eat meat or meat products.

vein—blood vessel that carries blood back to the heart.

venereal disease—a group of diseases usually transmitted by sexual contact with one having that disease.

verbal—transmitting messages using words.

virus—microorganism that lives and grows by feeding on living cells; the cause of many infections.

vital signs—measurements of temperature, pulse, respiration, and blood pressure.

vocational—related to the job or profession in which one is employed.

void—to release urine from the bladder.

voluntary movements—actions controlled by the brain after messages are sent by the senses through the nervous system; the body chooses the appropriate action.

vomitus—material vomited or brought up from the stomach.

wandering—moving around purposelessly, often seen in clients with dementia.

wellness—free of illness; a state of well-being free of psychological or physiological symptoms.

withdrawal—removing one's self physically or mentally from an uncomfortable or frightening situation.

xiphoid process—lower tip of the sternum.

Index

A

Abbreviations, **43–44**
  defined, 43
Abuse
  child, 100–101
  client, 35
Accidents, age group-related, **158**
Acne, **69**
Acute
  coronary occlusion, 76
  illness, defined, 6
Adjustment, in mental health, 135
Adolescence
  accidents during, **158**
  health problems during, 99–100
  home health aide, 97–100
Adulthood
  accidents during, **158**
  early, 104–5
  emotional needs of, 106–7
  exercise and, 105–6
  illness/disability, acceptance of, 106
  late,
    described, 110
    health/illness and, 112–16
    See also Aging
  middle, 105–6
  retirement and, 107
Advanced directives papers, 253
Aging
  body systems and, 110–12
  emotional/psychological effects of, 116–21
AIDS, 202–4
  AZT and, 203
  client with,
    care plan for, **205–6**
    caring for, 204–7
    working guidelines, **203**
  DDZ and, 203
  diet, 154
  protection against, 204
Airway, obstructed, clearing, 168, **175**
Allergies, food, 148–49

Alzheimer's disease, 121, 124–26
  guidelines for working with, **127–29**
  stages/symptoms of, **124**
    early, **125**
Anemia, 77
Angina pectoris, 76, 222–23
Anticoagulants, myocardial infarction and, 223
Anxiety, 137–38
Application form, employment, 406–8
Arterial system, **74**
Arteriosclerosis, 76–77, 225–26
Arthritis, 70–71, **114**
  defined, 236
  joint deformities due to, **237**
  management of, 238–41
  osteoarthritis, 236, 238
  rheumatoid, 236
Articulates, described, 247
Artificial eye, caring for, **348–49**
Assignments, variety in, 20
Assistive devices, **239**, 240
Asthma, 78–79
Atherosclerosis, 76–77
Attitude, described, 16
Auditory nerve, 73
AZT, AIDS and, 203

B

Back rub, procedure for, **328–29**
Bacteria, 192
Basement, safety in, **174**
Bath
  bed, assisting with, **326–28**
  partial, assisting with, **328**
  personal hygiene and, 16
  sponge, infants, **398–99**
  tub, assisting client with, **323–26**
Bathroom
  maintenance/cleaning of, 276–78
  safety in, 160–61, **172**
Bed
  assisting client, from chair to, **314**
  assisting client, to chair from, **313**

bath, assisting with, **326–28**
  making,
    occupied, **343**
    unoccupied, **340–42**
  moving client in, with drawsheet, **308**
  sores,
    care of, **330–31**
    integumentary system and, 66–67, **68**
Bedpan, giving/emptying, **354–56**
Bedroom, safety in, **171**
Birth, labor/delivery and, 93
Bladder, retraining the, **362–63**
Bland diet, **152**, 153
Blended family, 52
Blender, care/use of, **267**
Blindness, diabetes and, **217**
Blood
  disorders of, 77
  pressure,
    cardinal sign, 185–86
    taking, **371–73**
  vessels, disorders of, 76–77
Body
  alignment, maintaining, **306–7**
  mechanics,
    application of, 178–79
    defined, 175
    principles of, 175–79
  systems, aging and, 110–12
  See also Human body
Bonding, defined, 93
Bones
  aging and, **111**
  fractures of, 70
  skeletal, **70**
Bottle feeding, infants, **400–402**
Bowels, training/retraining, 382
Bradycardia, defined, 184
Brain, central nervous system and, **72**
Breast
  cancer of, 245–46
  feeding/care, assisting with, **397**

Note: Page numbers in **bold** type reference non-text material and client care procedures.

Breathing exercises, deep, assisting
    with, **394–95**
Briefs, adult, applying, **383**
Burns, preventing, **166–68**

C
Cabinets, cleaning, 276
Calorie
    controlled diet, 152–53
    empty, 145–46
Cancer
    client care, 244–45
    defined, 243
    gastrointestinal, 248–49
    larynx, 247–48
    reproductive system, female, 245–46
    respiratory system, 246–48
    skin, 249
    treatment of, 243–44
    warning signs of, 243, **249**
Cane, assisting client with, **319–21**
Carcinogen, defined, 243
Cardiac arrest, defined, 224
Cardinal signs
    blood pressure, 185–86
    height/weight, 186
    illness,
        pulse, 183–84
        respiration rates, 183–84
        temperature, 183
Career
    adjustments, 20–24
    defined, 20
Case studies
    client alone, 122–23
    client confidentiality, **34**
    communication, **45**
    job ethics, **35**
    spouse dependency, 119–20
Casts, caring for, **388–90**
Cataracts, 113
Catheterization, heart, 223
Central nervous system, **72**
Cerebral
    hemorrhage, 228
    infarction, 227
    palsy, **95**
Cerebral vascular accident (CVA), 77,
        114, 226–33
    aftereffects, 228
    communication problems after,
        230–33
    defined, 226
    rehabilitation after, 229–30
    risk factors, 226–27
    signs of, 227–29
Cesarean section, 93
Chair
    assisting client,
        to bed from, **314**

from bed to, **313**
CHAP (Community Health
        Accreditation Program),
        health care and, 8–9
Charting form, **28–29**
Chemotherapy, 244
Cheyne-Stokes respiration, 184
Child abuse, 100–101
Children
    discipline of, cultural differences,
        56
    with special needs, 53
Cholesterol, 144
Chronic
    bronchitis, 78
    illness, defined, 6
Circulation, collateral, defined, 223
Circulatory system, 73–77
    arterial system, **74**
    changes in, **111**
    disorders of, 76
        angina pectoris, 222–23
        arteriosclerosis, 76–77, 225–26
        congestive heart failure, 76,
            224–25
        myocardial infarction, 223–24
        stroke, 77, **114**, 226–30, 233
    risk factors concerning, 222
    venous system, **75**
Cleaning
    cabinets/drawers, 276
    floors, 276
    supplies, storage of, 276
    surfaces, 276
Cleaning tasks
    daily, 271–72
        bathroom, 277
    periodic, 272–73
    weekly, 272
        bathroom, 278
Cleanliness, personal, need for, 16
Clear-liquid diet, **152**
Cleft lip/palate, **95**
Client
    AIDS. *See* AIDS
    care services, **22**
    changes in, reportable, 25–26
    communication with, 43–48
    confidentiality, 27–30
        case study, **34**
    conscious, 186–87
    hearing/speech impaired, commu-
        nication guidelines for, **47**
    nonambulatory, care of, 116
    observations, documenting, 26–27
    rights of, 33–34
    transferring, bed to wheelchair,
        161–62
    unconscious, 186–87
        needs of, **188**

Client abuse, 35
Client alone case study, 122–23
Client care procedures
    artificial eye, 348–49
    assisting,
        from bed to chair, **313**
        from chair to bed, **314**
        from wheelchair to toilet/
            commode, **314–15**
        with crutches, walker, cane,
            319–21
    back rub, **328–29**
    bath,
        bed, giving a, **328–28**
        partial, giving a, **328**
        tub, assisting with, **323–26**
    bed,
        making occupied, **343**
        making unoccupied, **340–42**
        sores, **330–31**
    bedpan, giving/emptying, **354–56**
    bladder, retraining the, **362–63**
    blood pressure, taking, **371–73**
    body alignment maintaining, **306–7**
    bowels, training/retraining, **382**
    breast feeding/breast care,
        assisting with, **397**
    briefs, applying adult, **383**
    casts, caring for, **388–90**
    cough/deep breathing exercises,
        assisting with, **394–95**
    denture care, **334–36**
    described, 295
    drainage unit, emptying, **361–62**
    dressing/undressing client, **338–39**
    elasticized stockings, applying,
        339–40
    enema, giving a commercial,
        380–81
    feeding client, **351–53**
    fluid intake/output, measuring/
        recording, **353–54**
    Fowler's position, **312**
    gloving, **301–2**
    guidelines, 295, 297
    hair, shampooing in bed, **344–46**
    handwashing, **300–301**
    hearing aid, inserting, **347–48**
    ice bag/cap, collar, applying, **376**
    infants,
        assisting in breast feeding, **397**
        bottle feeding, **400–402**
        sponge bathing, **398–99**
    K-pad, applying, **377**
    lateral/side-lying position, **310–11**
    leg bag, connecting, **360–61**
    log rolling client, **309**
    mechanical life use, **321**
    medications, self-administered,
        346–47

moving client with drawsheet, **308**
nail care, **344**
oral hygiene, **333–34**
ostomy bag, changing, **390–92**
oxygen therapy, assisting with, **392–93**
passive range of motion exercises, **315–18**
perineal care,
    female, **329**
    male, **330**
personal protective equipment, **302–4**
procedures, **296**
prone position, **311–12**
pulse, taking radial/apical, **369–70**
rectal suppository, giving a, **381–82**
respirations, counting, **371**
shaving, **337–38**
skin, applying unsterile dressing/
    ointment to, **386–88**
specimen collecting, **304**
sputum specimen, collecting, **363**
stool specimen, collecting, **383–84**
supine position, **310**
temperature,
    taking,
        axillary, **368–69**
        oral, **365–66**
        rectal, **367–68**
turning client toward you, **307**
urinal, giving/emptying, **356**
urinary catheter, caring for, **359–60**
urine specimen, clear-catch
    collecting, **358**
warm foot soak, performing, **378**
weight/height, measuring, **374**
Clostridium tetani, **192**
Clothes dryer, care/use of, **267**
Coffee maker, care/use of, **267**
Colds, late adulthood and, **115**
Collateral circulation, defined, **223**
Coma, defined, **187**
Commode, transferring patient to, **314–15**
Communication
    board, **231–32**
    case study, **45**
    clients and, **43–48**
    components of, **39–40**
    guidelines, **44**
        hearing/speech impaired
            clients, **47**
    nonverbal, **41–42**
    situations, **46**
    therapy, **126–30**
    verbal, **40–41**
    written, **42**
Community Health Accreditation
    Program (CHAP) and, **8–9**

Compensation, defense mechanism, **137**
Components, defined, **12**
Conception, **93**
Confidentiality
    client, **27–30**
        case study, **34**
    defined, **27**
Congestive heart
    disease, **95**
    failure, **76, 224–25**
        diet and, **223**
        late adulthood and, **115**
Constipation, **79–80**
Contractures, **226**
    defined, **186**
Coronary occlusion
    acute, **76**
    late adulthood and, **115**
Cough exercises, assisting with, **394–95**
Crutches, assisting client with, **319–21**
Culture
    differences in, **56**
    minority, **54–55**
Customs, minority cultures, **54–55**
CVA. *See* Cerebral vascular accident
Cyanotic, defined, **219**
Cystic fibrosis, **95**
Cystitis, **82**

D

Daily cleaning tasks, **271–72**
    bathroom, **277**
DDZ, AIDS and, **203**
Deafness, **113**
Death
    adjustment stages to, **253–54**
    postmortem care, **254**
    religious/cultural influences and, **254–55**
    signs of approaching, **254**
Deep breathing, exercises, assisting
    with, **394–95**
Degenerative diseases, nutrition and, **146**
Delivery, in birth, **93**
Dementia
    Alzheimer's disease, **121, 125–26**
    reality orientation and, **130–31**
    validation therapy and, **126–30**
Denial defense mechanism, **137**
Denture care, **334–36**
Dermatitis, **69**
Diabetes mellitus, **85, 211**
    classification of, **211**
    client care procedure, testing
        blood, **213**
    complications of, **216–17**
    diet for, **151, 152, 214–15**

drug therapy,
    type I diabetes, **215**
    type II diabetes, **216**
    emergency treatment of, **212–14**
    exercise and, **215**
    identification tag and, **219**
    nursing care,
        foot care, **217–18**
        infection prevention, **218–19**
        neuropathy and, **217**
    signs/symptoms of, **211–12**
    testing for, **212**
Diabetic diet, **151, 152, 214–15**
Diagnostic related groupings, (DRGs), **6–7**
Diarrhea, **80**
Diastolic blood pressure, **185**
Diet
    congestive heart failure and, **224**
    diabetes, **214–15**
    food guide pyramid, **142–45**
    therapy, **151–55**
    See also specific type of diet
Digestive system, **79–81**
    disorders of, **79–81**
Dining room, safety in, **169**
Discrimination, racial, **57–58**
Disease
    home cleanliness and, **194–95**
    infectious. *See* Infectious disease
    transmission methods, **193**
    universal precautions against, **195–96**
    See also Illness
Dishwasher, care/use of, **266**
Dishwashing, **275**
Disorders
    congestive heart failure, **76, 224–25**
    heart,
        angina pectoris, **222–23**
        arteriosclerosis, **76–77, 225–26**
        myocardial infarction, **223–24**
        stroke, **77, 114, 226–30, 233**
    mental, **182**
Displacement defense mechanism, **137**
Diversion, need for, **189**
Divorce, **52–53**
Documenting, observations, **26–27**
Down syndrome, **95**
Drainage unit, emptying, **361–62**
Drawers, cleaning, **276**
Drawsheet, moving client with, **308**
Dressing, applying, **386–88**
Dressing/undressing client, **338–39**
DRGs (diagnostic related groupings), **6–7**
Drying clothes, **290–91**
Durable power of attorney, **253**
Dying, adjustment stages to, **253–54**
Dyspnea, defined, **184**

E

Ear, internal view of, **73**
Early adulthood, 104–5
Eating habits, developing good, 145–48
Egg crate mattress, **69**
Elasticized stockings, applying, **339–40**
Electric fry pan, care/use of, **267**
Emboli, late adulthood and, **115**
Emotional needs, adults, 106–7
Emotions
    defined, 135
    health and, 138–39
    understanding, 135–37
Employment
    application form, 406–8
    job interview, 409–11
    prospective employers, contacting,
        405–6
    trends affecting, 405
Empty nest syndrome, 105
Endocrine system, 85
    glands of, **86, 87**
Enema, giving, commercial, **380–81**
Environment, defined, 56
Equipment, variety of, 20
Erikson, Erik, personality
        development, stages of, **136**
Ethical
    dilemmas, 32–33
    standards, 31
Ethics, 31–33
    case study, **35**
Exercise
    effects of, 105-6
    range of motion, passive, **315–18**
External stimulus, defined, 135

F

Falls, 159–63
Family unit
    cultures of, 54–55
    current perspectives of, 52–54
    historic perspective of, 51–52
    religious practice and, 56–57
Fantasizing defense mechanism, 137
Fat
    saturated, 144
    total, 144
Fat-controlled diet, 151
Feeding, client, **351–53**
Fetal alcohol syndrome, 95
Fire safety, 163–68
    fire extinguishers, 164–65
Floors, cleaning, 276
Fluid intake/output, measuring/
        recording, 353–54
Food
    allergies, 148–49
    guide pyramid, 142–45

preparation of, 282–85
    appealing, 149–51
    purchasing, 280–82
    storing, 282
Foot soak, warm, **378**
Form, charting, **28–29**
Fowler's position, positioning client
        in, **312**
Fractures, 70
    late adulthood and, **114**
Freezer, care/use of, **265**
Full-liquid diet, **152**
Fungi, 193

G

Gangrene, 77
    diabetes and, **217**
    preventing, 218–19
Garbage
    compactor, care/use of, **266**
    disposal, care/use of, **266**
    disposing of, 274–75
Gas gangrene. *See* Gangrene
Gastrointestinal system, cancer of,
        248–49
Geriatrics, defined, 118
Germs, 192
    destroying, **194**
    dishwashing and, 275
Gestation period, 93
Glaucoma, **113**
Gloving procedure, **301–2**
Gonorrhea, 84
Gout, described, 236, 238
Grief, responses to, 56
Grooming, need for, 16

H

Hair
    aging and, **111**
    shampooing, in bed, **344–46**
Handwashing procedure, 300–301
Health, personal, 15–16
Health care
    Community Health Accreditation
        Program (CHAP) and, 8–9
    Medicare/Medicaid and, 9
    OBRA and, 9
    team, described, 16–17
Hearing
    aging and, **111**
    aid, inserting, **347–48**
Heart
    aging and, **111**
    attack, symptoms of, **224**
    block fibrillation, late adulthood
        and, **115**
    disorders of, 76
        angina pectoris, 222–23

arteriosclerosis, 76–77, 225–26
    congestive heart failure, 76,
        224–25
    myocardial infarction, 223–24
    external view of, **76**
    late adulthood and, **115**
Heartburn, 80–81
Height, measuring, 186, **374**
Heimlich maneuver, 168, **175**
Hemiplegia, 71
Hemophilia, 77
Hepatitis B, 200
Herbs, meal preparation and, **285**
Herpes, 84
Hierarchy of needs, 15
High-calorie diet, **152**
High-fiber diet, **153**, 154
High-potassium diet, **153**, 153–54
HIV, 202
Home care aide, defined, 5
Home care services
    growing need for, 5–6
    history of, 5
Home cleanliness, disease and, 194–95
Home health aide
    adolescence and, 97–100
    Alzheimer's disease and, **126**
    approved functions of, **23**
    client care limitations, **24**
    defined, 5
    ethics and, 31–33
    infants and, 96
    liability, 30–31
    observing, importance of, 24–25
    preschoolers and, 96
    rights of, 34
    role of, 7–8
    school-age children and, 96
    toddlers and, 96
Homemaker, defined, 5
Hormones, aging and, **111**
Household management
    appliances, use/care of, **265–67**
    bathroom, 276–78
    cleaning tasks,
        daily, 271–72, 277
        periodic, 272–73
        weekly, 272, 278
    client care and, 268
    discussed, 263–64
    injury prevention, 267–68
    kitchen, maintenance/cleaning,
        273–76
    planning/organization of, 264–67
Human body, **63**
    changes in, **111**
    circulatory system, 73–77
        arterial system, **74**
        disorders of, 76

venous system, **75**
development of, factors
    influencing, 87–88
digestive system, 79–81
  disorders of, 79–81
endocrine system, 85
  glands of, **86, 87**
integumentary system, 64–67
  bedsores and, 66–67, **68**
musculoskeletal system, 67–71
  disorders of, 70–71
nervous system, 71–73
  disorders of, 72–73
reproductive system, 82–84
respiratory system, 77–79
  disorders of, 78–79
systems of, **64**
urinary system, 81–82
Human development
  Erik Erikson's theory of, **136**
  infancy, 93–94
  labor/delivery and, 93
  pregnancy and, 93
Human immunodeficiency virus. *See*
  HIV
Hydrocephalus, **95**
Hygiene
  oral, 16
  personal, 15–16
Hyperthyroidism, 85
Hypothyroidism, 85

I
Ice bag/cap/collar, applying, **376**
Ileostomy, described, 248
Illness
  acute, defined, 6
  chronic,
    aging and, 112–16
    defined, 6
  controlling spread of, 195
  internal disorders, 182
  isolation and, 196–97
  signs/symptoms,
    cardinal, 183–86
    observing, 183
  See also Disease
Immune
  deficiencies, 202–4
  system, aging and, **111**
Immunizations, infancy and, 94
Incontinence, 81
Incubation period, defined, 192
Infancy, 93–94
  health problems during, 94–96
Infants
  accidents of, **158**
  bathing, sponge, **398–99**
  bottle feeding, **400–402**

breast feeding, assisting with, **397**
Infections
  control,
    gloving, **301–2**
    handwashing, **300–301**
    methods, 197–98
    personal protective equipment,
     302–4
    specimen collection in isolation,
     304
  preventing, diabetes and, 218–19
Infectious diseases
  control methods, 197–98
  hepatitis B, 200
  immune deficiencies and, 202–4
  list of, **200**
  precautions against, 201–2
  tuberculosis, 200–201
Injury prevention, 267–68
Instructions, following, 20–22
Insulin, diabetes and, 211
Integumentary system, 64–67
  aging and, 112
  bedsores and, 66–67, **68**
  cancer of, 249
Interaction, interpersonal, defined, 13,
  14
Internal
  disorders, 182
  stimulus, defined, 135
Interpersonal relationships, 13–14
Interracial family, 52
Intervention, defined, 25
Ironing clothes, 290–91
Irrigation, defined, 248
Ischemia, defined, 222
Isolation, illness and, 196–97

J
Job interview, 406
Joints, aging and, **111**

K
K-pad, applying, **377**
Kidneys
  aging and, **111**
  diabetes and, **217**
  stones in, 82
Kitchen
  maintenance/cleaning of, 273–76
  safety, **170**
Kübler-Ross, Elisabeth, death/dying
  and, stages of acceptance,
  253–54

L
Labor, in birth, 93
Language, differences in, 55–56
Laryngectomy, described, 247

Larynx, cancer of, 247–48
Late adulthood
  described, 110
  health/illness and, 112–16
  See also Aging
Lateral position, positioning client in,
  310–11
Laundry
  drying/ironing/mending, 290–91
  sorting clothes/lines, 288
  stain removal from, **289**
  washing machine loading, 288–90
Learning, procedures, 12
Leg bag, connecting, **360–61**
Leukemia, 77, **95**
Liability, 30–31
Licensed practical nurse (LPN),
  defined, 5
Licensed vocational nurse (LVN),
  defined, 5
Lift, mechanical, lifting client with,
  321
Ligaments, 68
Liquid diet, 154
Living room, safety in, 169
Living will, 253
Lobectomy, described, 247
Log rolling client, **309**
Long-term care facility, defined, 6
Low-calorie diet, **152**
Low-fat diet, 151, **152**
Low-residue diet, 153
Low-sodium diet, **152**, 154
LPN (Licensed practical nurse),
  defined, 5
Lungs, aging and, **111**
LVN (Licensed vocational nurse),
  defined, 5

M
Malnutrition, nutrition and, 146,
  148
Maltreatment, child, 100–101
Mammogram, described, 245
Marketing
  food purchasing, 280–82
  menus/shopping lists and,
  280
Maslow, Abraham, human needs
  identified by, **15**
Mastectomy, defined, 245
Mattress, egg crate, **69**
Meals
  herbs and, **285**
  planning, nutrition and, 148–51
  preparation, seasonings/spices
    and, **284**
  preparation of, 282–85
Meals on Wheels, 148

Mechanical lift, lifting client with, **321**
Medic alert tags, 219
Medicaid
    DRGs and, 6–7
    health care and, 9
Medical terminology, 42–43
Medicare, health care and, 9
Medications, self-administered, assisting with, **346–47**
Mending clothes, 290–91
Menopause, 105
Mental
    disorders, 182
    health,
        defense mechanisms and, 137–38
        emotions and, 135–37
        illness, defined, 139
Menus, marketing and, 280
Metastasize, defined, 245
Microorganisms, 192–94
Microwave oven
    care/use of, **266**
    cooking with, 283, 285
Middle adulthood, 105–6
Minority cultures, 54–55
    food and, **150–51**
Moles, cancer and, warnings signs, **249**
Multiple sclerosis, 106
Muscles, aging and, **111**
Musculoskeletal system, 67–71
    disorders of, 70–71
Myocardial infarction, 76, 223–24
Myocardium, 222

N
Nail care, **344**
Needs, hierarchy of human, **15**
Neglect, child, 100–101
Neisseria gonorrheae, **192**
Nerves, degeneration, diabetes and, **217**
Nervous system, 71–73
    aging and, **111**
    disorders of, 72–73
Nitroglycerin, angina and, 223
Nonambulatory client, care of, 116
Nonverbal communication, 41–42
Nutrition
    diet therapy and, 151–55
    eating habits and, 145–48
    food guide pyramid, 142–45
    meal planning and, 148–51
    terms used in, **145**

O
OBRA, 5
    health care and, 9

Observations, documenting, 26–27
Observing, 24–25
Obstructed airway, clearing, 168, **175**
Ointment, applying, **386–88**
Omnibus Budget Reconciliation Act (OBRA). *See* OBRA
Oral hygiene, 16
    assisting with, **333–34**
Osteoarthritis, 236, 238
Osteoporosis, late adulthood and, **116**
Ostomy bag, changing, **390–92**
Otosclerosis, 73
Overeating, nutrition and, 146
Oxygen therapy, assisting with, **392–93**

P
Pain, responses to, 56
Paraplegia, 71
Parkinson's disease, **113**
Partial bath, assisting with, **328**
Passive range of motion exercise, **315–18**
Pathogens, 192
    dishwashing and, 275
Patient. *See* Client
Patient Self-Determination Act, 252
Percolator, care/use of, **267**
Perineal care
    female, **329**
    male, **330**
Periodic cleaning tasks, 272–73
Permanent press fabrics, 290
Personal
    care worker, defined, 5
    health/hygiene, 15–16
    protective equipment, putting on/removing, **302–4**
Personality development, stages of, **136**
Phenylketonuria, **95**
Phlebitis, 77
Phobia, 138
Physical restraints, 179
PKU, **95**
Pneumonectomy, described, 247
Pneumonia, 78
    late adulthood and, **115**
Policies, following, 20–22
Practice, defined, 12
Pregnancy, 93
    teenage, 99–100
Prejudice, racial, 57–58
Preschoolers
    accidents during, **158**
    home health aide and, 96
Pressure sores. *See* Bed sores
Procedure, defined, 295

Professional, standards, 31–32
Projection defense mechanism, 137
Prone position, positioning client in, **311–12**
Protozoa, 192
Psoriasis, **69**
Psychology, 135
Puberty, physical changes during, 98–99
Pulse
    defined, 184
    illness and, 183–84
    taking, radial/apical, **369–70**

Q
Quadriplegia, 71

R
Racial prejudice/discrimination, 57–58
Rales, defined, 184
Range of motion exercises, 186
    passive, **315–18**
Rationalization defense mechanism, 137
Reality orientation, 130–31
Recreation, need for, 189
Rectal care
    adults briefs, applying, **383**
    bowels, training/retraining, **382**
    enema, giving a commercial, **380–81**
    stool specimen, collecting, **383–84**
    suppository, giving a, **381–82**
Refrigerator, care/use of, **265**
Registered nurse (RN), defined, 5
Rehabilitation
    defined, 187
    need for, 187, 189
Relationships, interpersonal, 13–14
Religious practices, 56–57
Remission, defined, 243
Reporting
    changes in clients, 25
    described, 26
Reproductive system, 82–84
    aging and, 112
    female,
        cancer of, 245–46
        external, **82**
        lateral view, **83**
        male, lateral view, **83**
Respiration
    Cheyne-Stokes, 184
    counting, **371**

defined, 184
  rates, illness and, 183–84
Respiratory system, 77–79
  cancer of, 246–48
  disorders of, 78–79
Responsibilities, knowledge of, 22–24
Restorative care, body alignment, maintaining, **306–7**
Restraints, physical, 179
Retirement, 107
Rheumatoid arthritis, 236, 106
RN (Registered nurse), defined, 5
Role, knowledge of, 22–24

S

Safe sex, 204
Safety
  accidents by age, **158**
  basement, **174**
  bathroom, 160–61, **172**
  bedroom, **171**
  dining room, 169
  falls, 159–63
  fire, 163–68
    fire extinguishers, 164–65
  injury prevention, 267–68
  kitchen, **170**
  living room, 169
  outside the home, **173**
  stairway, **174**
Salt, use of, 154–55
Saturated fat, 144
Scabies, **69**
School-age children
  accidents during, **158**
  home health aide and, 96
Seasonings, meal preparation and, **284**
Self-esteem, retirement and, 107
Self-understanding, developing, 14–15
Semicoma, defined, **187**
Sensory deficits, 72–73
Separation, 52–53
Sexuality, aging and, 112
Sexually transmitted diseases, 84
Shaving, male clients, **337–38**
Shopping lists, marketing and, 280
Shower, assisting with, 323–26
Sibling rivalry, 96
Sickle cell anemia, 77, **95**
Side-lying position, positioning client in, **310–11**
Single parent family, 52
Skeleton, bones of, **70**
Skin, 64–67
  aging and, **111**
  cancer, 249

cross section of, 65
disorders of, 66–67, **69**
  bed sores, 66–67, **68**, **330–31**
  pressure sores, care of, **330–31**
  unbroken, applying unsterile dressing/ointment to, **386–88**
Slicing machine, care/use of, **267**
Small appliances, care/use of, **267**
Soft diet, **153**, 154
Somnolence, defined, **187**
Special diets, 151–55
Specimen
  collection, in isolation, **304**
  sputum, collecting, **363**
  stool, collecting, **383–84**
  urine, clear-catch collecting, **358**
Speech, communication and, 40–41
Sphygmomanometer, 185
Spices, meal preparation and, **284**
Spinal cord
  central nervous system and, **72**
  injuries, 72
Sponge bath, infant, **398–99**
Spouse dependency case study, 119–20
Sputum specimen, collecting, **363**
Stains, removal, **289**
Stairway, safety on, **174**
Standards
  ethical, 31
  professional, 31–32
Staphylococcus aureus, **192**
Steroids, arthritis and, 239
Stockings, elasticized, applying, **339–40**
Stoma, described, 247
Stool specimen, collecting, **383–84**
Stove, care/use of, **266**
Streptococcus hemolyticus, **192**
Stress, described, 138
Stroke, 77, **114**, 226–33
  aftereffects, 228
  communication problems after, 230–33
  defined, 226
  rehabilitation after, 229–30
  risk factors, 226–27
  signs of, 227–29
Study habits, forming, 12
Stupor, defined, **187**
Subcutaneous, defined, 215
Sublingually, defined, 223
Substance abuse, adolescence, 100
Sudden infant death syndrome, 95
Supine position, positioning client in, **310**
Supplies, cleaning, storage of, 276
Surfaces, wiping, 276

Syphilis, 84
Systolic blood pressure, 185

T

Tay-Sachs, **95**
Teenage. *See* Adolescence
Teeth, brushing, hygiene and, 16
Temperature
  illness and, 183
  taking,
    axillary, **368–69**
    oral, **365–66**
    rectal, **367–68**
Terminally ill
  adjustment stages, 253–54
  culture and, 252–53
Terminology, medical, 42–43
Thalassemia, **95**
Theory, defined, 12
TIA (Transient ischemic attack), 227
Toddlers, home health aide and, 96
Toilet, transferring patient to, **314–15**
Tophi, defined, 238
Total fat, 144
Tracheostomy, described, 247
Transient ischemic attack (TIA), 227
Tuberculosis, 200–201
Turning
  client,
    log rolling, **309**
    toward you, **307**
    with drawsheet, **308**
Two-career families, 53

U

Unconsciousness, levels of, **187**
Understanding, self, developing, 14–15
Universal precautions against disease, 195–96
Urinal, giving/emptying, **356**
Urinary
  catheter, caring for, **359–60**
  system, 81–82
Urine specimen, clear-catch collecting, **358**

V

Validation therapy, 126–30
Vascular disease, diabetes and, **217**
Vegetarian, 57
  diet, 154
Venous system, **75**
Verbal communication, 40–41
Viruses, 193
  late adulthood and, **115**

Vision, aging and, **111**
Vital signs
  blood pressure, taking, **371–73**
  pulse, taking radial/apical,
      369–70
  respirations, counting, **371**
  temperature,
      taking axillary, **368–69**
      taking oral, **365–66**
      taking rectal, **367–68**
  weight/height, measuring, **374**

Vitamins, foods containing more than
    one, **146–47**

W
Walker, assisting client with, **319–21**
Washing machine
  care/use of, **267**
  loading of, 288–90
Water, importance of, 148
Weekly cleaning tasks, 272
  bathroom, 278

Weight, 186
  infancy and, 94
  measuring, **374**
Wellness, 182
  described, 138–39
Withdrawal defense mechanism, 137
Words, meaning/use of, 39–40
Working
  hours, described, 20
  with others, 12–14
Written communication, 42–43